Manual of
TRAVEL
MEDICINE
and HEALTH

Third Edition

...en, MD
of Travel Medicine

Head, Division of Epidem. Communicable Diseases
Institute of Socia. Medicine, University of Zurich
Director, World Health Organ. ollaborating Centre for Travelers' Health
Zurich, Switzerland
Adjunct Professor, University of Texas School of Public Health
Houston, Texas

Herbert L. DuPont, MD
Chief, Internal Medicine
St. Luke's Episcopal Hospital
Director, Center for Infectious Diseases
University of Texas, Houston School of Public Health
Mary W. Kelsey Chair, University of Texas, Houston
Department of Medicine, Baylor College of Medicine
H. Irving Schweppe Jr, Chair and Vice Chair
Houston, Texas

Annelies Wilder-Smith, MD, PhD, MIH, FACTM
Director, Travellers Screening and Vaccination Clinic,
National University Hospital
Associate Professor, National University Singapore
Adjunct Associate Professor, Centre for International Health,
Curtin University, Perth, Australia
Editor, WHO *International travel and health* 2007

2007
BC Decker Inc
Hamilton

BC Decker Inc
P.O. Box 620, L.C.D. 1
Hamilton, Ontario L8N 3K7
Tel: 905-522-7017; 800-568-7281
Fax: 905-522-7839; 888-311-4987
E-mail: info@bcdecker.com
www.bcdecker.com

07 08 09/GP/9 8 7 6 5 4 3 2 1

ISBN 978-1-55009-369-8

Printed in India by Gopsons Papers

Sales and Distribution

United States
BC Decker Inc
P.O. Box 785
Lewiston, NY 14092-0785
Tel: 905-522-7017; 800-568-7281
Fax: 905-522-7839; 888-311-4987
E-mail: info@bcdecker.com
www.bcdecker.com

Canada
BC Decker Inc
50 King St. E.
P.O. Box 620, LCD 1
Hamilton, Ontario L8N 3K7
Tel: 905-522-7017; 800-568-7281
Fax: 905-522-7839; 888-311-4987
E-mail: info@bcdecker.com
www.bcdecker.com

Foreign Rights
John Scott & Company
International Publishers' Agency
P.O. Box 878
Kimberton, PA 19442
Tel: 610-827-1640
Fax: 610-827-1671
E-mail: jsco@voicenet.com

Japan
Igaku-Shoin Ltd.
Foreign Publications Department
1-28-23 Hongo
Bunkyo-ku, Tokyo,
Japan 113-8719
Tel: 3 3817 5611
Fax: 3 3815 4114
E-mail: fd@igaku-shoin.co.jp

UK, Europe, Middle East
McGraw-Hill Education
Shoppenhangers Road
Maidenhead
Berkshire, England SL6 2QL
Tel: 44-0-1628-502500
Fax: 44-0-1628-635895
www.mcgraw-hill.co.uk

**Singapore, Malaysia, Thailand,
Philippines, Indonesia, Vietnam,
Pacific Rim, Korea**
Elsevier Science Asia
583 Orchard Road
#09/01, Forum
Singapore 238884
Tel: 65-737-3593
Fax: 65-753-2145

Australia, New Zealand
Elsevier Science Australia
Customer Service Department
Locked Bag 16
St. Peters, New South Wales 2044
Australia
Tel: 61 02-9517-8999
Fax: 61 02-9517-2249
E-mail: customerserviceau@
elsevier.com
www.elsevier.com.au

Mexico and Central America
ETM SA de CV
Calle de Tula 59
Colonia Condesa
06140 Mexico DF, Mexico
Tel: 52-5-5553-6657
Fax: 52-5-5211-8468
E-mail:
editoresdetextosmex@prodigy.net.mx

Brazil
Tecmedd Importadora E Dis-
tribuidora De Livros Ltda.
Avenida Maurílio Biagi, 2850
City Ribeirão, Ribeirão Preto –
SP – Brasil
CEP: 14021-000
Tel: 0800 992236
Fax: (16) 3993-9000
E-mail: tecmedd@tecmedd.com.br

**India, Bangladesh, Pakistan, Sri
Lanka**
Elsevier Health Sciences Division
Customer Service Department
17A/1, Main Ring Road
Lajpat Nagar IV
New Delhi – 110024, India
Tel: 91 11 2644 7160-64
Fax: 91 11 2644 7156
E-mail: esindia@vsnl.net

CONTENTS

PART 3 **NONINFECTIOUS HEALTH RISKS AND THEIR PREVENTION**

PART 4 **DIAGNOSIS AND MANAGEMENT OF ILLNESS AFTER RETURN OR IMMIGRATION**

APPENDICES

DEDICATION

To the early researchers and promoters in international and environmental medicine and public health who set the stage for the evolution of travel medicine.

J.C. Alary
David Bradley
Otto Gsell
Sir Edmund Hillary
Ben Kean

PREFACE TO THE FIRST EDITION

Life is risky, and travel is even more so. The aim of this manual is to offer health professionals all they need to know to keep travelers in good health. The purpose is therefore to raise the standard of practice of preventive travel medicine.

Part 1 contains the basics necessary for every newcomer to the field. The subsequent parts contain epidemiologic data required for risk assessment, supported by numerous maps. They not only provide information about various diseases and risks encountered by travelers but also advice on avoidance of exposure to risk, immunization, drug prophylaxis, and recommendations for self-assessment and self-treatment while abroad. Also, the agents used in travel health, vaccines, drugs, and others, are described here in detail. There are innumerable information sources available on the diagnosis and therapy for some illnesses experienced by travelers or imported by migrants. For such, only the very basic information to be known by every general practitioner is included in this manual, with the focus on prevention and self-treatment.

Progress has been made toward a consensus on advice in travel medicine as this is of utmost importance to avoid confusion and resultant lack of compliance in travelers. However, there remains variation of opinion in some fields. Wherever this occurs, we describe the different positions; otherwise, we adhere to the advice published by the World Health Organization (WHO), the Centers for Disease Control and Prevention (CDC), other international expert groups, or universally accepted individual experts.

Travel medicine is a dynamic field. Any information provided in this manual will need continuous updating from other sources as new information becomes available. We plan to revise the book regularly and therefore invite all users to inform us about inadequacies or missing data to allow us to make subsequent editions even more valuable.

Robert Steffen
Herbert L. DuPont

PREFACE TO THE SECOND EDITION

This manual has become a standard reference among travel health professionals and others interested in the field. Even after multiple printings, the first edition is now sold out. Less than four years after having completed the first edition, the rapid, emerging field of travel medicine requires that we provide the second edition.

The fundamental concept remains the same. Our primary aim is one that provides clear answers to the many questions—fundamental and complex—that we face today. Just as the first edition did, this manual focuses on preventive measures for consideration by travelers. Obviously, the recommendations are based on recent epidemiologic data. Therapy is included insofar as it is relevant for self-treatment abroad and to address problems and questions that primary care physicians are frequently confronted with by returning travelers. For more complex therapeutic questions, consult sources on infectious diseases or on tropical medicine.

Throughout this second edition, we included a short bibliography with each chapter. You will find several additional summary tables and updated maps. In Part 1, Basics, the segments on travel advice for pregnant women, for infants and children, for patients with chronic medical conditions and senior travelers, and for persons with HIV infection have been expanded. We have added new segments on pilgrimage to Saudi Arabia, fundamentals of migration medicine, screening immigrants and refugees, and adoption of children from developing countries. In Part 2, Infectious Health Risks and Their Prevention, an update became necessary—the epidemiologic situation has evolved, and many new products have or soon will be marketed. Although we should not exaggerate the actual threat of biologic weapons on the traveling population, we also added a range of new topics that cover aspects related to bioterrorism. Part 3, Noninfectious Health Risks and Their Prevention, has also been expanded, mainly by a new chapter entitled "Deep Vein Thrombosis and Pulmonary Embolism." Part 4, Diagnosis and Management of Illness after Return or Immigration, needed a thorough update. In addition, we have added one chapter each on the fundamentals of diagnosis and treatment of malaria and on diagnosis and treatment of sexually transmitted diseases.

Most of our readers are health professionals; however, a few are initiated travelers. Whether this manual is used in daily work or to prepare a certificate of knowledge, initiated by the International Society of Travel Medicine, we wish you all good luck and great satisfaction. May your clients and your own travels be healthy and happy! We plan to continue to revise this manual regularly, and we continue to invite all users to inform us about inadequacies or missing data, allowing us to make subsequent editions even more valuable.

Robert Steffen
Herbert L. DuPont
Annelies Wilder-Smith
April 2003

PREFACE TO THE THIRD EDITION

Third edition means success, it illustrates that this manual has become a companion to many health care professionals caring for the well-being of travelers. The world has changed in the four years since the past edition was published. Although the fundamental concept of the manual remains the same, major updates and additions were needed.

These include a revision of the epidemiologic data, basing it on the experience from Geosentinel, national monitoring, and recent surveys. New chapters were added on networks in travel medicine and on legal aspects reflecting the adopted revision of the International Health Regulations. In Part 1, Basics, chapters on food hygiene and on maritime medicine are now included.

In Part 2, a range of additional infectious have been included, reflecting, for instance, that chikungunya has recently become a problem to travelers, and that we now live in a stage of pandemic influenza alert.

The final part on diagnosis and management still contains no more than basic information to be known by any primary care physician or nurse who may see returning travelers presenting with health problems. For those having to treat ill travelers in a specialized setting, there are numerous textbooks on tropical medicine, infectious diseases, internal medicine already available. Finally, annexes and maps have been updated, and since the latter have not only been printed on a larger scale, but also in color, they are far more comprehensive.

Robert Steffen
Herbert L. DuPont
Annelies Wilder-Smith
May 2007

ACKNOWLEDGMENTS

We wish again to acknowledge the excellent advice and support we received in preparing this fundamentally revised manuscript. Dr. Hans Bock and his team reviewed data on vaccines, Dr. Ziad Memish assisted us in updating the chapter on the Hajj. Dr. Christina Vogel did a thorough proofreading, Cordy Kuederli gave valuable secretarial assistance. Last but not least, Brian Decker and his team, notably Petrice Custance and Norm Reid, made it possible that the draft became this handy booklet full of colors you are now holding in your hands.

R.S.
H.L.D.
A.W-S.

INTRODUCTION

Basic Concepts

Travel medicine is an interdisciplinary field that has been developed over the past two decades (Figure 1). The primary goal of travel medicine is to protect travelers from disease and death; the secondary one is to minimize the impact of illness and accidents through principles of self-treatment. Many health professionals in the field also care for returned ill travelers; here, obviously, travel medicine overlaps mainly with the disciplines of infectious diseases and tropical medicine.

To achieve these goals, it is first necessary to quantitate health risks through epidemiologic research. Based on such evidence, it becomes possible to determine priorities for preventive measures. The art of travel medicine lies in the careful selection of necessary preventive strategies, avoiding measures that may cause unnecessary fear, adverse events, expense, or inconvenience. One basic precept is that potential travelers need not be given protective therapy against rare diseases while simultaneously being exposed to more frequently occurring diseases of comparable severity. Only in exceptional circumstances should travelers be advised to abandon their travel plans.

Travel medicine is not merely a luxury service for individual travelers; it also benefits public health. Repeatedly, outbreaks of

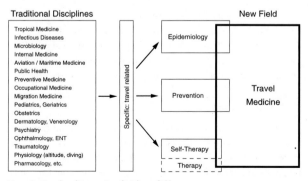

Figure 1   Travel medicine: an interdisciplinary field

malaria or other infections have only become known to local health authorities after a traveler returned home, was diagnosed, and reported through one of the surveillance systems, such as Geosentinel.

Collaboration between tourist-generating and tourist-receiving countries may result in improved hygienic conditions in resorts, and when health measures are copied and practiced, they will improve the situation for the local population, as well. New drugs and vaccines developed for travelers, although initially costly, later become available on the market everywhere at affordable prices.

The Travelers

Exposure of travelers to health risks depends on the destination, travel characteristics, and duration of stay. The importance of travel medicine is greatest for those venturing into the developing countries in tropic and subtropic regions where health standards and the health system are markedly substandard and there is minimal regard for public safety. The travel health community must give special attention to ethnic groups visiting friends and relatives in their native countries and to low-budget travelers, who often do not go through a travel agent and use the cheapest means of travel—these groups are at highest risk.

Travelers must carry the responsibility for their own health. If they neglect to seek advice or if they are noncompliant, they face a higher risk of accident, disease, or even death. Health of travelers also depends on the level of protection they purchase at the travel clinic or other medical institutions. It is an arbitrary decision as to what degree a traveler is willing to accept health risks; few will go as far as to carry their own blood supply, as some very important persons do. Experience often shows that those most intensely exposed to risks are on the tightest budget and believe they cannot afford travel health measures.

Travel Industry

Travel industry professionals should inform potential travelers about health measures at the earliest opportunity. This may be done through brochures or guide books, which must be reviewed by competent travel health professionals. In some countries, it is now possible for travelers to receive travel advice when booking an airline ticket through a computerized reservation system.

Travel industry professionals (travel agents, tour operators, and airlines) are the ones who most often have the earliest knowledge of an individual's travel plans. It should be travel industry policy to routinely refer for medical advice travelers who plan to visit areas with an elevated health risk. This should be done in a timely manner; some preventive measures need a few days or even weeks to become effective. This does not mean, however, that travel health consultation is useless and late for last-minute travelers. Travel industry collaborators need to be instructed accordingly. Only travel health professionals should provide detailed travel advice, not employees in travel agencies.

Ideally, tour operators' brochures and tour guides will use the opportunity to make a significant contribution by going beyond health issues and encourage travelers to respect the people, the environment, and the culture at their destination.

Travel Health Professionals

Specialized travel clinics or vaccination centers in Europe are consulted by up to 50,000 potential travelers to developing countries in one year. In contrast, in North America, many travel clinics will advise fewer than 1,000 travelers yearly. To provide travel health advice, any health professional should have extensive travel experience and, ideally, should have visited the continent under discussion.

The initiated family practitioner—and in some countries, nurses under supervision—can issue travel health advice to an individual with a low-risk profile and one who is visiting a developed nation. Often, he only needs to ascertain whether the potential traveler is still up-to-date on immunity against tetanus and diphtheria. Depending upon the frequency of travel to high-risk destinations from a travel-generating country, practicing physicians should have the opportunity to develop the expertise to give travel health advice to healthy travelers planning to stay on the "usual tourist trails." They should, however, refer persons with a high-risk profile to experienced centers. Inclusion of the basic concepts of travel medicine in the curriculum of medical schools and continuing medical education is essential to ensure a high quality of service in travel medicine as part of general practice.

Even if most recommendations are amended less than once yearly, travel health professionals must have access to a rapid up-to-date information system and they should regularly attend targeted courses and meetings.

The Institutions

Various institutions play a significant role in travel medicine. International (World Health Organization), and national public health (eg, Centers for Disease Control and Prevention) institutions carry the burden of data dissemination. The International Society of Travel Medicine (ISTM), various national associations of travel medicine, and other regional and national societies of tropical medicine contribute to the advancement of travel medicine mainly by promoting the exchange of information among those working in this field. Academic institutions and other travel clinics are the driving forces in mainly epidemiologic research, while the pharmaceutical industry develops and distributes—not always in sufficient quantities—various products to protect travelers' health. Other private sectors play a part by selling, for example, travel health software packages.

Final Remark

Everyone in travel medicine depends on the regular receipt of up-to-date information and recommendations on important destination-specific risks and disease-prevention strategies for travelers. All need to be up-to-date with the characteristics of the products they use. First steps have been taken on international, national, and local levels to urge travel health and travel industry professionals to collaborate. These efforts certainly need to be intensified.

PART 1

BASICS

TRAVELERS AND THEIR DESTINATIONS

Travelers

According to data provided by the World Tourism Organization (WTO) in Madrid, there is an almost continuous increase in the number of travelers (Figure 2). In 2006, there were 842 million recorded international tourist arrivals (Figure 2), the majority in the developed countries. Among them, 52% travel for leisure, recreation, and holidays, 16% for business or professional reasons, 24% are visiting friends or relatives (VFR) or they travel for health, religion, or other purposes, while the other 8% did not specify. About 10 million passengers travel on cruise ships annually, which represents an increase of over 1,000% in the last few decades. The worlds eight most frequently visited countries were France, Spain, the United States, China, Italy, the United Kingdom, the Hong Kong Special Administrative Region, and Mexico.

Each year, approximately 100 million travelers from a developed country visit a developing country (Table 1). The health systems at their destinations, particularly the hygiene conditions, are of poor standards in most places, which poses considerable health risks for the traveler; this manual emphasizes these particular destinations of the traveling population. Destinations in industrialized nations may also present travel risks (eg, reaching high altitudes, traveling on long flights that may increase the risk of deep vein thrombosis, and experiencing motion sickness, and also influenza may occur anywhere).

The projections show a substantial annual increase in travel from the developed to the developing countries and even more from developing countries to industrialized ones (Table 2). The economic crisis has been alleviated and the fear of terrorism has decreased, although terrorist acts continue to occur in many parts of the world.

According to the WTO definitions, the word "tourist" includes a broad variety of travelers, including business travelers, expatriates, crew members, etc., while according to Webster's Dictionary most "tourists" travel "especially for pleasure." We accept the latter definition and use the term "tourist" only for vacationers or similar.

International tourism receipts total US$623 billion yearly. The top tourism earners were the United States ($74 billion [US]), Spain ($45 billion [US]), France ($40 billion [US]), and Italy ($36 billion [US]).

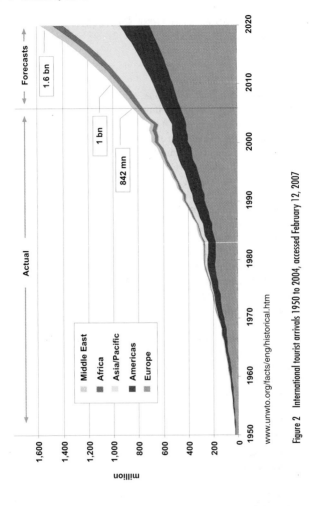

www.unwto.org/facts/eng/historical.htm

Figure 2 International tourist arrivals 1950 to 2004, accessed February 12, 2007

Destinations

Within a country, the risk profile may vary greatly, depending on whether the destination is on or off the "usual tourist trail." The terms "urban" and "rural" may be misleading, as people staying in a youth hostel in a suburb may be more exposed to a variety of pathogens, not only as compared to guests in a multistar hotel

Table 1 International Tourist Arrivals by Generating Region den Destination Region, 2004 (thousand) (including estimations for countries with missing data)

To:	From:						
	World	Africa	Americas	Asia and the Pacific	Europe	Middle East	Origin not specified
World	763,876	18,610	130,504	146,437	433,269	20,516	14,538
Africa	33,436	13,290	1,104	958	11,582	1,695	4,807
North Africa	12,770	1,248	164	88	6,006	1,579	3,685
West Africa	3,142	1,305	190	183	1,218	48	199
Central Africa	729	226	55	23	225	6	193
East Africa	7,597	4,093	372	367	2,583	45	137
Southern Africa	9,199	6,419	323	298	1,550	16	594
Americas	125,739	388	93,027	8,283	21,681	196	2,165
North America	85,854	298	64,718	7,775	12,747	185	131
Caribbean	18,091	11	12,162	66	4,336	3	1,513
Central America	5,740	3	4,933	83	579	0	142
South America	16,054	76	11,215	359	4,018	8	378
Asia and the Pacific	145,491	837	9,470	114,765	17,382	880	2,156
North-East Asia	79,412	301	4,839	67,296	6,020	124	833
South-East Asia	48,309	315	2,624	37,905	6,030	441	992
Oceania	10,157	82	1,101	6,918	1,883	47	124
South Asia	7,613	139	906	2,646	3,448	268	207
Europe	422,937	2,585	25,827	16,282	372,894	1,879	3,469
Northern Europe	48,373	710	6,447	3,262	37,276	384	293
Western Europe	138,821	1,328	9,559	6,732	119,464	529	1,209
Central/Eastern Europe	86,296	133	2,903	3,465	79,206	181	409
Southern Europe	149,447	414	6,919	2,823	136,949	784	1,558
Middle East	36,272	1,510	1,076	6,149	9,731	15,865	1,942

United Nations World Tourism Organization, Tourism Market Trends, World Overview and Tourism Topics chapter II.2, page 73

in the same city, but also compared to those staying in luxury resorts located in the countryside. Detailed assessment of the planned type of accommodation is thus essential.

Those advising potential travelers must have comprehensive knowledge of world geography time zones (Figure 3), the location of various countries and their capital cities (Figures 4A to K), and the climates and altitudes of at least the most frequently visited destinations.

Table 2 Travel market forecasts by region

	Base Year 1995	Forecasts 2010	2020	Market Share (%) 1995	2020	Average annual growth rate (%) 1995–2020
		(Million)				
World	565	1006	1561	00	100	4.1
Africa	20	47	77	3.6	5.0	5.5
Americas	110	190	282	19.3	18.1	3.8
East Asia and the Pacific	81	195	397	14.4	25.4	6.5
Europe	336	527	717	59.8	45.9	3.1
Middle East	14	36	69	2.2	4.4	6.7
South Asia	4	11	19	0.7	1.2	6.2

www.unwto.org/facts/eng/vision.htm (accessed February 15, 2007)

Environment

Environment plays an important role in most travels, from the developed to the developing countries. Travelers may find the climate of the country that they visit differs greatly from that of the home country. Changes in climate can cause diseases and other problems, directly or indirectly. Temperature, humidity, and rainfall have a direct impact on a traveler's health. Heat and humidity often lead to loss of energy and malaise, initially, and later to rapid exhaustion. Electrolyte and fluid depletion may lead to dangerous conditions, particularly in elderly travelers and those with preexisting illness. Excessive exposure to the sun rapidly results in sunburns, particularly at high altitudes. Some destinations in desert areas may be extremely dry and very cold at night. A traveler who experiences extreme differences in temperature and humidity may experience undesired clinical symptoms.

Excessive heat and humidity alone, or combined with inappropriate activities under such conditions, may lead to heat exhaustion due to salt and water losses. Heat stroke and hyperthermia may result. Morbidity and mortality from cardiovascular (including cerebrovascular) accidents are clearly increased after sudden and prolonged exposure to heat. Heat, humidity, and overcrowding, especially in the poorer sections of cities, pro-

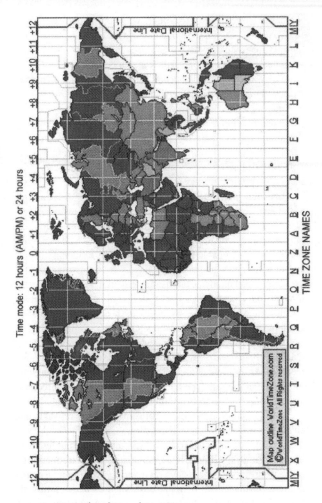

Figure 3   Coordinated Universal Time (UTC) zones

mote the survival, multiplication, and spread of infectious agents and their vectors. Air pollution is a significant problem in many large cities in the world (eg, Beijing, Mexico (Federal District), and Athens). The air may become polluted after bush and forest fires. Dust from unpaved roads or in arid areas may cause increased susceptibility to infections of the upper respiratory tract. Travel on rough roads may aggravate back pain. Food and beverages abroad may harbor pathogenic agents (see "Traveler's Diarrhea in Infectious Health Risks and Their Prevention"). Food may also be more spicy and cause gastric irritation or gastritis. Fish may contain toxins that are not eliminated by cooking or cleaning.

Excessive cold may cause hypothermia, possibly followed by the common cold and its complications—or frostbite. Other than bad weather conditions, contributing factors to frostbite (eg, in high altitude trekking) are inadequate clothing, inadequate judgment, immobility, fatigue, and hunger.

Particular meteorologic conditions, such as El Niño currents in the Pacific, sometimes influence global weather causing prolonged heavy rains with subsequent floods and epidemics. However, highly efficient early warning systems with long-term predictions now enable public health officers to identify at-risk populations.

Many travel agencies publish information on climatic conditions at frequently visited tourist destinations. Similarly, many airlines and other institutions (eg, media) have such information available in print or on their Web sites.

At high altitudes, trekkers and climbers with preexisting cardiac or pulmonary disease (see Table 3) face a risk. Above 2,400 meters, there is a risk of high-altitude illness for any person staying for several hours (see "Altitude" in Part 3, "Noninfectious Health Risks and Their Prevention").

Cosmic radiation, a concern in some frequent travelers and aircrew, is rather a theoretical concern.

Acclimatization and avoiding exertion for the first few days in an unfamiliar climate lessens the risk of environmentally induced problems. Mainstays of frostbite prevention are adequate clothing and footwear, avoidance of bad weather by respecting forecasts, sufficient food, and descent when needed. As often stated, gastrointestinal infection could be avoided by the basic rule "boil it, cook it, peel it, or forget it"—however, compliance is very low.

Additional Readings

O'Sullivan D. Medical considerations for wilderness and adventure travelers. Med Clin North Am 1999;83:885–902.

**Table 3 Altitudes of Important Tourist Destinations
(Most Above 1220 m/4000 ft)**

Cities and Countries	Meters	Feet
Addis Ababa, Ethiopia	926	3038
Albuquerque, USA	1620	5314
Andorra La Vella, Andorra	1080	3543
Antananarivo, Madagascar	1372	4500
Arieiro, Madeira Island, Portugal	1610	5282
Arusha, Tanzania	1387	4550
Asmara, Ethiopia	2325	7628
Aspen, USA	2369	7773
At Ta'if, Saudi Arabia	1471	4826
Banff, Canada	1397	4583
Bioemfontein, South Africa	1422	4665
Bishop, USA	1253	4112
Bogotá, Colombia	2645	8678
Boulder, USA	1611	5288
Bulawayo, Zimbabwe	1342	4405
Butte, USA	1693	5554
Byrd Station (Antarctica), USA	1553	5095
Cajamarca, Peru	2640	8662
Calgary, Canada	1079	3540
Caracas, Venezuela	1042	3418
Carson City, USA	1448	4751
Cherrapunji, India	1313	4309
Cheyenne, USA	1876	6156
Chihuahua, Mexico	1423	4669
Coban, Guatemala	1306	4285
Cochabamba, Bolivia	2550	8367
Colorado Springs, USA	1881	6172
Cuenca, Ecuador	2530	8301
Cuernavaca, Mexico	1560	5118
Cuzco, Peru	3225	10,581
Cyangugu, Rwanda	1529	5015

Table 3 (Continued)

Cities and Countries	Meters	Feet
Darjeeling, India	2265	7431
Davos-Platz, Switzerland	1588	5210
Denver, USA	1625	5331
Durango, Mexico	1889	6198
Erzurum, Turkey	1951	6402
Esfahan (Isfahan), Iran	1773	5817
Flagstaff, USA	2137	7012
Fort Portal, Uganda	1539	5049
Gangtok, India	1812	5945
Gilgit, Kashmir	1490	4890
Grand Canyon NP, USA	2015	6611
Grand Junction, USA	1481	4858
Guadalajara, Mexico	1589	5213
Guanajuato, Mexico	2500	8202
Guatemala, Guatemala	1480	4855
Gyumri (Leninakan), Armenia	1529	5016
Harare (Salisbury), Zimbabwe	1472	4831
Ifrane, Morocco	1635	5364
Iringa, Tanzania	1625	5330
Jasper, Canada	1061	3480
Jinja, Uganda	1172	3845
Johannesburg, South Africa	1665	5463
Jungfraujoch, Switzerland	3475	11,467
Kabale, Uganda	1871	6138
Kabul, Afghan	1815	5955
Kampala, Uganda	1312	4304
Kathmandu, Nepal	1337	4388
Kermanshah, Iran	1320	4331
Kerman, Iran	1859	6100
Ketama, Morocco	1520	4987
Kigali, Rwanda	1472	4828
Kisumu, Kenya	1149	3769

Table 3 (Continued)

Cities and Countries	Meters	Feet
Kitale, Kenya	1920	6299
La Paz, Bolivia	3658–4018	12,001
Lake Louise, Canada	1534	5032
Laramie, USA	2217	7272
Leh, India	3506	11,503
Lhasa, Tibet, China	3685	12,090
Lichinga (Vila Cabral), Mozambique	1365	4478
Lubumbashi (Elisabethville), Zaire	1230	4035
Lusaka, Zambia	1260	4134
Macchu Picchu, Peru	2380	7854
Marsabit, Kenya	1345	4413
Maseru, Lesotho	1528	5013
Mbabane, Swaziland	1163	3816
Mbala (Abercorn), Zambia	1658	5440
Medellin, Colombia	1498	4916
Merida, Venezuela	1635	5364
Mexico, Mexico	2308	7572
Morella, Mexico	1941	6368
Mt. Kilimanjaro, Tanzania	5890	19,340
Nairobi, Kenya	1820	5971
Nanyuki, Kenya	1947	6389
Ndola, Zambia	1269	4163
Nova Lisboa, Angola	1700	5577
Nuwara Eliya, Sri Lanka	1880	6188
Oaxaca, Mexico	1528	5012
Pachuca, Mexico	2426	7959
Petrified Forest NP, USA	1653	5425
Pretoria, South Africa	1369	4491
Puebla, Mexico	2162	7093
Queretaro, Mexico	1842	6043
Quetta, Pakistan	1673	5490
Quito, Ecuador	2879	9446

Table 3 (Continued)

Cities and Countries	Meters	Feet
Reno, USA	1344	4411
Rock Springs, USA	2058	6752
Sa da Bandeira, Angola	1786	5860
Salt Lake City, USA	1288	4226
San Antonio de los Banos, Cuba	2509	8230
San Jose, Costa Rica	1146	3760
San Luis Potosi, Mexico	1859	6100
San Miguel de Allende, Mexico	1852	6076
San'a, Yemen Arab Republic	2377	7800
Santa Fe, USA	1934	6344
Seefeld, Austria	1204	3950
Shiraz, Iran	1505	4938
Simla, India	2202	7224
South Pole Station (Antarctica), USA	2800	9186
Srinagar, India	1586	5205
St. Anton am Arlberg, Austria	1304	4278
St. Moritz, Switzerland	1833–3451	6013
Tabriz, Iran	1366	4483
Tamanrasset, Algeria	1400	4593
Tegucigalpa, Honduras	1004	3294
Tehran, Iran	1220	4002
Toluca, Mexico	2680	8793
Tsavo, Kenya	1462	4798
Tsumeb, Namibia	1311	4301
Ulaanbaatar (Ulan Bator), Mongolia	1325	4347
West Yellowstone, USA	2025	6644
Windhoek, Namibia	1728	5669
Yosemite NP, USA	1210	3970
Zacatecas, Mexico	2446	8025
Zermatt, Switzerland	1616–3900	5310–12,700

Time Zones

Time differences can affect travelers' health. Desynchronization of various physiologic and psychologic rhythms occurs after rapid passage across several time zones. Figure 3 shows the Coordinated Universal Time (UTC) zones (see "Jet Lag" in Part 3, "Noninfectious Health Risks and Their Prevention').

▌ Potential Health Hazards to Travelers by Region

This section intends to provide a general description of the health risks that travelers may face in various areas of the world and not encounter in their home countries. It is impractical to try and identify problem areas accurately and to define the degree of likely risk in each of them. For example, although viral hepatitis A is ubiquitous, the risk of infection varies not only according to area but also according to eating habits. Hence, there may be more risk from communal eating in an area of low incidence than from eating in a private home located in an area of high incidence. Generalizations would therefore be misleading.

Tourism is an important source of income for many countries, and labeling any country as high risk for a disease may cause serious economic repercussions. The national health administrations of these countries, however, would have a responsibility to provide travelers with an accurate picture of the risks that may be encountered from communicable diseases. In the past, some countries deliberately withheld information (eg, on the endemicity of cholera).

Africa (Figures 4A and 4B)

Northern Africa (Algeria, Egypt, Libyan Arab Jamahiriya, Morocco, and Tunisia) is characterized by a generally fertile coastal area and a desert hinterland, with oases that are often the foci of infections.

Arthropod-borne diseases are unlikely to be a major problem to the traveler, although filariasis (focally in the Nile delta), leishmaniasis, malaria, relapsing fever, Rift Valley fever, sand-fly fever, typhus, and West Nile fever do occur in some areas.

Food-borne and waterborne diseases are endemic, with the most common being dysenteries and other diarrheal diseases. Hepatitis A occurs throughout the area, and hepatitis E is endemic in some regions. Typhoid fevers, alimentary helminthic infec-

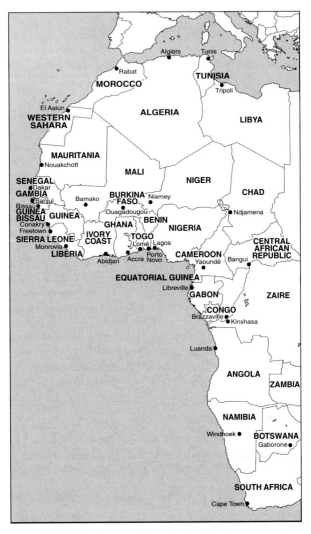

Figure 4A   Western Africa

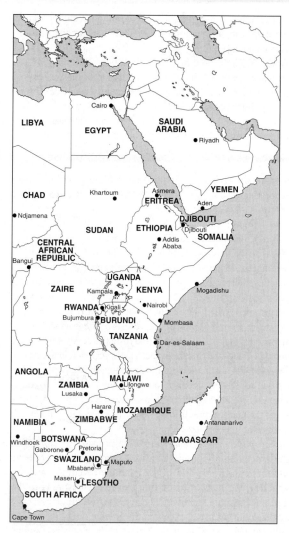

Figure 4B Eastern Africa

tions, brucellosis, and giardiasis are common. Echinococcosis (hydatid disease) and sporadic cases of cholera are also encountered occasionally.

Other Hazards. Poliomyelitis eradication efforts in northern Africa have been very successful, and virus transmission in most of the area has ceased. Egypt is the only country where confirmed cases of poliomyelitis were still reported in 2004. In addition, trachoma, rabies, snakes, and scorpions are hazards in certain areas. Schistosomiasis (bilharziasis) is prevalent both in the Nile delta and in the Nile valley; it occurs focally elsewhere in the area.

Sub-Saharan Africa comprises Angola, Benin, Burkina Faso, Burundi, Cameroon, Cape Verde, Central African Republic, Chad, Comoros, Congo, Cote d'Ivoire, Democratic Republic of the Congo, Djibouti, Equatorial Guinea, Eritrea, Ethiopia, Gabon, Gambia, Ghana, Guinea, Guinea-Bissau, Kenya, Liberia, Madagascar, Malawi, Mali, Mauritania, Mauritius, Mozambique, Niger, Nigeria, Reunion, Rwanda, Sao Tome and Principe, Senegal, Seychelles, Sierra Leone, Somalia, Sudan, Togo, Uganda, United Republic of Tanzania, Zambia, and Zimbabwe.

In this area, which lies entirely within the tropics, the vegetation varies from the tropical rain forests of the west and center to the wooded steppes of the east, and from the desert of the north through the Sahel and Sudan savannas to the moist orchard savanna and woodlands north and south of the equator. Many of the diseases that we discuss occur in localized foci and are confined to rural areas. We include them, however, so the international traveler and the medical practitioner concerned become aware of the diseases that may occur.

Arthropod-borne diseases are a major cause of morbidity. Malaria occurs throughout the area, except in places at above 2,600 meters altitude and in the islands of Reunion and the Seychelles. Various forms of filariasis are widespread in the region, and endemic foci of onchocerciasis (river blindness) exist in all the countries listed, except in the greater part of Kenya and in Djibouti, Gambia, Mauritania, Mozambique, Somalia, Zambia, Zimbabwe, and the island countries of the Atlantic and Indian Oceans. However, onchocerciasis exists in the island of Bioko in Equatorial Guinea. Individuals may encounter both cutaneous and visceral leishmaniasis, particularly in the drier areas. Visceral leishmaniasis is epidemic in eastern and southern Sudan. Human trypanosomiasis (sleeping sickness), in discrete foci, is reported from all countries except Djibouti, Eritrea, Gambia, Mauritania, Niger, Somalia, and the island countries of the Atlantic and Indian Oceans. The transmission rate of human trypanosomiasis is high in Sudan and Uganda and very high in Angola and the Democratic Republic of the Congo, and there is a significant risk of infection for travelers visiting or working in rural areas. Relapsing fever and louse-, flea-, and tick-borne typhus occur. Angola, the Democratic Republic of the Congo, Kenya, Madagascar, Mozambique, Uganda, the United Republic of Tanzania, and Zimbabwe have reported natural foci of plague. There is widespread incidence of tungiasis. Many viral diseases, some presenting as severe hemorrhagic fevers, are transmitted by mosquitoes, ticks, sandflies, and other insects that are found throughout this region. A substantial outbreak of chikungunya has in 2006 been reported from many islands and countries bordering the Indian Ocean. Large outbreaks of yellow fever occur periodically in the unvaccinated population, mainly in Western Africa. The natural focus of plague is a strictly delimited area, where ecological conditions ensure the persistence of plague in wild rodents (and occasionally other animals) for long periods of time and where epizootics and periods of quiescence may alternate.

Food-Borne and Waterborne Diseases. These are highly endemic in this region. Alimentary helminthic infections, dysenteries, diarrheal diseases such as giardiasis, typhoid fevers, and hepatitis A and E are widespread. Cholera is actively transmitted in many countries in this area. Dracunculiasis occurs in isolated foci. Paragonimiasis (oriental lung fluke) has been reported from Cameroon, Gabon, Liberia, and, most recently, from Equatorial Guinea. Echinococcosis (hydatid disease) is widespread in animal-breeding areas.

Other Diseases. Hepatitis B is hyperendemic. Poliomyelitis (also a food-borne or waterborne disease) since 2003 has again spread throughout many countries of the African continent; in 2007 cases still mainly occur in Nigeria. Schistosomiasis (bilharziasis) is present throughout the area, except in Cape Verde, Comoros, Djibouti, Reunion, and the Seychelles. Trachoma is widespread throughout the region. Among other diseases, certain arenavirus hemorrhagic fevers that are often fatal have attained notoriety. Lassa fever has a virus reservoir in a commonly found multimammate rat. Studies have shown that an appreciable reservoir exists in some rural areas of West Africa, and people visiting these areas should take particular care to avoid rat-contaminated food or food containers, but the extent of the disease should not be exaggerated. Ebola and Marburg hemorrhagic fevers are present but are reported only infrequently. Epidemics of meningococcal meningitis may occur throughout tropical Africa, particularly in the savanna areas during the dry season.

Other hazards include rabies and snake bites.

Southern Africa (Botswana, Lesotho, Namibia, Saint Helena, South Africa, and Swaziland) has varied physical characteristics, ranging from the Namib and Kalahari deserts, to the fertile plateaus and plains, to the more temperate climate of the southern coast.

Arthropod-borne diseases, such as Crimean-Congo hemorrhagic fevers, malaria, plague, relapsing fever, Rift Valley fever, tick-bite fever, and typhus (mainly tick-borne) have been reported from most of this area, excepting Saint Helena. Apart from malaria in certain areas, however, they are unlikely to be a major health threat for the traveler. Trypanosomiasis (sleeping sickness) may occur in Botswana and Namibia.

Food-borne and waterborne diseases, particularly amebiasis and typhoid, are common in some parts of this region. Hepatitis A is also prevalent, and an outbreak of poliomyelitis occurred in Namibia in 2006.

Other Diseases. The Southern African countries are on the verge of becoming poliomyelitis free, thus making the risk of poliovirus infection low. Hepatitis B is hyperendemic. Schistosomiasis (bilharziasis) is endemic in Botswana, Namibia, South Africa, and Swaziland. In addition, snakes may be a hazard in some areas.

The Americas

In 1994, an international commission certified the eradication of endemic wild poliovirus from the Americas. Ongoing surveillance in formerly endemic Central and South American countries confirms that poliovirus transmission remains interrupted.

North America (Bermuda, Canada, Greenland, Saint Pierre and Miquelon, and the United States [with Hawaii]) extends from the Arctic to the subtropical cays of the Southern United States (Figure 4C).

The incidence of communicable diseases is so low that it is unlikely to pose any more of a hazard to international travelers than that found in their own countries. There are, of course, certain health risks, but in general, only minimal precautions are required. Certain diseases, such as plague, rabies in wildlife including bats, Rocky Mountain spotted fever, tularemia, and arthropod-borne encephalitis occur on rare occasions. Rodent-borne hantavirus has been identified, predominantly in the Western United States and the western provinces of Canada. West Nile virus had rapidly spread mainly through the United States, but the incidence is now decreasing. Lyme disease is endemic in the northeastern, mid-Atlantic, and the US upper Midwest, with occasional cases reported from the Pacific Northwest. During recent years, the incidence of certain food-borne diseases (eg, salmonellosis) has increased in some regions. Other hazards include poisonous snakes, poison ivy, and poison oak. In the northernmost parts of the continent, exposure to very low temperatures in the winter can be a hazard.

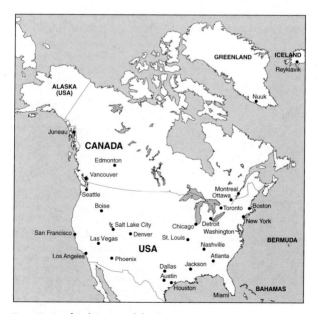

Figure 4C Map of North America, excluding Mexico.

Mainland Middle America (Belize, Costa Rica, El Salvador, Guatemala, Honduras, Mexico, Nicaragua, and Panama) ranges from the deserts of the north to the tropical rain forests of the southeast (Figure 4D).

Of the *arthropod-borne diseases*, malaria and cutaneous and mucocutaneous leishmaniasis occur in all eight countries of this region. Visceral leishmaniasis is encountered in El Salvador, Guatemala, Honduras, and Mexico. Onchocerciasis (river blindness) is found in two small foci in the south of Mexico and four dispersed foci in Guatemala. American trypanosomiasis (Chagas' disease) has been reported to occur in localized foci in rural areas in all eight countries. Bancroftian filariasis is present in Costa Rica. Dengue fever and Venezuelan equine encephalitis may occur in all these countries.

Food-borne and waterborne diseases (including amebic and bacillary dysenteries and other diarrheal diseases) and typhoid are very common throughout the area. All countries except Panama reported cases of cholera in 1996. Hepatitis A occurs throughout the area, and hepatitis E has been reported in Mexico. Helminthic infections are common. Paragonimiasis (oriental lung fluke) has been reported in Costa Rica, Honduras, and Panama. Brucellosis

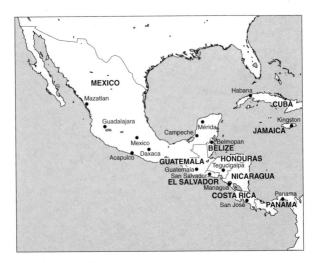

Figure 4D   Map of Middle America

occurs in the northern part of the area. Many *Salmonella typhi* infections from Mexico and *Shigella dysenteriae* type 1 infections from mainland Middle America have generally been caused by drug-resistant enterobacteria.

Other Diseases. Rabies in animals (usually dogs and bats) is widespread throughout the area. Snakes may be a hazard in some areas.

Caribbean Middle America (Antigua and Barbuda, Aruba, Bahamas, Barbados, British Virgin Islands, Cayman Islands, Cuba, Dominica, Dominican Republic, Grenada, Guadeloupe, Haiti, Jamaica, Martinique, Montserrat, Netherlands Antilles, Puerto Rico, Saint Kitts and Nevis, Saint Lucia, Saint Vincent and the Grenadines, Trinidad and Tobago, Turks and Caicos Islands, and the Virgin Islands [US]). The islands, of which several are mountainous with peaks 1,000 to 2,500 meters high, have an equable tropical climate with heavy rainstorms and high winds at certain times of the year (Figure 4E).

Of the *arthropod-borne diseases*, malaria occurs in endemic form only in Haiti and in parts of the Dominican Republic. Diffuse cutaneous leishmaniasis was recently discovered in the Dominican Republic. Bancroftian filariasis is seen in Haiti and some other islands, and other filariases may occasionally be found. Human fascioliasis, due to *Fasciola hepatica*, is endemic in Cuba. Outbreaks of dengue fever occur in the area, and dengue hem-

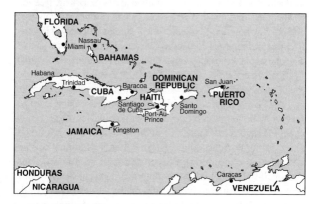

Figure 4E   Map of Carribean

orrhagic fever has also been encountered. Tularemia has been reported from Haiti.

Of the *food-borne and waterborne diseases*, bacillary and amebic dysenteries are common, and hepatitis A is reported, particularly in the northern islands. No cases of cholera have been reported in the Caribbean.

Other Diseases. Schistosomiasis (bilharziasis) is endemic in the Dominican Republic, Guadeloupe, Martinique, Puerto Rico, and Saint Lucia; control operations are in progress in these countries, and it may also occur sporadically in other islands. Other hazards may occur from spiny sea urchins, coelenterates (corals and jellyfish), and snakes. Animal rabies, particularly in the mongoose, is reported from several islands.

Tropical South America (Bolivia, Brazil, Colombia, Ecuador, French Guiana, Guyana, Paraguay, Peru, Suriname, and Venezuela) consists of the narrow coastal strip on the Pacific Ocean, the high Andean range with numerous peaks 5,000 to 7,000 meters high, and the tropical rain forests of the Amazon basin, bordered on the north and south by savanna zones and dry tropical forest or scrub (Figure 4F).

Arthropod-borne diseases are an important cause of ill health in rural areas. Malaria occurs in all 10 countries or areas, as do American trypanosomiasis (Chagas' disease) and cutaneous and mucocutaneous leishmaniasis. There has been an increase of the latter in Brazil and Paraguay. Visceral leishmaniasis is endemic in northeast Brazil, with foci in other parts of Brazil; it is less frequent in Colombia and Venezuela, rare in Bolivia and Paraguay, and unknown in Peru. Endemic onchocerciasis occurs in isolated foci in rural areas in Ecuador, Venezuela, and northern Brazil. The bite of blackflies may cause unpleasant reactions. Bancroftian filariasis is endemic in parts of Brazil, Guyana, and Suriname. Plague has been reported in natural foci in Bolivia, Brazil, Ecuador, and Peru. Among the arthropod-borne viral diseases, jungle yellow fever may be found in forest areas in all countries of this region except Paraguay and areas east of the Andes; in Brazil, it is confined to the northern and western states. Epidemics of viral encephalitis and dengue fever occur in some countries. Bartonellosis (which begins with Oroya fever), a sandfly-borne disease, occurs in arid river valleys on the western slopes of the Andes in altitudes up to 3,000 meters. Louse-borne typhus is often found in the mountainous areas of Colombia and Peru.

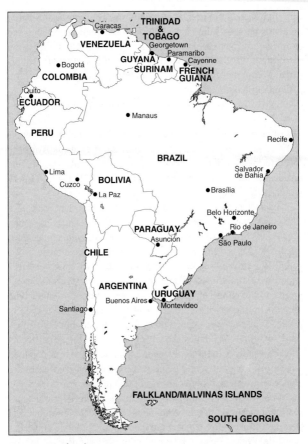

Figure 4F   Map of South America

Food-borne and waterborne diseases are common and include amebiasis, diarrheal diseases, helminthic infections, and hepatitis A. Paragonimiasis (oriental lung fluke) has been reported from Ecuador, Peru, and Venezuela. Brucellosis is common, and echinococcosis (hydatid disease) occurs particularly in Peru. Bolivia, Brazil, Colombia, Ecuador, Peru, and Venezuela all reported autochthonous cases of cholera in 1996.

Other diseases include rodent-borne arenavirus hemorrhagic fever in Bolivia and Venezuela, and rodent-borne pulmonary syndrome in Brazil and Paraguay. Hepatitis B and D (delta hepatitis) are highly endemic in the Amazon basin. The intestinal form of schistosomiasis (bilharziasis) is found in Brazil, Suriname, and north-central Venezuela.

Rabies has been reported from many of the countries in this area. Meningococcal meningitis and dengue occurs in the form of epidemic outbreaks in Brazil.

Snakes and leeches may be a hazard in some areas.

Temperate South America (Argentina, Chile, Falkland Islands [Malvinas], and Uruguay). The mainland extends from the Mediterranean climatic area of the western coastal strip, over the Andes divide, on to the steppes and desert of Patagonia in the south, to the prairies of the northeast (see Figure 5F).

Arthropod-borne diseases are relatively unimportant, except for the occurrence of American trypanosomiasis (Chagas' disease). Outbreaks of malaria occur in northwestern Argentina; cutaneous leishmaniasis is also reported from this part of the country.

Of the *food-borne and waterborne diseases*, gastroenteritis (mainly salmonellosis) is relatively common in Argentina, especially in the suburban areas and among children younger than 5 years. Some cases of cholera were reported from Argentina in 1996. Typhoid fever is uncommon in Argentina, but hepatitis A and intestinal parasitosis are widespread, with the latter occurring especially in the coastal region. Taeniasis (tapeworm), typhoid fever, viral hepatitis, and echinococcosis (hydatid disease) are reported from the other countries of this region.

Other Diseases. Anthrax is an industrial or agricultural occupational hazard in the three mainland countries. Meningococcal meningitis is reported to occur in the form of epidemic outbreaks in Chile. Rodent-borne hantavirus pulmonary syndrome has been identified in the north-central and southwestern regions of Argentina and in Chile.

Asia (Figures 4G and 4H)

East Asia (China [including Hong Kong Special Administrative Region], the Democratic People's Republic of Korea, Japan, Macao, Mongolia, and the Republic of Korea). This region includes the high mountain complexes, the desert and the steppes of the west, and the various forest zones of the east, down to the subtropical forests of the southeast.

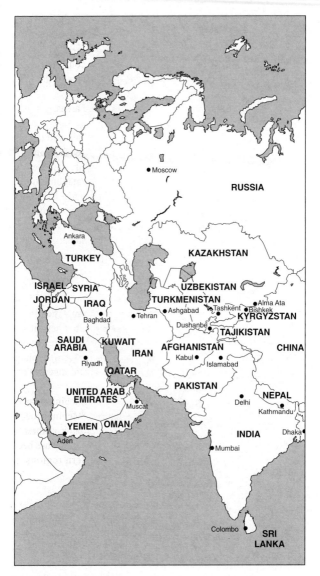

Figure 4G   Map of Western Asia

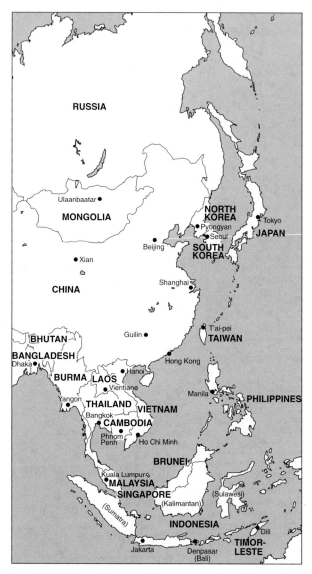

Figure 4H   Map of Eastern Asia

Of the *arthropod-borne diseases*, malaria occurs in China, and in recent years, cases have also been reported from the Korean peninsula. Although reduced in distribution and prevalence, bancroftian and brugian filariasis are still reported in southern China. There has been a resurgence of visceral leishmaniasis in China. Cutaneous leishmaniasis was reported from Xinjiang in the Uygur Autonomous Region. Plague may be encountered in China and Mongolia. Rodent-borne hemorrhagic fever with renal syndrome and Korean hemorrhagic fever is endemic, except in Mongolia, and epidemics of dengue fever and Japanese encephalitis may occur in some countries. Mite-borne or scrub typhus may be found in scrub areas in southern China, certain river valleys in Japan, and in the Republic of Korea.

Food-borne and waterborne diseases such as the diarrheal diseases and hepatitis A are common in most countries. Hepatitis E is prevalent in western China. Clonorchiasis (oriental liver fluke) and paragonimiasis (oriental lung fluke) are reported in China, Japan, Macao, and the Republic of Korea. Fasciolopsiasis (giant intestinal fluke) and brucellosis occur in China. Cholera may occur in some countries in this area.

Other Diseases. Hepatitis B is highly endemic. The present endemic area of schistosomiasis (bilharziasis) is in the central Chang Jiang (Yangtze) river basin in China; active foci no longer exist in Japan. Poliomyelitis eradication activities have rapidly reduced poliovirus transmission in east Asia. Reliable surveillance data indicate that poliovirus transmission has been interrupted in China since 1994. Likewise, Mongolia no longer reports cases. Trachoma and leptospirosis occur in China. Rabies is endemic in some countries. There are reports of outbreaks of meningococcal meningitis in Mongolia.

Eastern South Asia (Brunei Darussalam, Cambodia, Indonesia, Lao People's Democratic Republic, Malaysia, Myanmar, the Philippines, Singapore, Thailand, and Vietnam). From the tropical rain and monsoon forests of the northwest, the area extends through the savanna and the dry tropical forests of the Indochina peninsula, and down to the tropical rain and monsoon forests of the islands bordering the South China Sea.

The *arthropod-borne diseases* are an important cause of morbidity and mortality throughout the area. Malaria and filariasis are endemic in many parts of the rural areas of all the countries.In

Brunei Darussalam and Singapore, however, normally only imported cases of malaria occur. Foci of plague exist in Myanmar; cases of plague also occur in Vietnam. Japanese encephalitis, dengue, and dengue hemorrhagic fever can occur in epidemics in both urban and rural areas of this region. Mite-borne typhus has been reported in deforested areas in most countries.

Food-borne and waterborne diseases are common. Cholera and other watery diarrheas, amebic and bacillary dysentery, typhoid fever, and hepatitis A and E may occur in all countries in the area. Among helminthic infections, fasciolopsiasis (giant intestinal fluke) may be acquired in most countries in the area, clonorchiasis (oriental liver fluke) in the Indochina peninsula, opisthorchiasis (cat liver fluke) in the Indochina peninsula, the Philippines, and Thailand, and paragonimiasis (oriental lung fluke) in most countries. Melioidosis can transpire sporadically throughout the area.

Other Diseases. Most cases of H5N1 influenza (commonly known as bird flu) observed in humans have been diagnosed in this region. Hepatitis B is highly endemic in the region. Schistosomiasis (bilharziasis) is endemic in the southern Philippines and in central Sulawesi (Indonesia) and occurs in small foci in the Mekong delta in Vietnam. Poliovirus transmission most likely has been interrupted in Eastern South Asia. Trachoma exists in Indonesia, Myanmar, Thailand, and Vietnam.

Other hazards include rabies, snake bites, and leeches.

Middle South Asia (Afghanistan, Armenia, Azerbaijan, Bangladesh, Bhutan, Georgia, India, Islamic Republic of Iran, Kazakhstan, Kyrgyzstan, Maldives, Nepal, Pakistan, Sri Lanka, Tajikistan, Turkmenistan, and Uzbekistan). Bordered for the most part by high mountain ranges in the north, the area extends from the steppes and desert in the west to monsoon and tropical rain forests in the east and south.

Arthropod-borne diseases are endemic in all these countries; malaria, however, is not endemic in Georgia, Kazakhstan, Kyrgyzstan, the Maldives, Turkmenistan, and Uzbekistan. There are small foci of malaria in Armenia, Azerbaijan, and Tajikistan. In some of the other countries, malaria occurs in urban, as well as rural areas. Filariasis is common in Bangladesh, India, and the southwestern coastal belt of Sri

Lanka. Sandfly fever is on the increase in the region. A sharp rise in the incidence of visceral leishmaniasis has been observed in Bangladesh, India, and Nepal. In Pakistan, it is mainly reported from the north (Baltistan). Cutaneous leishmaniasis occurs in Afghanistan, India (Rajasthan), the Islamic Republic of Iran, and Pakistan. There are small foci of cutaneous and visceral leishmaniasis in Azerbaijan and Tajikistan. Natural foci of plague exist in India and Kazakhstan. Afghanistan, India, and the Islamic Republic of Iran report tick-borne relapsing fever, and typhus occurs in Afghanistan and India. Outbreaks of dengue fever may occur in Bangladesh, India, Pakistan, and Sri Lanka, and the hemorrhagic form has been reported from eastern India and Sri Lanka. Japanese encephalitis has been reported from the eastern part of the area and Crimean-Congo hemorrhagic fever from the western part. Another tick-borne hemorrhagic fever has been reported in forest areas in Karnataka State in India and in a rural area of Rawalpindi District in Pakistan. Large chikungunya epidemics were reported from India 2006/07.

Food-borne and waterborne diseases are common throughout the area—in particular, cholera and other watery diarrheas, dysenteries, typhoid fever, hepatitis A and E, and helminthic infections. Large epidemics of hepatitis E can happen. Giardiasis is common in the area. Brucellosis and echinococcosis (hydatid disease) are found in many countries in the area.

Other Diseases. Hepatitis B is endemic. A limited focus of urinary schistosomiasis (bilharziasis) persists in the southwest of the Islamic Republic of Iran. Outbreaks of meningococcal meningitis have been reported in India and Nepal. Poliomyelitis eradication activities are pursued in all countries in the area. Surveillance data are incomplete, however, and we should still assume poliovirus transmission to be a risk to travelers in most countries, especially in the Indian subcontinent. Trachoma is common in Afghanistan and in parts of India, the Islamic Republic of Iran, Nepal, and Pakistan. Snakes and the presence of rabies in animals are hazards in most of the countries in the area.

Western South Asia (Bahrain, Cyprus, Iraq, Israel, Jordan, Kuwait, Lebanon, Oman, Qatar, Saudi Arabia, Syrian Arab Republic, Turkey, the United Arab Emirates, and Yemen). The area ranges from the mountains and steppes of the northwest to the large deserts and dry tropical scrub of the south.

Arthropod-borne diseases, except for malaria in certain areas, are not a major hazard for the traveler. Malaria does not exist in Kuwait and no longer occurs in Bahrain, Cyprus, Israel, Jordan, Lebanon, or Qatar. Its incidence in the Syrian Arab Republic and United Arab Emirates is low, but elsewhere, it is endemic in certain rural areas. Cutaneous leishmaniasis is reported throughout the area; visceral leishmaniasis, although rare throughout most of the area, is common in central Iraq, in the southwest of Saudi Arabia, in the northwest of the Syrian Arab Republic, in Turkey (southeast Anatolia only), and in the west of Yemen. Murine and tick-borne typhus, as well as tick-borne relapsing fever, can occur in certain countries. Crimean-Congo hemorrhagic fever has been reported from Iraq, and limited foci of onchocerciasis are reported from Yemen.

Food-borne and waterborne diseases are, however, a major hazard in most countries in the area. Typhoid fevers and hepatitis A exist in all countries. Dracunculiasis occurs in isolated foci in Yemen. Taeniasis (tapeworm) infestation is reported from many countries in the area. Brucellosis is reported from most countries, and there are foci of echinococcosis (hydatid disease).

Other Diseases. A few cases of H5N1 influenza (bird flu) have been diagnosed in Turkey. Hepatitis B is endemic in the region. Schistosomiasis (bilharziasis) occurs in Iraq, Saudi Arabia, the Syrian Arab Republic, and Yemen. The risk of poliovirus infection is low in most countries in the area, with the exception of Yemen. Trachoma and animal rabies are found in many of the countries. The greatest hazards for pilgrims to Mecca and Medina are heat stroke and dehydration if the period of the Hajj coincides with the hot season.

Europe (Figures 4I and 4J)

Northern Europe (Belarus, Belgium, Czech Republic, Denmark [including Faroe Islands], Estonia, Finland, Germany, Iceland, Ireland, Latvia, Lithuania, Luxembourg, Netherlands, Norway, Poland, Republic of Moldova, Russian Federation, Slovakia, Sweden, Ukraine, and the United Kingdom [including Channel Islands and the Isle of Man]). The area comprising these countries extends from the broadleaf forests and the plains of the west to the boreal and mixed forests, as far east as the Pacific Ocean.

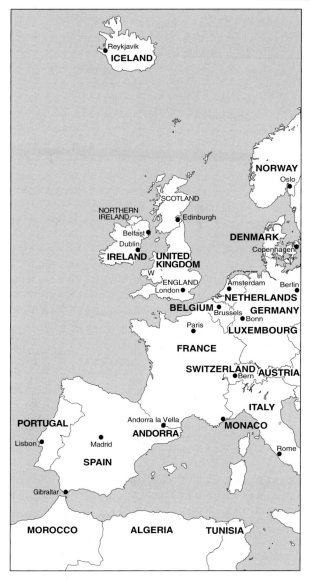

Figure 4I Map of Western Europe

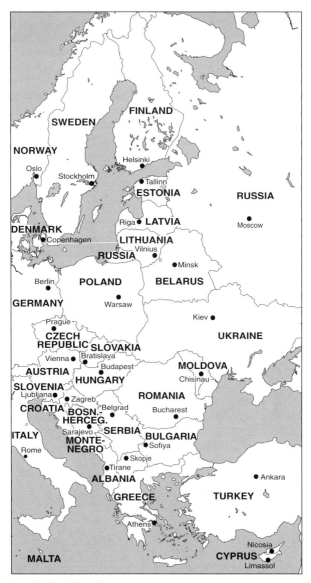

Figure 4J   Map of Eastern Europe

The incidence of communicable diseases in most parts of the area is such that these diseases are no more likely to prove a hazard to international travelers than those found in their own countries. There are, of course, some health risks, but in most of the area, few precautions are required.

Of the *arthropod-borne diseases*, there are very small foci of tick-borne typhus in east and central Siberia. Tick-borne encephalitis and Lyme disease may occur throughout forested areas where vector ticks are found. Rodent-borne hemorrhagic fever with renal syndrome is now recognized as occurring at low endemic levels in this area.

Food-borne and waterborne diseases reported, other than the ubiquitous diarrheal diseases, are taeniasis (tapeworm) and trichinosis in parts of northern Europe, and diphyllobothriasis (fish tapeworm) from the freshwater fish around the Baltic Sea area. *Fasciola hepatica* infection can occur. Hepatitis A is encountered in the eastern European countries; outbreaks associated with *Giardia lamblia* still occur in Northeast Europe. The incidence of certain food-borne diseases (eg, salmonellosis and campylobacteriosis) is increasing significantly in some countries.

Other Diseases. All countries in the area where poliomyelitis was endemic are now making intense efforts to eradicate the disease. Rabies is endemic in wild animals (particularly foxes) in rural areas of northern Europe. In the previous decade, Belarus, the Russian Federation, and Ukraine have experienced extensive epidemics of diphtheria. Diphtheria cases, mostly imported from these three countries, have also been reported from neighboring Estonia, Finland, Latvia, Lithuania, Poland, and the Republic of Moldova.

In parts of northern Europe, the extreme cold in the winter can be a climatic hazard.

Southern Europe (Albania, Andorra, Austria, Bosnia and Herzegovina, Bulgaria, Croatia, France, Gibraltar, Greece, Hungary, Italy, Liechtenstein, Malta, Monaco, Portugal [including Azores and Madeira], Romania, San Marino, Slovenia, Spain [including the Canary Islands], Switzerland, the Former Yugoslav Republic of Macedonia, and Yugoslavia). The area extends from the broadleaf forests in the northwest and the mountains of the Alps to the prairies and, in the south and southeast, the scrub vegetation of the Mediterranean.

Among the *arthropod-borne diseases*, sporadic cases of murine and tick-borne typhus and mosquito-borne West Nile fever occur in some countries bordering the Mediterranean littoral. Both cutaneous and visceral leishmaniasis and sandfly fever are also reported from this area. Leishmania and human immunodeficiency virus (HIV) coinfections have been reported from France, Italy, Portugal, and Spain. Tick-borne encephalitis, for which a vaccine exists, Lyme disease, and rodent-borne hemorrhagic fever with renal syndrome may occur in the eastern and southern parts of the area.

Food-borne and waterborne diseases—bacillary dysentery, diarrhea, and typhoid fever—are more common in the summer and autumn months, with a high incidence in the southeastern and southwestern parts of the area. Brucellosis can occur in the extreme southwest and southeast, and echinococcosis (hydatid disease) in the southeast. *Fasciola hepatica* infection has been reported from different countries in this area. Hepatitis A occurs in the eastern European countries. The incidence of certain food-borne diseases (eg, salmonellosis and campylobacteriosis) is increasing significantly in some countries.

Other Diseases. The last continental foci of poliomyelitis were in southern Europe, but subsequent to eradication activities, no more cases have been observed since 1996. Hepatitis B is endemic in the southern part of eastern Europe (Albania, Bulgaria, and Romania). Rabies in animals exists in many countries of southern Europe.

Oceania (Figure 4K)

This comprises Australia, New Zealand, and the Antarctic. In Australia, the mainland has tropical monsoon forests in the north and east; dry tropical forests, savanna, and deserts in the center; and Mediterranean-like scrub and subtropical forests in the south. New Zealand has a temperate climate, with the North Island characterized by subtropical forests, and the South Island by steppe vegetation and hardwood forests.

International travelers to Australia and New Zealand will, in general, not be subjected to the hazards of communicable diseases to any extent greater than those found in their own countries.

Arthropod-borne disease (mosquito-borne epidemic polyarthritis and viral encephalitis) may occur in some rural areas of Australia. Occasional outbreaks of dengue have occurred in northern Australia in recent years.

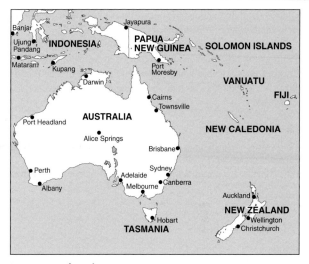

Figure 4K   Map of Australasia

Other Hazards. Coelenterates (corals, jellyfish) may prove a hazard while bathing in the sea, and heat during summer is a hazard in the northern and central parts of Australia.

Melanesia and Micronesia-Polynesia (American Samoa, Cook Islands, Easter Island, Fiji, French Polynesia, Guam, Kiribati, Marshall Islands, [Federated States of] Micronesia, Nauru, New Caledonia, Niue, Palau, Papua New Guinea, Samoa, Solomon Islands, Tokelau, Tonga, Tuvalu, Vanuatu, and the Wallis and Futuna Islands). The area covers an enormous expanse of ocean, with the larger, mountainous, tropical, and monsoon–rain–forest-covered islands of the west giving way to the smaller, originally volcanic peaks and coral islands of the east.

Arthropod-borne diseases occur in most islands. Malaria is endemic in Papua New Guinea, Solomon Islands, and Vanuatu. Filariasis is widespread but its prevalence varies. Mite-borne typhus has been reported from Papua New Guinea. Dengue fever, including its hemorrhagic form, can occur in epidemics in most islands.

Food-borne and waterborne diseases, such as the diarrheal diseases, typhoid fever, and helminthic infections, are commonly reported. Biointoxication may occur from raw or cooked fish and shellfish. Hepatitis A is reported in this area, as well.

Other diseases. Hepatitis B is endemic in the region. Poliomyelitis cases have not been reported from any of these areas for more than 5 years. Trachoma occurs in parts of Melanesia. Hazards to sea bathers include the coelenterates, poisonous fish, and snakes.

Additional Reading

Wilson M. A world guide to infections. Oxford University Press: New York, Oxford; 1991.

World Health Organization. International travel and health. Geneva, Switzerland; 2007.

EPIDEMIOLOGY OF HEALTH RISKS IN TRAVELERS

Mortality

There are limited data on deaths of travelers occurring abroad. On first sight, the few existing mortality data look contradictory. In fact, some studies claim that accidents, particularly in small children and young adults, are the leading cause of death, while others demonstrate the predominance of cardiovascular events. These differences are primarily due to differences in examined populations and destinations. Southern Europe, Florida, and parts of the Caribbean are favorite destinations of elderly travelers in whom elevated mortality rates associated with various natural causes are to be expected; age-specific cardiovascular mortality rates are similar to the population remaining at home. At developing destinations, the risk of fatal accidents is clearly higher.

Overall, among 1,262 French corpses repatriated from 2000 to 2004, about half had died abroad of accidents and half from illness—just 1.4% died of infections. The mortality rate of Swiss travelers in developing countries is 0.8 to 1.5 per 100,000 per month, whereas among those traveling in North America, it is only 0.3 per 100,000. Trekking in Nepal is associated with a particularly high mortality rate of 15 per 100,000.

Accidents

Deaths abroad due to injury are higher by a factor of two to three in travelers aged 15 to 44 years, compared with rates for nontravelers.

Fatalities are mostly due to traffic accidents. In 10,000 registered vehicles, 1.4 road traffic fatalities yearly are reported in the United Kingdom, compared to 20 to 118 in sub-Saharan Africa and 9 to 67 in Asia. Motorbikes are frequently implicated, partly because in many countries, individuals are not obliged to wear a helmet. Alcohol often plays a role and a lack of seatbelts in rental cars, chaotic traffic conditions in the developing countries, particularly at night, are decisive factors (see "Accidents" in Part 3, "Noninfectious Health Risks and Their Prevention"). Tourists are reported to be several times more likely than local drivers to have accidents. British Airport Authority statistics report that air travel is 2,200 times safer than cycling, 165 times safer than traveling by car, and 27 times safer than rail travel.

Drowning is another major cause of accidental death and accounts for 16% of all deaths because of injuries among US travelers. Again, alcohol appeared to be a factor in the outcome. Other factors include the presence of unrecognized currents or undertow and being swept out to sea. Small children may drown in foreign swimming pools, just as they might at home.

Assaults and terrorism are statistically less important, although there is significant concern mainly among travelers from the United States. Americans are frequently political targets of terrorism, which causes this feeling of apprehension that many experience. Among other countries, murder rates exceeding 20 per 100,000 are observed in Colombia (62), South Africa (50), Jamaica and Venezuela (32 each), and Russia (20). Kidnapping and killing have recently increased, but this is mainly targeted at employees of international and nongovernmental organizations, and at journalists. Fatal assaults on tourists and terrorism may occur anywhere, not only in developing countries.

Being killed by animals is an uncommon cause of death among travelers. There were 105 confirmed shark attacks worldwide in 2005 (58 not provoked, 4 fatal), with the number rising, possibly owing to neoprene wetsuits that allow the wearer to stay longer in cooler water where the risk is greater. Among safari tourists in South Africa, wild mammals killed 3 foreigners; in fact, two were killed by lions when the individuals left their vehicle to approach them. The number of fatalities due to snakebites is estimated at 40,000 worldwide (mainly in Nigeria, India), but few are travelers.

In addition, a broad variety of toxins may be a risk to travelers. Ciguatoxin leading to ciguatera syndrome after the consumption of tropical reef fish is probably the most important one—the case fatality rate is 0.1 to 12%. "Body-packing" of heroin, cocaine, and other illicit drugs in the gastrointestinal tract or in the vagina may result in the death of travelers when the condoms or other packages break. Fatal toxic reactions and life-threatening neurologic symptoms after applying highly concentrated N,N,diethyl-methyl-toluamide (DEET) in small children have rarely been observed. Lead-glazed ceramic that is purchased abroad may result in lead-poisoning, which may remain undetected for a long time.

Infections

Infections claim a lower toll than many would expect; to a large extent, they may be effectively prevented. Data on mortality after travel abroad, however, are limited to infections with mandatory reporting. According to a French survey, almost 7% were due to malaria, few to typhoid and paratyphoid, amebiasis, viral encephalitis, etc. Malaria, certainly the most frequent cause of infectious death among travelers abroad, has a mortality rate exceeding 1 in 100,000 in travelers who visit tropical Africa. In the 1989 to 1995 period, 373 fatalities had been reported in nine European countries and 25 reported in the United States. Obviously, this was almost exclusively due to *Plasmodium falciparum*, with the case fatality rate ranging from 0 to 3.6%. The mortality among those using chemoprophylaxis was lower as compared to those without such prevention at least in high risk destinations.

No information is available on travelers' deaths that occur after return as a consequence, for example, of acquired immunodeficiency syndrome (AIDS) many years after human immunodeficiency virus (HIV) infection or accidents during the stay abroad. It was, a few years ago, estimated that 6 in 100,000 travelers ultimately died of AIDS, owing to HIV transmission mostly through unprotected, casual sex during a stay in a developing country before effective therapy was possible. In Switzerland, 10% of infections are acquired abroad; in the United Kingdom, the risk of acquiring HIV was considered 300 times higher while abroad, compared with staying home. All travelers may be exposed to risk. However, seamen, military personnel, and those visiting friends and relatives in high endemicity countries are likely exposed more often than businessmen or tourists. HIV patients who are traveling have a higher risk of complications that, ultimately, may be fatal.

There is a multitude of other infections that may result in the death of a traveler, ranging from the usual harmless traveler's diarrhea and influenza to rabies. Almost every year there are anecdotal reports on rabies-associated deaths in travelers. The latter is associated with a case fatality rate of almost 100% unless postexposure prophylaxis is given promptly. Overall, other than those already mentioned, it appears that fatal consequences of infections in travelers are quite effectively avoided by prevention or adequate therapy, but concise epidemiologic data on mortality in this population are scarce. Other emerging infections that often make headlines only rarely affect travelers, but anecdotal cases of fatal Ebola and West Nile virus have been reported. Fatalities associated with imported severe acute respiratory syndrome

(SARS) had been noted in the first days of that outbreak in 2003. No traveler in the past decade has been a victim of bioterrorism or avian influenza. Equally, there is no known case of variant Creutzfeldt-Jacob disease acquired during traveling.

Noninfectious Illness

Senior travelers, in particular, may experience new or complications of preexisting illness. We are mostly concerned about cardiovascular conditions; in fact, recently, evidence has been generated that pulmonary embolism associated with long distance air travel may occur at a rate of 5 in 1 million, and many are fatal. Risk factors have been clearly identified (see "Deep Vein Thrombosis and Pulmonary Embolism" in Part 3, "Noninfectious Health Risks and Their Prevention"). Few data exist on fatal travel health risks in infants, small children, and pregnant women.

Additional Readings

Cornall P, et al. Drowning of British children abroad. Child Care Health Dev 2005;31:611–3.

Dahl E. Passenger mortalities aboard cruise ships. Int Marit Health 2001;52:19–23.

Hargarten SW, et al. Overseas fatalities of United States citizen travelers: an analysis of deaths related to international travel. Ann Emerg Med 1991;20:622–6.

Jeannel D, Allain-Ioos S, Bonmarin I, et al. Les décès de français lors d'un séjour à l'étranger et leurs causes [French]. Bull epid hebdo 2006;23-24:166–8.

Krause G, et al. Chemoprophylaxis and malaria death rates. Emerg Infect Dis 2006;12:447–51.

McInnes RJ et al. Unintentional injury during foreign travel. J Travel Med 2002;9:297–307.

▌ Morbidity

Health problems in travelers are frequent. As many as 75% of short-term travelers to the tropics or subtropics report some health impairment or use of self-medication. Short-term transatlantic travelers report a 50% rate of health impairment, most often constipation. However, even in travelers to developing countries, only a few of these self-reported health problems are severe: of these travelers, 7% need medical attention abroad, 16% upon return, and 4% both abroad and upon return. Of travelers, 14% are incapacitated while abroad, and 2% of their time abroad is lost due to illness or accidents. Less than 2% of individuals are unable to go back to work upon return; in all studies, about 1% of travelers require admission to a hospital but usually for a few days only. In contrast, less than 1% among visitors to Paris required emergency medical care. Among 2,000 travelers, only one required emergency aeromedical evacuation, either by scheduled or ambulance flight (Figure 5).

A survey conducted among World Bank employees illustrates that travel is associated with increased morbidity and that this is not attributable only to infections. The risk per trip is greatest for first-time travelers; experienced travelers know how to diminish risks (Figure 6). It is instructive that the greatest claim ratio increase in travelers was for psychological reasons.

Infections

Since the initiation of epidemiologic surveys in the 1970s, transmission of some infectious diseases has been reduced; for instance, traveler's diarrhea or typhoid fever in southern Europe and Thailand. Also, in Jamaica and Tunisia, joint actions by the min-

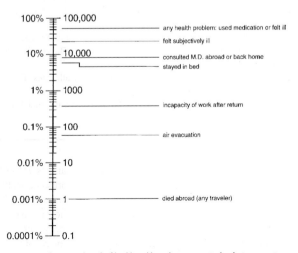

Figure 5 Incidence rate/month of health problems during a stay in developing countries

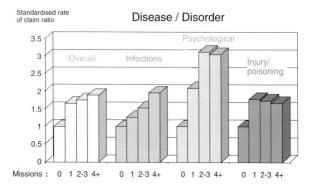

Figure 6   International business travel and insurance claims (5,672 male World Bank employees)

istries of Health and Tourism resulted in reducing the incidence of traveler's diarrhea. Conversely, the incidence rates of most infections affecting travelers in the developing countries have remained fairly constant. Some, such as dengue, are clearly increasing. The Geosentinel study has demonstrated that dengue now is more frequently diagnosed, compared to malaria, in travelers having returned from the Caribbean, South America, or Asia.

Importantly, be aware of what infections in travelers are frequent and which ones are rare (Figure 7). Traveler's diarrhea remains the most frequent ailment encountered in those traveling from the developed nations to developing countries. Second are upper respiratory tract infections, either without fever or, less frequently, with fever; the monthly incidence of influenza is 1%. Among the life-threatening infections in tropical Africa, Papua New Guinea, and on some islands in the Pacific, malaria occurs most often. Besides enterotoxigenic *E. coli* (ETEC) infection caused by LT-toxins and influenza, hepatitis A and hepatitis B are the most frequent among the vaccine-preventable diseases. Concerns about exposure to rabies after animal bites are fairly frequent. Regional and seasonal variations to these worldwide data are listed under the respective headings.

Sexually transmitted diseases, including HIV infection, continue to cause great concern, because even in the presence of risk of possible HIV transmission, not all casual sexual encounters include the use of condoms. Human papillomavirus (HPV) infection can be transmitted, even if condoms are used correctly.

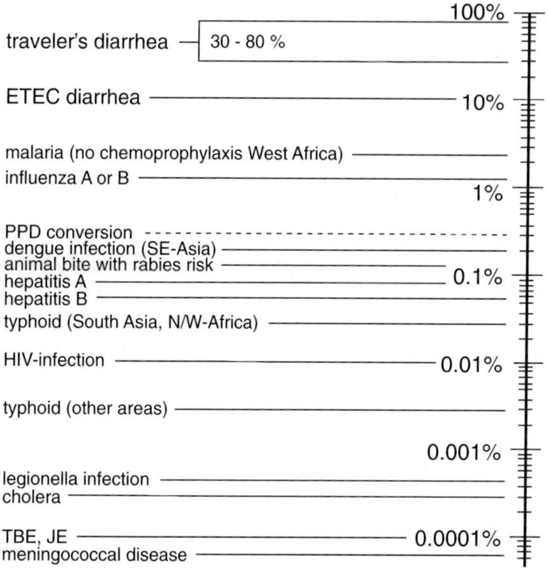

Figure 7 Incidence rate of health problems per month during a stay in developing countries

The media largely promote fears among travelers, one of which is the fear of becoming affected by emerging infections, such as Ebola and other filoviruses, Lassa, or West Nile virus. Part 2 describes these infections; however, except for dengue and HIV, these infections are extremely rare. Similarly, in the past few years, not a single traveler has been affected by pathogens spread in bioterrorist actions.

Additional Readings

Ansart S, et al. Pneumonia among travelers returning from abroad. J Travel Med 2004;11:87–91.

Leder K, et al. Respiratory tract infections in travelers; a review of the GeoSentinel Surveillance Network. Clin Infect Dis 2003;36: 399–406.

Liese B, et al. Medical insurance claims associated with international business travel. Occup Environ Med 1997;54:499–503.

Steffen R. Travel epidemiology—a global perspective. Int J Antimicrob Agents 2003;21:89–95.

▌ Risk Behavior And Compliance

Travelers may choose not to consult travel health professionals prior to departure, owing to their fear of needles or side effects of medication, to their apprehension about high costs, or to their psychological reasons. A proportion of both high- and low-risk travelers decide against travel health consultations for lack in confidence in conflicting recommendations. Many want to be "free" from rules and regimented behavior during their stay abroad. Others consider themselves not at risk, despite their knowledge about some basic epidemiologic features. Some travelers prefer to use alternative medical methods, such as herbal medicine or homeopathy, in spite of their lack of safety or effectiveness. Homeopathic malaria prophylaxis, for example, has been demonstrated to pose a considerable health risk that results in fatalities and in prolonged intensive care.

Behavior is hypothesized to originate from two factors: (1) the value that an individual places on the behavior, and (2) the individual's estimate of the likelihood that a given action will lead to the desired goal. The following cognitive dimensions play a role: perceived susceptibility of an illness or accident, its severity, benefits from prevention, and disadvantages owing to the preventive action, such as cost, adverse reactions, or discomfort.

Travel health professionals must recognize that travelers often will not follow given recommendations. More than 90% of travelers from Europe and North America succumb to gastronomic temptations and forget the old rule "boil it, cook it, peel it, or forget it." A multicenter survey reported that the risky food and beverage items most often ingested are salads, ice cubes, and ice cream. This may increase the risk of gastrointestinal disorders.

With respect to malaria, almost all travelers (> 95%) are informed about the risk in high transmission areas. Most travelers use medication as prescribed for the chemosuppression of malaria while abroad; however, only about 50% will use the medication regularly, and, when indicated, continue up to 4 weeks upon return. Most use some form of personal protection against mosquito bites, but less than 5% systematically attempt to completely avoid such bites by using all possible methods available. Most travelers, although aware of the risk of malaria, decide not to consult a doctor within 24 hours of developing a febrile illness as instructed, and if unable to find a health professional within that time, they refuse to use the standby medication obtained prior to departure. This mistake has cost numerous lives.

Approximately 5% of British, German, Swiss, or Canadian tourists—more often men than women—have casual sex abroad. According to one survey, when men travel alone, this rate may be 20%. These travelers are not all "sex tourists," who travel with the goal of having sex, but many just stumble into a romantic affair, more often with locals than with fellow travelers. The rate of unprotected contacts has recently decreased from one-half to one-third, with men above age 40 years being significantly more careless than are young men, perhaps because of fear of impotence if using a condom. Similarly, women often fail to protect themselves or have their partners use condoms, even when their partners are natives of tropical Africa where HIV prevalence is particularly high.

Noncompliance has been associated with low quality of consultation prior to the journey, long duration of stay, multiple journeys, lower age, and adverse reactions. Businessmen, who are the least well informed, and those who visit relatives or friends in a developing country are less compliant than tourists, particularly when they travel in groups. Noncompliant travelers often forget preventive measures or consider them unnecessary. Moreover, other travelers or friends often encourage them to disregard travel health advice.

Additional Readings

Abdullah ASM, et al. Sexually transmitted infections in travelers. Clin Infect Dis 2004;39:533–8.

Livingston MR, et al. Human immunodeficiency virus acquired heterosexually abroad. J Travel Med 2005;12:19–25.

Lobel HO, et al. Use of malaria prevention measures by North American and European travelers to East Africa. J Travel Med 2001;8:167–72.

von Sonnenburg F, et al. Risk and aetiology of diarrhoea at various tourist destinations. Lancet 2000;356;133–4.

Van Herck K et al. Knowledge, attitudes and practices in travel related infectious diseases. The European airport survey. J Travel Med 2004;11:3–8.

PRINCIPLES OF PRETRAVEL COUNSELING

Standardized Pretravel Questioning

In pretravel consultations, first and foremost, remember that potential travelers are not usually patients but healthy persons. Most often, initially, they will register and indicate name, address, and birth date. Learning the nationality of the individual may enable the travel health professional to find out what language the individual communicates in and then to obtain background on immune status. Potential travelers should then indicate their travel plans, according to a minimum checklist as follows:

- Destination(s): countries, city, resort, or off-the-tourist trail, and itinerary
- Purpose: tourism, business, or other professional (what type?), visit (to natives/expatriates), or other (military, airline crew, adoption)
- Hygiene standard expected: high (eg, multistar hotels and restaurants) or low-budget travel (street vendors, youth hostels)
- Special activities: high-altitude trekking, diving, hunting, or camping
- Date of departure
- Duration of stay abroad

Potential travelers should answer the following set of questions about their health status and medical history:

- Do you currently use any medication? If yes, which ones?
- Do you currently have a fever?
  If yes, what temperature?
- Do you suffer from any chronic illnesses?
  If yes, which ones?
- Are you allergic to eggs or medication?
  If yes, describe.
- Are you pregnant or nursing?
  Provide details.
- Have you ever had seizures?
  Provide details.
- Have you ever had psychiatric or psychological problems?
  Provide details.

- Have you ever had jaundice or hepatitis?
  Provide details.
- Are you or anybody in your household infected by HIV? Do you have any other immunodeficiencies?
- Have you been operated on your thymus or spleen?
  Provide details.

With future use of antimalarials, it may become essential to question travelers about glucose-6-phosphate dehydrogenase (G-6-PD) deficiency; however, this has not yet become routine.

Often, travelers are unable to provide accurate information about their immunization status; this is best discussed while reviewing the vaccination certificates. In addition, immunizations may have been performed during armed service duty; for this reason, discuss the possibility of military documents. Inviting all visitors to a travel health consultation to bring these documents is a useful standard procedure.

Whenever medical problems are indicated, discuss and, if necessary, assess those carefully. Otherwise, a medical checkup or further examinations are usually not warranted unless the traveler plans to become a long-term resident abroad or if extreme exertion is expected, such as mountaineering at high altitudes. A psychological and dental evaluation may be particularly important in both these circumstances.

Additional Readings

CATMAT. Guidelines for the practice of travel medicine. Canada Communicable Dis Rep 1999;25:ACS-6,7.

Eidex RB. History of thymoma and yellow fever vaccination. Lancet 2004;364:936.

Spira A. Preparing the traveler. Lancet 2003;361:1368–81.

Zuckenman JN. Travel medicine. Brit Med J 2002;325:260–4.

Pretravel Health Advice: Minimizing Exposure To Risks

Principles in the Practice of Travel Health Advice

To minimize exposure to risks—among others, the German language has the useful term "exposure prophylaxis"—the traveler needs to acquire some knowledge and some discipline. Intelligent behavior reduces risks. Ideally, the travel health professional should provide potential travelers with counsel that is tailored to suit the specific trip planned and to the individual's health status.

Large travel clinics often elect to use video programs that provide basic instructions to their customers. Such programs allow the travel staff to target the interview to specific items. Video programs should be based on "edutainment" rather than on rigid and strict dos and don'ts, and although the health professional must provide all necessary advice, avoid overloading the customer with unnecessary, or far too theoretical, information. Studies have shown that only a limited amount of information can be absorbed in such consultations. The counseling medical professional should ensure that all the important messages have been understood. The goal is to avoid discouraging customers from travel or to have them travel full of fears. Counseling families with children, long-term travelers, and persons with preexisting medical conditions is usually time-consuming.

To follow the basic rules of thoughtful behavior abroad, the traveler should be aware of the risks inherent in the 4 F and the 4 S (Table 4). They should become aware about the risks, as well as obtain knowledge about the preventive measures.

Avoiding Environmental Risks

Travel involves a considerable amount of physical effort. Various forms of environmental stress may impair a person's sense of well-being, may reduce resistance to disease, or may even cause disease. To a great extent, such stress can be avoided (Table 5).

To begin with, advise travelers to avoid stress by packing early, not in the last hour and then having to rush to the airport. As

Table 4 Main Instruction Targets for Travelers

Food	Boil it, cook it, peel it, or forget it
Fluids	Avoid tap water, drink plenty
Flies	Measures against mosquito bites
Flirts	No unprotected casual sex
Safe cars	Wear safety belt, no night driving
Swimming	Check currents, no alcohol
Sun	Don't get burned
Stress	Get rest, don't overload program

Table 5 How to Minimize Exposure to Risks

Risk Category	Type	Preventive Action
Psychological environment	Stress	Allow sufficient time
During travel	Claustro- and agoraphobia	Seat selection, cognitive therapy: avoid small boats and planes,
	Motion sickness	Seat selection, relaxed position of rest, preventive medication
	Jet lag	Melatonin or short-acting sleeping pill?
At destination	Climate	Clothing, fluids, minerals, frequent showers, avoid exertion
	Sun	Sun screen, minimal exposure
	Freshwater	Do not touch if risk of schistosomiasis, pools safe (?)
	Saltwater	Avoid currents, avoid bruises
	Soil	Do not walk barefoot or lie on soil
	Altitude	Slow ascent, warn high-risk subjects
	Traffic	Avoid night travel, motorbikes
Human to human	STD	Avoid unprotected casual sex
	Assault	Avoid risky areas, night strolls
Animal to human	Rabies	Do not pet unknown animals, do not touch cadavers
	Snakes (rare), scorpions	Wear shoes, check clothing
	Jellyfish, poisonous fish	Ask locals, wear goggles
Vectorborne	Malaria, dengue, etc	Measures against mosquito bites
Foodborne	Traveler's diarrhea, etc	"Boil it, cook it, peel it, or forget it"—as far as possible
Intoxicating drugs	Alcohol, marijuana, etc	Abstain before casual sex, swimming, diving

described in the Air Travel section (see "Essentials of Aviation Medicine"), it may be beneficial to select special seats while booking. At the destination, one should take necessary precautions to cope with the climate; specifically, in hot, dry places, it is important to maintain sufficient fluid balance. In particular, remind senior travelers, whose thirst reflex is vastly reduced, to consume many fluids. An excellent indicator is the color of the urine, which should be light. Salt tablets are usually not indicated, but after excessive sweating, travelers should take care to replenish their electrolytes by salt-containing food items or soups. Appropriate clothing (eg, cotton that is highly absorbent), will contribute to well-being. Gradual acclimatization over the initial days by avoiding exertion also benefits.

It is unrealistic to advise travelers to "avoid the sun." However, recommending that they avoid the sun at its highest intensity and to use ultraviolet (UV) blockers is practical. This is discussed in detail in Part 3 (see "Ultraviolet Rays" in Part 3, "Noninfectious Health Risks and Their Prevention").

There are many risks associated with large bodies of water. Swimmers and divers should beware of currents. (Check warning signs and flags—and ask the locals!) Sewage or industrial effluents can cause contamination. The visitor should find out if there is risk of schistosomiasis infection before swimming in lakes, ponds, and swamps; fast-flowing rivers pose lower risk of schistosomiasis. Pools are safe only if they are properly chlorinated. In all beach sports, accident prevention is paramount. Even a small bruise may result in a serious infection and pain; the traveler may be incapacitated for any physical activity. Advise individuals to use life jackets in potentially dangerous water sports.

Part 3 details the prevention of accidents related to the environment.

Avoiding Human Risks

If travelers cannot abstain from casual sex, they should at least avoid unprotected sex. More than half of British medical students do not practice safe sex on holiday! Travel health professionals (eg, tour guides) who know the plans of individuals in their group must learn to raise the subject, particularly in persons who are likely lonely or under the influence of alcohol or drugs. Even though sexual encounters are not always deliberately planned, all travelers should be warned of risks associated with casual, unprotected sex. Often, women do not convince their partners to wear a condom, and frequently men over age 40 are afraid of being rendered impotent while using a condom.

To avoid assaults, it is wise to abstain from walks, particularly alone and at night, in areas that are considered unsafe. It may help to hire a taxi even, for short distances in such situations, and to lock the doors during the ride. A few people need to be explicitly reminded not to wear jewelry and not to show money in poor countries.

Avoiding Animal Risks

Most animals avoid human beings. The danger from animals often arises following unnecessary intrusion from humans. Local guides who accompany trekking safaris to watch bears, elephants, and gorillas usually direct individuals in their group about the best behavior methods, both under normal circumstances and then when being charged by an animal. Travelers must obey these directives. To prevent the risk of rabies, one should not pet, terrify, or tease unknown animals. Travelers should keep a safe distance from dogs and other animals, whenever possible. If bitten, the individual must assume that the animal may be rabid and take appropriate measures (unless the country is certified to be rabies-free) (see "Rabies" in Part 2, "Infectious Health Risks and Their Prevention"). Accompanying animals (dogs and, for many countries, cats) must be immunized against rabies before they are allowed to cross international frontiers.

While walking anywhere, including the beach, one should wear strong, thick shoes. This will protect against snake bites and scorpion stings as well as jigger fleas, Tunga penetrans, sandflies (phlebotomes), and thus Leishmania infection, fungal infections, and plantar warts.

Before putting on any clothing or shoes, one should first check for small animals or poisonous insects.

Avoiding Vector-borne Diseases

Female mosquitoes use visual, thermal, olfactorial (carbon dioxide, butanoic acid, etc.) and visual stimuli to locate a human host required for their reproduction cycle. Male mosquitoes feed primarily on the nectar in flowers.

Dark colors attract the Anopheles mosquitoes, light ones attract the Aedes mosquitoes. The mosquitoes prefer to target male adults usually more than women and children, but there are is important individual variations in attraction. Anopheles gambiae place 80% of the bites on the ankles, whereas other mosquitoes prefer the neck and face areas. Fragrances from perfumes, soaps, or lotions may attract mosquitoes.

To avoid arthropods transmitting a wide variety of communicable diseases, first and foremost, tourists should prevent mosquito bites between dusk and dawn to avoid malaria infection by Anopheles and Japanese encephalitis by Culex. Aedes mosquitoes, however, transmit dengue fever during daytime.

Therefore, personal protection measures (PPM) are paramount at all times, especially when increased mosquito activity is noted, such as after rainy periods.

Screened Rooms, Air-Conditioning, Clothing

Staying in air-conditioned rooms or rooms that are protected by wire meshes (screens with 6 to 8 meshes per cm2) are quite safe, but few tourists will renounce outdoor activities just to avoid mosquito bites. While outdoors, they should use clothing to cover arms, legs, and particularly the ankles. Mosquito bites may penetrate thin clothes (< 1 mm thick and openings > 0.02 mm), which obviously are preferred in a tropical climate.

Repellents

Thus, it is recommended to spray clothing with repellents or, even better, with insecticides. Individuals should protect the uncovered skin with a repellent.

Repellents are chemicals that cause insects to turn away. Most contain DEET (N,N-diethyl-3-methylbenzamide), an effective substance that has been used for more than 40 years. Some others contain ethyl-buthylacetyl¬aminopropionate (EBAAP), picaridin (1-piperidinecarboxylic acid 2-(2-hydroxyethyl)-1-methyl-propylester, Bayrepel), DMP (dimethylphtalate, reduced effect when temperature > 23 °C), ethylexanediol, indalone, or a mixture of these. Synthetic repellents are effective for several hours (most 3 to 4 hours; microencapsulated products may last longer), and thus requiring reapplication in prolonged exposure. Although older-generation DEET formulations are rapidly lost through sweating, newer ones containing polymers or other additives last longer but are frequently considered too sticky. The duration of protection depends on:

- Environment: temperature (each 10 °C increase may result in up to 50% reduction in protection time), humidity, sunlight, wind
- Formulation: concentration, solvent (eg, polymers), encapsulation
- Host factors: sweating, individual odor, percutaneous penetration of repellent in the skin
- Part of the skin exposed: body vs. head
- Abrasion by clothing

- Behavior: swimming, washing off repellent
- Targeted insects: blood feeders vs. stinging insects

There is a low risk of DEET toxicity, which usually occurs when the product is misused. This is due to absorption of 9% to 56% of the chemical through the skin, with higher rates in alcohol-based solutions, especially in young children. This raises concerns in infants, in whom three cases of lethal encephalopathy using high concentrations (up to 100%) have been observed. The concentration is therefore limited to 35% in many countries. Any formulation with higher concentrations is not recommended for anyone. Repellents can be used in children > 2 months of age; in older infants and young children, the concentration for DEET and EBAAP should not exceed 10%, and mosquito nets should always be applied.

Travelers should be instructed to apply the repellent sparingly on all exposed areas. Unprotected skin areas just a few centimeters from a treated area may be attacked by hungry mosquitoes. Repellents should not be inhaled, ingested, applied on open wounds or irritated skin, or allowed to get into the eyes. For this reason, avoid applying repellents on children's hands, because the chemical is then likely to get into their eyes or mouth. Most repellents (with the exception of Bayrepel) are solvents of plastic materials; therefore, eyeglasses or lenses, plastic watches, or varnish, must be protected or removed before the repellent is applied. It is recommended to wash off the repellent when it is no longer needed.

Natural repellents, such as citronella oil or other plant extracts, are rarely used anymore; their effectiveness is usually limited to < 1 hour and such substances are more likely to cause allergic reactions.

Ethylhexamedial (Rutgers 612) apparently is the only agent that is effective against tsetse flies, known to transmit sleeping sickness.

Insecticides

Insecticides are poisons that target the nerves of insects and other cold-blooded animals and thus kill them. Synthetic pyrethroid insecticides (permethrin, deltamethrin, and others) are more photostable and less volatile than are the natural product pyrethrum (obtained from the flowers of Chrysanthemum cinerariaefolium). Pyrethrum acts as an insecticide and a repellent.

Use pyrethroid-containing sprays to eliminate mosquitoes from living and sleeping areas during evening and night-time hours. Such sprays are also used in aircraft for disinsection (ie, to avoid the importation of mosquitoes to countries non-endemic for malaria). Most experts consider them nontoxic. Occasionally, mosquitoes may enter even air-conditioned rooms. Mosquito coils containing pyrethroids may be used, although these coils last only a few hours. Many products are of questionable quality and may cause irritation of the mucous membranes.

Clothing sprayed with permethrin or deltamethrin provides residual protection for 2 to 4 weeks; the spraying causes no stains and minimal odor. For adults, this is considered nontoxic, whereas in infants and children this is questionable. Permethrin, however, should not be applied directly on the skin.

If an accommodation allows entry of mosquitoes, use sprays, dispensers, or pyrethroid mosquito coils, in addition to a mosquito net. Impregnation (soaking) of such nets with insecticide offers additional protection for 2 to 3 months, even when the net is slightly damaged. Nets should always be trussed under the mattress. For impregnation of nets (or clothing, used mainly by the military), use premixed Peripel, or measure 0.5 g/m2 of permethrin or 0.05 g/m2 of deltamethrin. Soak and squeeze the clothing to absorb the insecticide solution, wring gently, dry flat on a plastic sheet, avoiding direct sunlight, and after a while, hang up the clothing to speed up the drying process. Use gloves to do it and dispose of the rest of the solution with the garbage or directly into the soil. Avoid disposing into the water, because of long lasting toxic effect to cold-blooded animals like fish. Pre-impregnated bed nets are available and some bed nets use pre-impregnated fibers, that offer a long lasting insecticidal protection.

Other Ineffective Agents

Oral agents such as vitamin B, ultrasonic devices, and bug zappers that lure and electrocute insects are ineffective measures against mosquito bites.

Avoiding Contaminated Food and Beverage

Almost all travel counselors recommend avoiding contaminated food; however, few travelers consistently follow such advice. It is only rarely that travelers test the food with a thermometer and refuse it unless the core temperature is at least 60 °C. Careful behavior

Principles of Pretravel Counseling

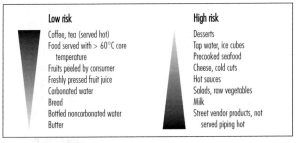

Figure 8 Food risk scale

will reduce the size of inoculum of infectious organisms that are ingested. However, it is not practical and will not completely protect from all gastrointestinal infections; sometimes, pathogens are found even in bottled water (Figure 8). Because it is impossible to convince all travelers to avoid cold buffets or other potentially contaminated food or ensure satisfactorily hygienic kitchens in all parts of the world, a new strategy is necessary. Travelers should be educated about the risk scale, and emphasis should be on abstaining from highly dangerous items and situations. All travelers are free to decide what risks they want to take, but the decision should be made on an informed basis.

Additional Readings

Fenton KA, et al. HIV transmission risk among sub-Saharan Africans in London travelling to their countries of origin. AIDS 2001;15:1442–5.

Fradin MS, Day JF. Comparative efficacy of insect repellents against mosquito bites. N Engl J Med 2002;347:13–8.

Gratz NG, et al. Why aircraft disinsection. Bull World Health Organ 2000;78:995–1004.

Kalapurakkal SM, Brown AM. Exposure of children to DEET and other topically applied insect repellents. Am J Industrial Med 2005;47:91–7.

Matteelli A, Carosi G. Sexually transmitted diseases in travelers. Clin Infect Dis 2001;32:1063–7.

Potasman I, et al. Infectious outbreaks associated with bivalve shellfish consumption: a worldwide perspective. Clin Infect Dis 2002;35:921–8.

van Netten C. Analysis and implications of aircraft disinfectants. Sci Total Environ 2002;293:257–62.

Legal Issues

International Health Regulations

Obviously, a manual used worldwide cannot address issues based on national legislation. Of regional interest, at least to Europeans, is the Council Directive of 13 June 1990 on package travel, package holidays and package tours (90/314/EEC), Article 4, 1. (a) "The organizer and/or the retailer shall provide the consumer, in writing or any other appropriate form, before the contract is concluded, ... with information on the health formalities required for the journey and the stay;..."

Of worldwide relevance is the fact that revised International Health Regulations (IHR) are gradually becoming effective. The World Health Assembly decided (WHA 59.2) that Member States should "comply immediately on a voluntary basis with provision of the IHR 2005 considered relevant to the risk posed by avian influenza and pandemic influenza." Ratification was scheduled to take place overall June 15, 2007. The new IHR are a tremendous advance over those of 1969, which were limited to three infections: cholera, plague, and yellow fever.

The purpose of the IHR remains "to prevent, protect against, control and provide public health responses to international spread of disease in ways that are commensurate with risks and threats to public health, and which avoid unnecessary interference with international traffic." Not the World Health Organization (WHO), but the national authorities within their respective jurisdictions are responsible for the health measures under these regulations. Under the new IHR, we can expect improved surveillance and information. In public health emergencies of international concern, WHO will issue temporary recommendations.

Similar, to the 1969 IHR, "State Parties shall designate specific yellow fever vaccination centers within their territories in order to ensure the quality and safety of the procedures and materials employed." (Annex 7, f). Yellow fever vaccination must be documented in "an international certificate of vaccination … in the form specified." (Annex 6, 2). "Certificates must be signed in the hand of the clinician, who shall be a medical practitioner or other authorized health worker, supervising the administration of the vaccine.… The certificate must also bear the official stamp of the administering center.... (Annex 6, 4).

"If the supervising clinician is of the opinion that the vaccination or prophylaxis is contraindicated on medical grounds, the supervising clinician shall provide the person with reasons, written in English or French, and where appropriate in another language in addition to English or French, underlying that opinion, which the competent authorities on arrival should take into account. The supervising clinician and competent authorities shall inform such persons of any risk associated with non-vaccination and with the non-use of prophylaxis in accordance with paragraph 4 of Article 23." (Annex 6, 9)

Health authorities in most countries usually respect such exemption certificates.

This is to certify that [name] ...., date of birth ....

sex ...., nationality ...., national identification document,

if applicable ...., whose signature follows

....

has on the date indicated been vaccinated or received prophylaxis against:

(name of disease or condition)..

in accordance with the International Health Regulations.

Vaccine or prophylaxis	Date	Signature and professional status of supervising clinician	Manufacturer and batch no. of vaccine or prophylaxis	Certificate valid from .... until	Official stamp of administering centre
1. *yellow fever*	*15 Jun 07*	*MᵢᵢᵢᵢL MD*	STAMARIL® PASTEUR Lot:A5255-10	*25 Jun 07* *24 Jun 17*	*stamp of center*
2.					

Figure 9 International Certificate of Vaccination or Prophylaxis (WHO 2007 edition).

Health Insurance

In countries where the usual health insurance does not cover treatment abroad and air evacuation, it may be recommendable to obtain special insurance coverage, particularly when a traveler has a preexisting illness. As there are vast differences in customary insurance contracts in various parts of the world, this cannot be discussed in this Manual. Travel health professionals should ascertain that their customers are aware of possible need for additional subscription.

Additional Readings

Colville J, et al. The cost of overseas visitors to an inner city accident and emergency department. J Accid Emerg Med 1996;13:16–7.

Leggat PA, Leggat FW. Travel insurance claims made by travelers from Australia. J Travel Med 2002;9:59–65.

BASICS OF IMMUNIZATION

The human immune system protects the body by eliminating or neutralizing materials recognized as foreign. The goal of immunization is to evoke an immune response in the vaccinee, for instance, by producing antibodies. This is based on the fact that the immune system is capable of remembering previous encounters with immunogenic substances, which results in stronger responses upon rechallenge. As a public health measure, the goal is to achieve herd immunity—interrupting transmission by immunizing a sufficient proportion of individuals in the population.

In active immunization (vaccination), an immunogenic substance (a vaccine) is administered. This is processed and modified by various cells of the human immune system until ultimately the B lymphocytes either differentiate into antibody-producing plasma cells specific for that vaccine or into long memory B lymphocytes. In passive immunization, antibodies produced by another (usually human) organism, mostly called immune globulins, are occasionally administered to provide immediate but short-lasting protection.

Live attenuated vaccines contain live microorganisms that have been attenuated (weakened) to induce active immunity without causing illness. Inactivated vaccines are composed of killed microorganisms or of components that will induce active immunity.

The individual vaccines are described in detail in Part 2. Because national standards for licensure differ, not all vaccines are available in all countries. Similarly, for vaccines against the same disease and for vaccine schedules, contraindications and other regulations may differ by product and by country. Recommendations issued by national authorities and manufacturer's instructions must therefore be consulted for up-to-date information and details.

Strategy for Application of Immunizations

Appropriate immunizations prior to travel not only reduce the risk of vaccine-preventable diseases for the recipient, but secondarily they also reduce the risk of international spread of the respective diseases. Consider several key factors when planning immunizations for individuals with travel plans as illustrated in this chapter. The essentials are as follows:

Travel related:
- Destination: country/countries, cities or resorts vs. rural or off the beaten track
- Duration of travel—not just for this journey, but also consider cumulative exposure over the individual's lifetime or at least the next years
- Characteristics: chaperoned luxury tour vs. backpacker; individual risk exposure, possibly depending on reasons for travel, such as certain professionals, personal hobbies, visiting friends and relatives (VFR)
- Legal obligations at destination: required immunizations

Host related:
- Personal immune status: previous immunizations, history of infection with resulting lifelong immunity
- Personal state of health with subsequent special risk (eg, travelers with splenectomy)
- Age (eg, infants, senior travelers with additional needs for vaccines (that is, routine immunizations against influenza)
- Specific contraindications in the vaccine recipient, such as pregnancy, lactation, altered immune competence, lower age limit

Vaccine related:
- Protective efficacy
- Safety profile
- Cost and financial constraints
- Contraindications
- Time restraints for useful protection

Most certainly, not all travel-related vaccines are indicated for all travelers. Ultimately, it is an arbitrary decision to what degree one wishes to recommend protection to a client. Decisions must primarily be based on a risk assessment. Some vaccines may be medically contraindicated, such as in pregnancy, or there may be time constraints (Figure 10). The travel health professional should be aware of priorities, with respect to incidence and severity of the various infections (Table 6). The health professional and the traveler should also take into account cost and risk of adverse reactions and decide on what and how much immunization is required. It is illogical to immunize travelers against rare diseases that have a low case fatality rate with modern

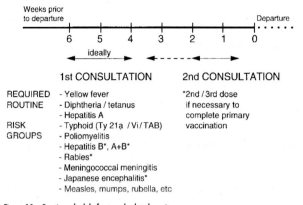

Figure 10   Routine schedule for travel-related vaccines

therapy and leave the travelers unprotected against more frequent and life-threatening infections for which no effective treatment is available.

Table 6   Rationale for Immunization of Travelers

Infection	Incidence	Impact	Total	Immunization	
				Yes	No
Hepatitis A	+++	++	+++++		
Hepatitis B	++	+++	+++++		
Rabies	++	++	++++		
Yellow fever	(+)	+++	+++(+)		
Typhoid fever	++	+	+++		
Influenza	++(+)?	(+)	+++		
Poliomyelitis	(+)	++	++(+)		
Diphtheria	(+)	++	++(+)		
Tetanus	(+)	++	++(+)		
Meningococcal disease	(+)	++	++(+)		
Japanese encephalitis	(+)	++	++(+)		
Cholera	+	+	++		
Measles	(+)	+	+(+)		

The overcautious physician or traveler, those unconcerned about adverse events — Rational / Illogical

The hazardous, the cost conscious

Rate per 100,000:   +++ = >100; ++ = 1–99; + = 0.1–0.9; (+) = < 0.1

Impact: +++ = high case fatality rate, serious residuals; ++ = > 5% case fatality rate or incapacitation > 4 weeks; + = low case fatality rate, brief incapacitation

Additional Readings

Berger A. How does herd immunity work. BMJ 1999;319:1466–7.

Shlim DR, Solomon T. Japanese encephalitis vaccine for travelers: exploring the limits of risk. Clin Infect Dis 2002;35:183–8.

Steffen R, Connor BA. Vaccines in travel health: from risk assessment to priorities. J Travel Med 2005;12:26–35.

General Immunization Rules

Vaccine Administration

Store vaccines as recommended by the manufacturer. In the case of vaccines in suspension form, verify the shelf life and shake the suspension well before use. Administer the vaccines as recommended by the manufacturer—intramuscularly (IM), subcutaneously (SC), or intradermally (ID). Some vaccines come with several options in the route of administration. Although it is important to observe the required minimum intervals between vaccine doses, it is irrelevant if too many months, years, or decades have elapsed since the last dose, except that there may be inadequate immunity during the interval before the next dose. There is a fundamental principle: "Every dose counts!" It is unnecessary to restart an interrupted series of vaccination or to add extra doses.

The skin at the injection site (deltoid region in adults and in children age > 1 year, anterolateral thigh in infants age < 1 year, quadriceps muscle if intramuscular) should be cleansed with an antiseptic agent, such as 70% isopropyl alcohol, povidone-iodine, or simply soap and water. Ideally, wait 5 minutes for optimal germicidal effect before the vaccine is administered. Use a new needle and a new syringe for each injection. The only exceptions to this are live vaccine scarifications (smallpox, some bacille Calmette-Guérin) where antiseptic agents would inactivate the vaccine; cleansing with a dry pad is sufficient. Some health professionals find it useful to ask the traveler to take a deep breath just when the injection is administered; this may reduce the pain by distracting the patient. For children, Eutetic Mixture of Local Anesthetics (EMLA) patches may be applied at the site of injection about 15 minutes prior to injection to desensitize the skin.

Vaccination Rules and Requirements

The required vaccinations, based on the International Health Regulations (IHR) are provided in Appendix B.

As a condition for entry, various countries require proof of vaccination administered at an approved vaccination center; this must be documented on the International Certificate of Vaccination or Prophylaxis (Figure 9). Many countries require such proof only from travelers arriving from infected or potentially endemic areas, whereas others require such evidence from all travelers, sometimes even those in transit. For international travel, the only certificate that is required now is the International Certificate of Vaccination or Prophylaxis as defined by the new IHR. As listed below, additional requirements exist, particularly for immunizations against cholera, diphtheria, and meningococcal disease. The latter applies mainly to pilgrims visiting Saudi Arabia to participate in the Hajj or Umra, where proof of immunization with the quadrivalent vaccine is now required. When immunizations are not required as a condition for entry, it is unnecessary to transfer information on national or provincial vaccination documents to the International Certificate of Vaccination.

Travelers who have a contraindication to a required vaccination should obtain a validated waiver from the proper authorities. In addition, waivers obtained from embassies or consulates of the countries to be visited may be useful. In fact, on rare occasions the health authorities of some countries have refused to accept medical waivers.

Mainly in the United States, proof of immunization against diphtheria, measles, poliomyelitis, and rubella is now universally required for entry into educational institutions. Likewise, school-entry requirements of most states include immunization against tetanus (49 states), pertussis (44 states), mumps (42 states), and hepatitis B (34 states). Increasingly also proof of vaccination against hepatitis A is required. Some institutions also need proof of varicella (chicken pox) vaccine. Many colleges in the United States and the United Kingdom now request, or at least recommend, meningococcal vaccination for students.

All developed countries have national plans and programs for routine childhood immunizations, with minor differences. They are therefore not described in detail in this manual, as this would be beyond the scope of international travel.

Travel brochures often refer only to vaccinations required by the IHR. It is of utmost importance to know and to convince travelers that generally recommended routine immunizations often play a more significant role in maintaining a traveler's health than those that are legally required.

Schedule, Simultaneous Administration, Combined Vaccines

In the past, travelers have received their immunizations on up to seven different dates. This certainly was not practical and may well have had a negative effect both on compliance and costs. Because there are few significant interactions between vaccines, all travel-related vaccines can be administered in one single session, except in cases where multiple doses are needed (Figure 10). This is, however, only needed in risk groups or in persons who failed to receive their routine childhood immunizations.

Most widely used antigens can be given on the same day without impairing antibody response or increasing the rate of adverse reactions. Use different injection sites in simultaneous vaccinations, with a distance of at least 2 cm between each site. Usually in right-handed adults, all simultaneously given vaccines are administered into the left deltoideus; the vaccinees will feel less pain at work and will not be inconvenienced by pain in both arms while lying in bed. Mixing vaccines in the same syringe or sequential injection through the same needle is clearly wrong, unless explicitly allowed by the manufacturer. For some travel-related vaccines (hepatitis A and hepatitis B, hepatitis A and typhoid) and mainly in the pediatric field (see "Infants and Children" in Part 1, "General Strategies in Host-Related Special Risks"), vaccine combinations exist, allowing a reduction in the number of injections.

When simultaneous administration is not performed, one should consider that the immune response to a live virus vaccine may theoretically be impaired if the vaccine is administered within 30 days of administration of another live virus vaccine. Thus, live virus vaccines should be given simultaneously or at least 1 month apart.

Contraindications

Part 2 lists the details on each vaccine. The following provides the general contraindications for vaccines:

1. Acute illness. Persons with acute illness are unlikely to present themselves for travel related immunization. Moderate or severe illnesses are a good reason to postpone immunization, whereas mild ones (eg, a common cold with low-grade fever) are no reason for delay.

2. Lower age limit. Infants may be unable to produce antibodies to some vaccines; they may, however, be protected by maternal antibodies.

3. Hypersensitivity to vaccine components. Some people may have experienced hypersensitivity during previous vaccine administration. Some individuals may be hypersensitive to thimerosal or trace amounts of antibiotics or proteins. No vaccine currently used in the developed nations contains penicillin or penicillin derivatives.

   Allergy to egg proteins (found in yellow fever, influenza, measles-mumps-rubella [MMR], measles, and mumps vaccines) is no contraindication for immunization, but perform vaccination in a setting where adverse reactions can be dealt with appropriately. Skin tests with a 1:20 to 1:100 saline diluted vaccine, whereby 0.1 mL is injected ID, or desensitization is obsolete.

4. Pregnancy. There are considerable differences when national recommendations are compared. Essentially, the risk in use of live vaccines during pregnancy is largely theoretical; thus, weigh the risk of infection against the risk of immunization (this also applies for the one- (previously three-) month period before pregnancy); take into consideration the concerns of the pregnant woman in the decision-making process. In most countries, there are also some reservations with respect to the use of inactivated vaccines during pregnancy (See individual vaccines.)

5. Lactation. Although the risk in the use of live vaccines in lactating women is largely theoretical, weigh the risk of infection against the risk of immunization, taking into account concerns of the lactating woman. (See individual vaccines.)

6. Altered immunocompetence. Congenital immunodeficiency, acquired immunodeficiency syndrome (AIDS), leukemia, lymphoma, generalized malignancy, therapy with antimetabolites or alkylating agents, radiation, and large doses (body weight 2 mg/kg/d or > 20 mg/d) of prednisone or equivalents alter immunocompetence. After systemic treatment with high-dose corticosteroids for a period of > 2 weeks, at least 3 months should elapse after stopping treatment before a live-virus vaccine is administered. In limited immune deficits such as asplenia or renal failure, higher doses of vaccines or additional vaccines may be indicated, but these subjects do not have contraindications for any particular vaccine.

Inactivated vaccines do not represent danger to immuno-compromised recipients, but the immune response may be suboptimal. In contrast, live vaccines may lead to serious complications and are often contraindicated. Sometimes, for example, with poliomyelitis or typhoid vaccines, there are options to select an inactivated vaccine, rather than a live one.

7. Anticoagulation. See Part 2.

Note that interferon medications and glatiramer acetate are not immunosuppressants; people who are taking these medications can be given all vaccines

Effectiveness of Vaccines

The effectiveness of vaccines varies greatly, from less than 50% (for instance, against influenza in a senior citizen) to close to 100% (eg, for hepatitis A and tetanus). Details are described under the separate vaccine headings in Part 2. Measurement of immune response is usually not indicated, particularly it is a misconception to try to assess anti-HAV (hepatitis A antibodies) after completed immunization as the usually performed assays are not sufficiently sensitive. Assessment of immune response is mainly indicated after immunization against hepatitis B in health professionals and other persons at high risk. For other vaccines, there are few additional indications, such as in persons who experienced hyperergic local reactions after diphtheria-tetanus booster injections, or professional exposure to rabies.

Reactions to Travel-Related Vaccines

Although severe reactions are extremely rare in vaccines required for travel, anaphylaxis or serious hypersensitivity reactions are possible. Every clinic must have the necessary therapeutic agents (epinephrine, antihistamines, corticosteroids) immediately available, and the personnel administering vaccines must be trained and be qualified to handle such an emergency. Most would agree that, in a travel clinic, a physician must be available on site within less than 5 minutes for such emergencies.

Local pain and swelling are common problems after a parenteral dose of vaccine; fever, rash, or other symptoms may rarely occur (see Part 2 for details). Illness resulting in long-term sequelae or death may occur after vaccination, but the incidence rate for the routine or travel-related vaccines is below 1 in 1 million.

Cost-Effectiveness of Travel Immunizations

No travel-related vaccination is considered beneficial with respect to cost; the cost of vaccination is greater than the cost of avoided infection and death. Nevertheless, immunization before travel remains vital for health reasons, and many travelers are willing to invest in safety, just as they elect to invest in comfort when choosing a more expensive hotel.

Recommendations for Immunizations

As Table 6 illustrates, there is considerable consensus with respect to immunization recommendations issued by the World Health Organization and other selected major national expert groups. On the basis of this consensus, the subsequent recommendations for specific vaccines for specific countries have been formulated. Details are provided in Part 2 of this manual, wherein individual vaccines are discussed.

Table 7 Recommended Immunizations in Nonimmune Travelers to a Developing Country

Expert Group	WHO (World)	CATMAT (Canada)	CDC (USA)	HPA (UK)	NHMRC (Australia)
REQUIRED					
• Yellow fever	**	**	**	**	**
ROUTINE					
• Diphtheria/tetanus	***	***	***	***	***
• Poliomyelitis	**	**	**	**	**
• Measles, usually MMR	***	***	***	***	***
RECOMMENDED					
• Hepatitis A	***	***	***	***	***
• Hepatitis B	***	*	*	*	*
• Rabies	*	*	*	*	*
• Influenza	*	*	*	*	*
• Typhoid fever	*	*	*	*	*
• Meningococcal disease	*	*	*	*	*
• Japanese encephalitis	*	*	*	*	*
• Tuberculosis	*	–/*	–	*	*
• Cholera	–	–	–	–	–

*** = all; ** = all when visiting endemic country; * = risk group only, – = none; N/A = not available

In Table 7, the term "risk group only" relates to different risk groups for each vaccine, and as described on page 66, mainly travel- and host-related aspects need to be considered. See "Recommendations for Vaccine Use" under each heading of vaccine-preventable infections in Part 2. As a rule of thumb, in addition to the short-term travel recommendations, long-term travelers to developing countries should get immunized against the following:

- Hepatitis B
- Typhoid fever
- Rabies (unless in a region with low endemicity, or there is a small risk [eg, for some diplomats])

Additional Readings

Ess SM, Szucz TD. Economic evaluation of immunization strategies. Clin Infect Dis 2002;35:294–7.

Plotkin SA, Orenstein WA, editors. Vaccines. 5th ed. Philadelphia (PA): WB Saunders; 2007.

BASICS OF MALARIA PROPHYLAXIS

Malaria, a protozoan disease, is caused by four species of the genus Plasmodium. *Plasmodium falciparum* is the most important, as it leads to malaria tropica, whereas *Plasmodium vivax* and the less frequently occurring *Plasmodium ovale* and *Plasmodium malariae* only rarely cause life-threatening disease. Plasmodia are mainly transmitted through the bite of infected female Anopheles mosquitoes, feeding almost exclusively between dusk and dawn. As described in detail in Part 2, the risk of malaria varies according to the region, altitude, and season.

Malaria infection results in partial immunity ("semi-immunity") that provides protection at least from serious disease. This immunity seems to be directed primarily against the erythrocytic stages of the parasite and decreases rapidly (within 6 to 12 months) once the person leaves the endemic area, leaving him or her as susceptible to the disease as any nonimmune individual.

Prophylaxis for malaria and its complications is based on four principles:

- Information
- Personal protection measures against mosquito bites (discussed earlier and in Part 2)
- Chemoprophylaxis (usually, chemosuppression), where appropriate
- Prompt assessment and treatment of symptoms suggestive of malaria, including emergency self-therapy in special circumstances

Information

Travelers visiting countries where malaria is endemic should obtain essential information on the following:
- Location of endemic regions and of areas free (or with negligible risk) of transmission (Figure 11; Appendix B)
- Mode and period of transmission: infected mosquitoes that bite almost exclusively at night, particularly around midnight
- Incubation period: minimum 6 days for *P. falciparum* and may be up to several months (occasionally even exceeding 1 year), particularly in other Plasmodium species

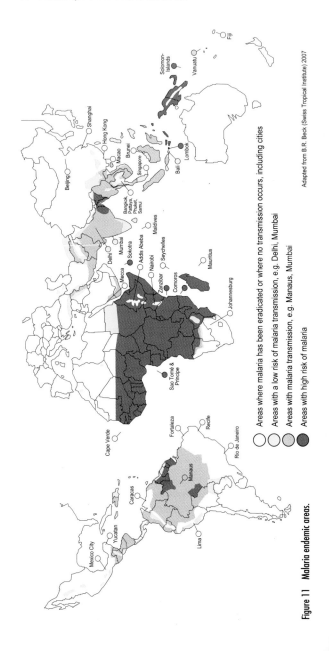

Adapted from B.R. Beck (Swiss Tropical Institute) 2007

○ Areas where malaria has been eradicated or where no transmission occurs, including cities

○ Areas with a low risk of malaria transmission, e.g. Delhi, Mumbai

○ Areas with malaria transmission, e.g. Manaus, Mumbai

● Areas with high risk of malaria

Figure 11 Malaria endemic areas.

- Early symptoms: usually flu-like, with fever, chills, headache, generalized aches and pains, and malaise. These symptoms may or may not occur with classic periodicity
- Options for prevention:
  1. Preventive measures against mosquito bites are the first line of defence.
  2. When indicated, use chemoprophylaxis, but also caution travelers
     - that this strategy is not 100% effective even when compliance is perfect, and
     - the chemoprophylactic agent may cause adverse reactions.
  3. Explain to travelers why their prophylactic regimen should be continued for 4 weeks after leaving the transmission area.
- Necessity of medical consultation within 24 hours when symptoms are suggestive of malaria, because complications may develop rapidly thereafter. The best advice is to "think malaria" when febrile symptoms occur.

Chemoprophylaxis

Chemoprophylaxis is essentially a misnomer; most currently marketed drugs do not prevent infection. Instead, these agents act by suppressing the proliferation and development of the malarial parasite and, thus, are better termed "chemosuppressive agents."

Mode of Action

Prevention of malaria symptoms requires a disruption of the plasmodial life cycle. Several agents are available, which act at one or more points in the parasite's cycle. Causal prophylactics (such as atovaquone) act on the hepatic (exoerythrocytic) cycle, interfering with early hepatic development of the plasmodium and, therefore, preventing the next stage, the erythrocytic cycle. Other drugs (chloroquine and mefloquine) are blood schizonticides, which act by destroying the asexual intraerythrocytic parasites. The terminal prophylactic, primaquine, prevents relapses of *P. vivax* and *P. ovale* infection by eliminating the latent hepatic hypnozoites (Figure 12).

Risk-Benefit Analysis

All antimalarial agents—when selected correctly—have a prophylactic efficacy exceeding 95%, but also have a potential for causing adverse events. It is logical to recommend chemopro-

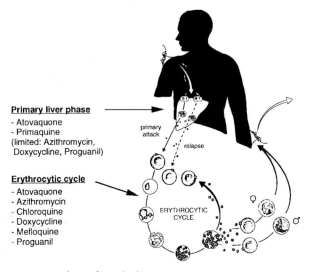

Primary liver phase
- Atovaquone
- Primaquine
(limited: Azithromycin,
 Doxycycline, Proguanil)

Erythrocytic cycle
- Atovaquone
- Azithromycin
- Chloroquine
- Doxycycline
- Mefloquine
- Proguanil

Figure 12   Site of action of antimalarials

phylaxis for travelers to endemic areas, whenever the benefit of avoided symptomatic infections exceeds the risk of serious adverse events (ie, events that require hospitalization). This is the case for most stays (except very short ones) in areas with high or intermediate transmission, such as tropical Africa, some Pacific areas, and certain provinces in Brazil (Figure 11; see also Appendix B). In contrast, at the most frequently visited destinations in Southeast Asia and Latin America, the risk of acquiring a malaria infection is low. The frequency of adverse experience with subsequent hospitalization associated with the use of prophylactic medication with chloroquine, chloroquine plus proguanil, or mefloquine clearly exceeds any expected benefit. With the atovaquone plus proguanil combination fewer hospitalizations have been reported. According to the World Health Organization (WHO) and various European expert groups, for trips to areas of low risk, it is more appropriate to insist on personal protection measures against mosquito bites and to recommend consulting a doctor within 24 hours of onset of suggestive symptoms than it is to prescribe malaria chemoprophylaxis. If the traveler stays in an area where competent medical infrastructure is not present, standby or presumptive treatment may constitute an alternative strategy. This approach is discussed

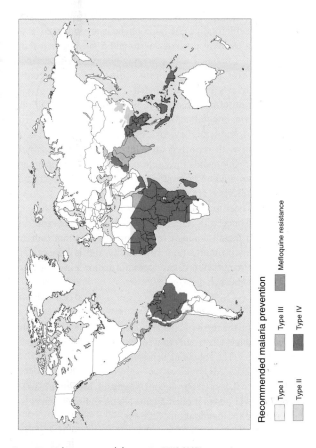

Recommended malaria prevention

Type I
Type II
Type III
Type IV
Mefloquine resistance

Figure 13 Malaria: recommended prevention (WHO 2007)

in detail in Part 2 of this manual; it is not, however, endorsed by the Centers for Disease Control and Prevention (CDC) in the United States nor by various other national expert groups.

Type I means very limited risk of malaria, thus mosquito bite prevention only is sufficient.

Type II means that there is only risk of *P. vivax* malaria or of fully chloroquine-sensitive *P. falciparum.* Mosquito bite prevention plus chloroquine chemoprophylaxis are indicated.

Type III areas have a risk of *P. vivax* and *P. falciparum* malaria transmission, combined with emerging chloroquine resistance. Mosquito bite prevention plus chloroquine+proguanil chemoprophylaxis are recommended.

Type IV describes areas with either high risk of *P. falciparum* malaria, in combination with reported antimalarial drug resistance; or moderate/low risk of P. falciparum malaria, in combination with reported high levels of drug resistance. WHO here recommends mosquito bite prevention plus mefloquine, doxycycline or atovaquone-proguanil chemoprophylaxis (details for selection are described in Part 2).

There is near-total consensus that travelers should be cautioned in advance with respect to possible side effects and how to deal with them, although few experts believe that overemphasis of this promotes poor tolerability and is unnecessary because the manufacturer's product information is available for those who want such details.

Schedules for Chemoprophylaxis

Depending on the regimen, malaria chemoprophylaxis is administered by tablets taken daily or weekly. Duration of prophylactic regimens vary. The following schedules are valid:

- Begin 1 to 2 days (if atovaquone/proguanil, Malarone is used) or 7 days (17 days if other agents are used) before travel.
- Continue for the duration of the stay
- Maintain for 1 week (if atovaquone/proguanil, Malarone is used) and 4 weeks (if other agents are used), respectively, after leaving the endemic area

Treatment in the pretravel period allows analysis of tolerability prior to departure and ensures protective plasma drug concentrations. This is essential when mefloquine 250 mg weekly or chloroquine 300 mg base/week is prescribed; a sufficient plasma concentration would be achieved within 2 days with chloroquine 100 mg base/day or with doxycycline. The 17/10/3 days predeparture scheme is particularly attractive to test tolerance to mefloquine; if three tablets are well tolerated, it is unlikely that additional doses will result in severe adverse reactions. If there are side effects, there is still time to prescribe atovaquone/ proguanil. Additionally, the customer will not travel on a day on which he takes medication; that results in the highest serum levels and in the highest risk of adverse events. In last-minute travelers, a loading dose is recommended (see Part 2). The continued intake after return ensures that late infections will be dealt with by effective plasma concentrations when the merozoites emerge from the liver to invade the erythrocytes. If an effective causal prophylactic drug is used, the duration of post-travel chemoprophylaxis could theoretically be shorter, because the parasite's development will already have been interrupted in the hepatic cycle.

When using doxycycline, it is sufficient to start chemoprophylaxis 2 days before arrival in the endemic zone, but continue for 4 weeks after leaving the endemic country. As for atovaquone plus proguanil, starting 1 to 2 days before arrival in the endemic zone is sufficient, and this combination drug (Malarone) may be discontinued 7 days after leaving the endemic country.

Choice of Agent

Selecting a prophylactic agent is often complex, and although there are generalized guidelines to minimize confusion, recommendations for travelers need to be tailored on an individual basis. Efficacy and tolerability are the most important factors to be considered.

Travel health professionals implementing WHO recommendations or national guidelines should be aware of

- Destination factors, such as the degree of endemicity
- Predominant Plasmodium species
- Extent of drug resistance (Figure 34), as this will define the efficacy of a particular agent
- Availability of drugs in the destination countries (beware of fake drugs)

The traveler's health and other characteristics (such as age and pregnancy) may also influence the choice of prophylaxis; certain regimens have clearly defined contraindications and precautions, which need to be observed to ensure tolerability. The duration and mode of travel have also been shown to be important, as well as medication factors such as compliance and acceptability.

█ Standby Emergency Treatment

When symptoms suggestive of malaria occur while abroad or after return, the traveler must obtain competent medical care within 24 hours of the onset of symptoms. Medical assessment must include blood sample screening, either by microscopic examination or with an appropriate rapid diagnostic test kit. Most travelers anywhere in the world have access to competent medical attention within the specified time frame. Only a minority may find themselves with symptoms suggestive of malaria in a location remote from established medical facilities. Advise these travelers to carry antimalarial medication for standby emergency treatment (SBET) and, if possible, to bring a malaria test kit. These emergency supplies can be used for self-diagnosis and self-therapy or made available to the consulted physician.

The disadvantage of this strategy is both over- and under-use of SBET. For travelers using this approach, it is imperative to provide the

- Precise instructions on how to recognize malaria symptoms
- Recommendation to seek local medical care, if possible
- Time frame to reach medical attention
- Precise use of the SBET medication
- Warning about the potential for adverse events
- Advice about the necessity to seek medical advice as soon as possible after initial treatment with SBET, which ensures that the therapy was successful or to obtain the proper treatment in case of erroneous self-diagnosis

Additional Reading

Schlagenhauf P. Traveler's malaria. Hamilton (ON): BC Decker; 2007.

OPTIONS FOR SELF-THERAPY AND TRAVEL MEDICINE KIT

Benefits of Self-Therapy

Travelers feel at a disadvantage when they fall ill while away from home and from customary medical care. At the place of visit, the desired medication may be unavailable or, when available, may be obsolete, past the expiry date, stored at the wrong temperature, unknown and explained in a foreign language, or it may just be a placebo. Whatever the reason, travelers are often reluctant to consult a local doctor in a developing country. Such hesitation may be perfectly justified. In the poorest countries, for instance, hepatitis B is often transmitted by injection because there is a lack of disposable materials. It may be impossible to contact their own physicians back home, and long-distance consultations, as well as telemedicine, have their own problems and limitations. Therefore, it is advisable to arm travelers to high-risk areas with medications to treat common health problems or accidents, such as:

- travelers' diarrhea
- the common cold
- malaria (low endemicity areas without access to medical care, see Part 2)
- insomnia due to jet lag
- frequent ailments in certain types of travelers (eg, constipation, bronchitis, low back pain)
- motion sickness
- small wounds
- sprained ankles

There are some basic rules with respect to self-therapy.

- Give proper verbal and written instructions on use and dosage of drugs.
- Set an upper time limit before a doctor is to be consulted.
- Inform travelers about possible adverse effects of therapeutic medication.

- Give preference to medications that the traveler has used previously.
- Avoid recommending self-therapy to the traveler who obviously cannot understand procedures and limitations.

Additional Readings

Newton PN, et al. Murder by fake drugs. BMJ 2002;324:800–1.

Shakoor O, et al. Assessment of the incidence of substandard drugs in developing countries. Trop Med Int Health 1997;2:839–45.

Simonsen L, et al. Unsafe injections in the developing world and transmission of bloodborne pathogens: a review. Bull World Health Organ 1999;77:789–800.

▌ Composition of the Travel Medical Kit

The content of the travel medical kit will be influenced by the destination (particularly if remote), the length of stay, the number of persons depending on the kit, potential health risks (eg, diving), and the health of the traveler.

The minimum requirements for a travel medical kit include:

- Medications regularly or occasionally used at home (including birth control)
- Malaria chemoprophylaxis, when indicated
- Medications for traveler's diarrhea (usually)
- Antimotility agents, preferably loperamide
- Antibiotics, preferably quinolone, rifaximin, or azithromycin for selected destinations
- Medications for the common cold, bronchitis (possibly levofloxacin, moxifloxacin, or azithromycin, which may be used for both gastrointestinal and respiratory tract infections, whereas older quinolones were limited for use in gastrointestinal infections)
- Analgesics/anti-inflammatories/antipyretics
- Sun block

Travelers should also consider taking

- condoms,
- a thermometer,
- material to treat cuts and bruises (disinfectants, dressings, scissors),
- elastic bandages.

Traveler's Health Center

Complete Address

City and Country

Telephone or Fax

Date: _____, 200___

Mr/Mrs

I, _____, MD, certify

that Mr/Mrs _____ carries with

him/her a medical kit that includes prescribed medication,

syringes, and needles to be used by a doctor, during

his/her trip in case of emergency. These are recommended

for personal use only to avoid the risk of accidental

transmission of infectious diseases. They are not to be sold.

_____

Medical Director

Traveler's Clinic

Figure 14 Sample of letter to accompany the travel medical kit

Some travelers may need or wish to take

- laxatives (if constipated during previous travels),
- rehydration powders,

- topical creams, such as steroids, anti-infectives, anti-inflammatories,
- ear and eye drops,
- motion sickness medication,
- altitude medication,
- jet lag medication, sleeping pills,*
- narcotics for analgesia,*
- syringes and needles.*

Additional Readings

A'Court CH. Doctor on a mountaineering expedition. BMJ 1995;310:1248–52.

Harper LA, et al. Evaluation of The Coca-Cola Company Travel Health Kit. J Travel Med 2002;9:244–8.

Goodyer L, Gibbs J. Medical Supplies for Travelers to Developing countries. J Travel Med 2004;11:208–12.

Welsh TP. Data-based selection of medical supplies for wilderness travel. Wilderness Environ Med 1997;8:148–51.

---

*To avoid problems with custom officers, it may be beneficial to have a letter of authorization that explains the reason for carrying these items (Figure 14). Many countries have strict laws with respect to importation of controlled substances; in some countries, benzodiazepines require special permits, although this is rarely enforced.

WATER DISINFECTION

Clean water is a scarce resource. Only 1% of the total water on earth (including the water in our atmosphere, lakes, rivers, streams, and the ground) is easily available. The rest is trapped in ice and glaciers or is saline. In many developing countries, the available raw water is virtually wastewater, contaminated with human feces. Tap water is frequently contaminated, and transmission of illness by water occurs often.

Safe beverages in such regions are boiled water, hot beverages, such as coffee or tea made with boiled water, canned or bottled carbonated beverages, beer, and wine. Most infectious agents are resistant to freezing, which means that ice in beverages is not safe either, even if the ice is in alcoholic drinks.

For consumption, water should first be cleaned from the rough particles by sedimentation (letting the particles settle) or filtration, disinfected, and then conserved.

Separating suspended particles large enough to settle rapidly by gravity (eg, sand and silt) takes an hour. The clear water should then be decanted or filtered from the top. This is not a disinfection method but helps to clarify water and simplifies further steps, such as halogenation.

Vigorous boiling for one minute is the quickest and most effective way to kill the waterborne pathogens. Boiling can kill even Cryptosporidium, one of the most resistant pathogens. The flat taste of boiled water can be improved by pouring it back and forth from one container to another (called aeration), by allowing it to stand for a few hours, or by adding a small pinch of salt. A disadvantage to boiling is that fuel sources may be unavailable and that the boiling point decreases with increasing altitude, which is 90 $^{\circ}$C at 3,000 m. In this situation, increase boiling time as a safety margin.

In a process called coagulation-flocculation, smaller suspended particles that are too small to settle by gravity can be removed. For coagulation, we use lime (alkaline chemicals, principally containing calcium or magnesium and oxygen) and alum (an aluminum salt) that causes particles to stick together as a result of electrostatic and ionic forces. Rapid mixing is important to obtain dispersion of the coagulant. The second stage, flocculation, is a physical process obtained by prolonged gentle mixing.

After settling, separate the water by decantation or filtration. This method removes 60 to 99% of the bacteria, viruses, Giardia, helminth ova, heavy metals and dissolved phosphates. Nevertheless, we advise a subsequent disinfecting step such as halogenation or filtration. One advantage of this method is that it also works with cold water, and toxicity is not an issue as long as the alum is not ingested. In an emergency, use normal baking powder or fine white ash.

Filtration is possible with rough filters and microfilters. Rough filters retain dirt. Microfilters may be single-layered or depth filters, which retain bacteria, protozoa, and parasites. Cryptosporidium cysts often pass through a standard size filter (a 1 μm pore size is recommended to hold them back), and viruses are too small to be trapped. Viruses can adhere to the walls of diatomite (ceramic) or charcoal filters by electrostatic chemical attraction. In heavily polluted water, they often aggregate in large clumps with the dissolved particles and are thus filtered. Generally, filters should not be considered adequate for complete removal of viruses, and additional treatment with heat or halogens is essential for effective virus removal.

Filters do not add an unpleasant taste to the water, and, in fact, often improve taste and odor by special granular-activated carbon. A silver layer on the filter improves the disinfecting rate but does not prevent contamination by microorganisms after prolonged use. A disadvantage is their weight and tendency to clog. The increased pressure that is needed can force microorganisms through the filter. Depth filters (eg, ceramic, fiber, or compressed granular-activated carbon) have a large capacity for holding particles, so they last longer than single-layer membrane filter. However, they are more difficult to clean effectively. Surface cleaning is only partially effective, and for this reason, microorganisms may grow in the depth. Reverse osmosis filters use high pressure to force water through a semipermeable membrane that filters out solids, molecules, and dissolved ions. It is effective in removing microbiologic contamination, but pressure can cause membrane breakdown, which renders them ineffective. For ocean travelers, it is an important survival item.

The germicidal activity of halogens, chiefly chlorine(Cl^-) and iodine(I^-), results from oxidation of essential cellular structures and enzymes. The impact of halogens depends on the concentration of the contamination and of the halogens, the time, the pH and temperature of the water, and the turbidity. The higher the concentration of the halogens, the better the disinfectant effect, but this also leaves "residual" halogen in the water, causing a bad taste and smell. Therefore, a prolonged contact time reduces the halogen concentration needed. The pH of the water should be neutral. If it is too acidic (eg, high mountain lakes) or too alkaline (eg, desert water), increase the contact time and concentration. The colder the water, the less germicidal activity halogens have. High turbidity can also shield the microorganisms from the impact of the halogens. To improve the taste of the halogens, the dose can be decreased and the contact time increased. Cloudy water can be filtered before adding the halogen, or dehalogenation like granular-activated charcoal, zinc brush, chlorination-dechlorination, and ascorbic acid can be used. Organisms, in order of increasing resistance to halogen disinfection, are bacteria, viruses, protozoan cysts, bacterial spores, and parasitic ova and larvae. Contact time varies from 2 hours for Giardia to 10 minutes for bacteria, with an average dose for average contaminated and dirty water of 1 to 2 mg per liter. Preference between iodine and chlorine varies. Chlorine has no known toxicity when used for water disinfection. The question of iodine toxicity remains controversial. Studies show that use of high levels of iodine (16 to 32 mg/day), as the recommended doses of iodine tablets, should be limited to a month. Iodine treatment that produces a low residual concentration of < 1 to 2 mg/L appears to be safe, even when given for long periods to individuals with healthy thyroids, but pregnant women, those with iodine hypersensitivity, and persons with thyroid problems should avoid iodine.

In addition, miscellaneous disinfectants can be used. Potassium permanganate is a strong oxidizing agent with some disinfectant properties but has been largely replaced by chlorine. It can be easily used for the purpose of washing fruit and vegetables. Hydrogen peroxide is a strong oxidizing agent but a weak disinfectant. Bacteria are inactivated within minutes to hours, depending on the level of contamination. Viruses require extremely high doses and longer contact times. Today, it is still popular as a wound cleanser and for odor control in sewage. Ultraviolet light (UV) can inactivate bacteria, viruses, and protozoa when administered at sufficient doses. Cysts should be removed by filtration. UV light does not require chemicals, does not affect the taste, and works rapidly. Because it has no residual disinfection power, water

Table 8 Temperature and time required for heat inactivation of microorganisms

Organism	Lethal temperature and time
Giardia species	70°C for 10 min (100% inactivation)
Cryptosporidium species	72°C heated up over 1 min
Bacterial Enteropathogens (ie, *E. coli*, *Salmonella*, *Shigella*, and *Campylobacter* species)	reaching 65°C
Enteric viruses	70°C for < 1 min
Hepatitis A virus	98°C for 1 min

Adapted from Backer (2002) and Bandres (1988).

can become recontaminated. Data are insufficient, so use this process only in emergency situations. Silver ions have a bactericidal effect when given in low doses, and these products have no impact on color, taste, and odor. However, available data on their use for disinfection of viruses and cysts show limited efficacy. The concentration is highly affected by adsorption onto the surfaces of the containers. This substance is probably best employed as a water preservative to prevent bacterial regrowth.

With respect to conservation, halogens are most suitable to prevent water from becoming recontaminated when stored. Maintain a residual concentration of 3 to 5 mg/L, and use iodine for short periods. Silver has also been approved for this purpose. For longtime storage, a tightly sealed container works best to decrease the risk of contamination.

Additional Reading

Backer H. Water disinfection for international and wilderness travelers. Clin Infect Dis 2002;34:355–64.

Bandres JC, Mathewson JJ, Dupont HL. Heat susceptibility of bacterial enteropathogens. Implications for the prevention of travelers' diarrhea. Arch Intern Med 1988; 148:2261–3.

General Strategies in Environment-Related Special Risks

DURATION OF EXPOSURE: FROM SHORT TRIPS TO EXPATRIATES

In this manual, we have defined "short trips" as stays in the developing countries lasting 1 to 6 days, and "long-term" stays as those that exceed 3 months. "Usual" stays abroad are for 7 days to 12 weeks.

Short Trips Abroad

Usually, individuals visiting the developing countries for just 1 to 6 days are business people, politicians or other VIPs, airline crews, or, less often, transit passengers, who use the airline of a developing country to obtain a cheaper fare. Among the short-term travelers, many are frequent travelers.

Epidemiology

Various studies illustrate that the attack rate (per stay) for illnesses, such as traveler's diarrhea, and the rate of accidents is lower for short-term travelers compared with usual or long-term travelers, but the incidence rate (per specified period of stay) is usually independent of the duration of stay. Exceptions with lower rates, such as for malaria, in short-trip travelers most often are due to travelers staying in urban centers, which, to some extent, are a protected environment with limited exposure to pathogenic agents. The rate of traveler's diarrhea among international corporate business travelers staying abroad for 1 week or less was < 6%, but the proportion of travelers who visited high-risk destinations is unknown. Several anecdotal cases of serious illness (including poliomyelitis and yellow fever) and accidents during and after short stays in the developing countries have been reported. A Swiss traveler apparently was infected by HIV during casual sex while awaiting his connecting flight at a Brazilian airport.

In long-haul airline crews, upper respiratory tract infections are the most common cause of lost work time, followed by gastrointestinal illness and trauma. Low back pain, fatigue, and insomnia, probably related to jet lag, are also frequently reported by airline crew members. Repeated travel results in mental stress on travelers and their families.

Some evidence exists that seasoned travelers are less susceptible, both to illness and to accidents abroad; conversely, business travelers are among the most negligent travelers. They avoid taking any preventive measures, or they follow outdated advice obtained during their first trip long ago. Often, business travelers rely on and use travel medical kits.

Pretravel Health Advice

The same basic rules for minimizing exposure and for immunizations apply for persons on short trips and for the usual travelers. Often, the total exposure time, over a year, may be similar to a more typical vacationer when travelers, e.g. airline crews, repeatedly expose themselves, but each time just for 24 to 48 hours. Recommendations for malaria chemoprophylaxis for such short-term travelers may differ from those offered to the usual travelers. First, the risk of adverse reactions from prophylactic medication (1 of 10,000) may be in a similar order of magnitude or even exceed the benefit of avoiding infection. In rural areas of tropical Africa where malaria is transmitted, the risk of infection is 1 in 3,000 daily, and probably no more than 1 in 10,000 daily in urban centers. In other parts of the world, the risk of malaria is usually much lower. The second factor for consideration is that, for many frequent travelers, the post-travel period of medication may overlap with the next trip. This means that the traveler would be taking chemoprophylaxis continuously, which often results in noncompliance. Many short-trip travelers will have returned home within the incubation period of malaria and thus need a reminder to consult a physician within a maximum of 24 hours if symptoms that are clinically compatible with those of malaria occur. From all this, one may decide to recommend measures against mosquito bites, but no chemoprophylaxis. Some airlines offer crews standby emergency medication to be carried everywhere in the event that a crew member, while off duty, stays in an area without access to medical facilities. This alternative strategy eventually needs to be considered in other short-term travelers, as well.

Because many short-term travelers, among them the VIPs, usually are unable to refuse the food and beverages offered by their hosts, chemoprophylaxis of traveler's diarrhea may be appropriate. This is not the case in airline crews, who often have organized, hygienically high-quality catering in the hotels, even in high-risk destinations. Medication to treat traveler's diarrhea is a must in travel medical kits.

It may be worthwhile to explicitly warn short-term travelers to avoid unprotected casual sex.

Additional Readings

Byrne NJ, Behrens RH. Airline crews' risk for malaria on layovers in urban sub-Saharan Africa: risk assessment and appropriate prevention policy. J Travel Med. 2004;11:359–63.

Dimberg LA, et al. Mental health insurance claims among spouses of frequent business travelers. Occup Environ Med 2002;59:175–81.

Long-Term Travelers And Expatriates

This is a heterogeneous group, including students on a very low budget, missionaries and relief workers, employees of multinational firms, and diplomatic staff—often accompanied by their families. A few epidemiologic data were presented earlier in Part 1 on the morbidity and mortality in this group of travelers (see "Epidemiology of Health Risks in Travelers"). In general, they have risks greater than those of "usual" travelers, both for the duration of exposure and because they often reside far from the usual "tourist tracks."

Pretravel Health Advice and Assessment

Travel health professionals need to devote more time to health advice for long-term travelers than for the usual travelers; part of the information is probably best given as written documentation. After having read such documentation, give these travelers the opportunity to have a second consultation to ask questions.

Persons who choose to live in another country must know that they will need to adjust to the new environment: climate, seasonal variations, and different kinds of food and beverages. The basic living conditions, the culture, the language, and the people's attitudes may all differ, which can be stimulating for some and stressful and depressing for others. A new job in a developing country will require new skills, including diplomatic ones; thus, individuals must prepare to take unusual responsibilities. Other members of the family may find life rather dull. Expatriates will often experience a sense of isolation. Cultural adaptation may be the most difficult, and the potential expatriate must know in advance that this is normal and to be expected.

Before departure, long-term travelers should ideally undergo a thorough medical assessment that includes the following:

- Medical history
- Physical examination and psychological evaluation
- Vision test and, if necessary, a prescription for new glasses
- Laboratory examination, particularly hematology, liver function tests, urinalysis, HIV test (see Appendix C), venereal disease research laboratory, and hepatitis serology
- Tuberculin test
- Chest radiography
- Dental assessment
- For women, a pap smear and, depending on age, mammography
- For older travelers, electrocardiography

The reports generated from the pretravel examination may be most useful when problems arise while abroad or upon return. On the basis of such examination, determine whether the candidate is fit enough to live in the country where he or she plans to move, whether to recommend additional tests, or whether to advise the person against a long stay in that region of the world. The reason for travel health professionals to advise individuals against prolonged stays abroad are as follows: if the individual suffers from chronic or recurrent illness that requires frequent and continuous medical monitoring (see Preexisting Health Conditions, page 127), if the person has an immunocompromised state, or if the individual has a serious handicap. It must be ascertained that persons posted abroad take adequate supplies of medication; unfortunately, drugs may be substandard—or even placebo—at the destination.

It is essential to consider the physical and psychological aptitude of all family members who are making the move to a new country. All family members will experience some culture shock, both upon arriving and when returning home. This may result in substance abuse, risky behavior, and depression.

Further, advise future expatriates about how to set up their kitchen: boiling water, for instance, does not eliminate all toxins (rarely a practical issue); charcoal filtration or even water distillers may be more appropriate in few situations. Water can be tested for chemicals, including pesticides, with commercially available test kits in industrialized countries. The samples, however, must arrive without much delay after collection. Wash fruits and vegetables first in water treated with a small amount of dish soap to eliminate pesticides and pollutants, then rinse with tap water, and finally soak in iodine solution (4 to 8 parts per million) to kill most microorganisms. The exceptions are Cryptosporidium and Cyclospora that are neither killed by iodine nor chlorine. Screen the kitchens—and specifically the food—to avoid fecal contamination by flies. In view of frequent power cuts, a fallback generator is often a good solution for refrigerators.

Ensure that future expatriates know, and are reassured, that it is common for their stools to be overall looser while staying in the developing country. Investigation is only indicated when they lose weight or lose energy. The safety of long-term use of malaria chemoprophylaxis is to some extent documented.

Additional Readings

Chen LH et al. Prevention of malaria in long-term travelers. JAMA 2006;296:2234–44.

Jones S. Medical aspects of expatriate health: health threats. Occup Med (Lond) 2000;50:572–8.

Riddle MS et al. Incidence, etiology, and impact of diarrhea among long-term travelers. Am J Trop Med Hyg 2006;74:891–900.

Shaffer MA, Harrison DA. Forgotten partners of international assignments: development and test of a model of spouse adjustment. J Appl Psychol 2001;86:238–54.

Shlim DR, Valk TH. Expatriates and long-term travelers. In: DuPont HL, Steffen R, editors. Textbook of travel medicine and health. 2nd ed. Hamilton (ON): BC Decker Inc; 2001. p. 414–21.

Uslan DZ, Virk A. Postexposure chemoprophylaxis for occupational exposure to human immunodeficiency virus in traveling health care workers. J Travel Med 2005;12:14–18.

Last-Minute Travelers

People who decide to, or need to, travel within a few days (or who neglect to get travel health advice until shortly before departure) should be made aware that it is never too late to obtain pretravel health advice. Provide the same recommendations for minimizing exposure to risks as those for the usual travelers.

For immunizations, some special aspects need to be observed. Booster doses usually grant protection almost immediately, and the same most likely applies for hepatitis A vaccines. Conversely, in a person leaving the same day for a 1-week trip to India, avoid immunizing against typhoid because it is effective only 14 to 19 days after application, depending on whether a parenteral or an oral vaccine is used. This last-minute traveler may already have returned home by then. For malaria chemoprophylaxis, particularly mefloquine, consider a loading dose for last-minute travelers (see "Malaria" in Part 2, "Infectious Health Risks and Their Prevention"). In short-term, last-minute travelers, chemoprophylaxis with the atovaquone, plus the proguanil combination, has clear advantages.

ESSENTIALS OF AVIATION MEDICINE

Undoubtedly, for most travelers, the destination itself is more hazardous than the process of getting there. In international travel, however, there is some evidence that the stress of going through all the procedures at airports is a greater health risk than the actual air travel itself. In Germany, for instance, the risk of a fatal aircraft accident is only 3.1 in 1 billion kilometers, compared with 10.6 in car travel.

Environmental Factors

Unlike small or obsolete aircraft, all modern aircraft now have pressurized cabins, with pressure equivalent to that at an altitude of < 2,500 m (8,000 ft) (usually 1,800 to 2,300 m). This compares with being a passenger in a bus on a mountain road, and healthy persons will experience a drop in hemoglobin saturation from 98% to between 92 and 94%. The reduction in the oxygen partial pressure is almost 30%.

Motion sickness is only rarely a problem in modern aircraft (see "Essentials of Maritime Medicine").

Air humidity within 2 hours of modern aircraft reaching cruising altitude decreases to 5% in first class and to 25% in the economy class, where the passengers are more closely seated—although that may improve with the introduction of the B787. This dryness may cause problems, primarily for contact lens wearers (irritation, corneal ulcer), who should therefore use glasses on long-range flights. Dry skin may be treated with moisturizing creams. There is a definite need on long flights for extra fluid consumption to avoid dehydration and to raise plasma viscosity, which may be detrimental, especially to patients with a history of arterial obstruction.

During and within 48 hours after long flights, there is a risk of venous stasis, thrombosis, and thromboembolism, inaccurately labeled "economy class syndrome" because it can also occur in those at the front of the cabin with more leg space. At the Heathrow Airport in London, United Kingdom, pulmonary embolism has been the second leading cause of in- or postflight death, with 81% of cases being women. Patients with a history of deep venous thrombosis and recent hospital admission, smokers, obese passengers, and women on contraceptives are at greater risk;

malignancy, pregnancy, congestive heart failure, presence of antiphospholipidantibodies, and familial thrombophilia are also risk factors. This is discussed in more detail in Part 3 (see "Deep Vein Thrombosis and Pulmonary Embolism").

Ozone may be an irritant but most ozone is converted to oxygen as the outside air is compressed before it enters the cabin; additionally, many aircraft are equipped with catalytic converters.

Ionizing radiation from cosmic sources, with higher levels occurring over the poles, have been noted. However, even frequent flyers, such as diplomatic couriers, hardly ever cross the 2,000 hours yearly limit (pregnant women, 200 hours) set by the International Commission on Radiation Protection.

Disease transmission in aircraft has been documented for influenza, severe acute respiratory syndrome, measles, meningitis and tuberculosis. Most likely, this was due to direct person-to-person transmission since the high-efficiency particle absorption filters in aircraft are reported to be effective in retaining bacteria, viruses, and aerosols; thus, recirculated air should be no risk to passengers. Microbiologic evaluation of airliner cabin air shows levels of colony-forming units and molds that are much less than in public areas on the ground.

Fitness To Fly

Traditionally, experienced airline medical directors had a rule of thumb: those who were able to climb the stairs into a plane were fit to fly. This rule is still valid when assessing travelers with respiratory disorders, anemias, or heart failure.

There are few contraindications for travel by air. Cardiovascular, pulmonary, and other serious conditions do not necessarily preclude air travel, although it must be kept in mind that more than 50% of in-flight deaths are attributed to a cardiac cause. Hypoxia most likely due to chronic obstructive airway disease is a major cause for concern. In those with this condition, if they are able to walk 100 meters on a flat surface without stopping or if they have an arterial oxygen pressure of 9 kPa (70 mm Hg), they do not normally require supplementary oxygen for airline travel. Often, it is not so much the cardiopulmonary condition but stress, fear, and excitement that result in problems. For this reason, emotional factors need to be seriously considered.

The following conditions are considered contraindications for flying:

- Severe congestive heart failure (note: oxygen is available on request)
- Myocardial infarction within the past 2 to 12 weeks, depending on severity (assessment by cardiologist)
- Psychosis that is obvious; possibly allowable when accompanied and sedated
- Gas trapped in body cavities (see also air ambulance, page 105), such as in the middle ear because of eustachian tube dysfunction
- Recent middle ear surgery (wait for healing of the eardrum)
- Recent inner ear surgery (wait 2 to 8 weeks)
- Pneumothorax: wait until lung has re-expanded, plus 10 days
- Mediastinal tumors
- Recent chest surgery (wait 21 days)
- Big intestinal hernias
- Recent abdominal surgery (wait more than 10 days)
- Plaster casts and, if air is trapped in plaster, split plaster
- Acute contagious diseases of relevance
- Repulsive dermatologic diseases
- Incontinence or other disorders causing bad odor
- Recent surgical wounds that are insufficiently healed
- Recent gastrointestinal bleeding (wait 21 days)
- Serious anemia (erythrocytes < 3 million/mm^3; no preflight transfusion)
- Pregnant women < 1 month before delivery for long-range flights
- Newborns (wait until 48 hours, preferably 2 weeks, as the lungs may not be fully expanded)

Additional Readings

Aw JJ. Cosmic radiation and commercial air travel. J Travel Med 2003;10:19–28.

Gendreau MA, DeJohn C. Responding to medical events during commercial airline flights. N Engl J Med 2002;346:1067–73.

WHO. Travel by air: health considerations. Weekly epid Records 2005;80:181–92.

▌ **Passengers with Special Needs**

It often helps, when booking, to reserve—if necessary, with a medical certificate—a specific seat in the aircraft. Those who suffer from claustrophobia or agoraphobia should try and book convenient seats ("a little cozy corner" or the first row of a section) in the aircraft. Senior travelers with an urgency to urinate are best served on an aisle seat close to the toilets. Those easily affected by motion sickness will suffer least in the center of an aircraft (see "Essentials of Maritime Medicine").

Patients with colostomies will have increased gas venting and may require extra bags and dressings. In epilepsy, it may be necessary to increase the drug dose because excitement, fear, sleep deprivation, hypoglycemia, alcohol intake, or hyperventilation can trigger seizures.

Each airline offers medical services that have varying criteria for acceptance and refusal of patients, depending on internal regulations and the duration of a flight. It is of utmost importance to complete and submit the Incapacitated Passengers Handling Advice form required by the International Air Transport Association (IATA) preferably 72 hours before departure. Obtain these forms from the airline office.

The airline office will relay the necessary information to the aircraft personnel and will outline the following special requirements for provision to the passengers (PAX):

- Special diets (about 20 different types, depending on the catering service)
- Special seating (with options for leg rest, adjacent seat for escort)
- Wheelchairs to bring the patient right up to the stairs of the plane (when PAX able to ascend and descend stairs)
- Ramps (when PAX can walk a few steps, but not up the stairs)
- Seats in the plane (when PAX completely immobile)
- Stretchers
- Oxygen (usually intermittent 2 to 4 L/min, with option for humidified oxygen)
- Medical/doctor's kit on board, many including a defibrillator
- Ambulance at departure or arrival airports

Note that patients flying without escorts must be able to care for themselves. Some patients may be holders of a Frequent Travelers' Medical Card with a specific number and duration of validity; this is valid on all IATA airlines, and no further formalities are required.

Additional Reading

Robson AG, et al. Laboratory assessment of fitness to fly in patients with lung disease: a practical approach. Eur Respir J 2000;16:214–9.

Ambulance Flights

There are few limitations for an ambulance flight, because resuscitation and defibrillation are possible even during the flight. The limitations are as follows:

- Gas trapped in body cavities, such as after pneumoencephalography (1 week)
- Vitrectomy with gas inflation
- Pneumothorax, unless in-flight treatment is possible
- Decompression sickness after a diving accident
- Infectious diseases that may pose a risk to crew members. The US and British Air Forces have special planes for the evacuation of few highly contagious patients, whereas other air ambulances cannot handle BL4 security level needs. If such evacuations are considered, requests from abroad most often require clearance through diplomatic channels.

Additional Reading

Patel D, et al. Medical repatriation of British diplomats resident overseas. J Travel Med 2000;7:64–9.

Fear Of Flying

According to surveys using different methods, 1 to 15% of the traveling population experience at least some degree of fear of flying. Among patients with stress disorders, 82% admitted to some degree of anxiety while flying. In the United States, some 15% of adults limit or completely avoid air travel.

Anticipatory anxiety is characterized by unease and somatic symptoms, tending to increase as the event draws closer. The dysphoric arousal tends to settle some time after take-off. Phobic anxiety—most frequently agoraphobia, claustrophobia, or social phobia—is more intense and may lead to panic reactions and, often, subsequent avoidance of flying. Typically, the attack has a rapid onset; patients feel that they have lost personal control and are preoccupied with anxiety about what others will think. Fear of heights is not really associated with flight phobia; one might find the former even in airline pilots.

Contributing factors to flight phobia are recent stress and an anxious, obsessional, depressive, or immature personality; inactivity and quietness during the flight also may play a part. Lack of information or knowledge is a major cause for fear in infrequent or novice passengers (eg, fear experienced when strange new noises are heard before landing). There are two basic treatments, which may be combined. Some airlines offer therapeutic courses to persons suffering from fear of flying. These courses provide information about aircraft on the ground and all the noises made by an aircraft during a flight, provide a short demonstration flight during which the captain is particularly careful to explain all his moves, and include discussion about environmental factors. Cognitive and behavioral therapies may also be useful. Many passengers get relief from anticipatory anxiety or slight to moderate phobic anxiety by administering alcohol or tranquilizers before and during the flight.

Additional Reading

Van Gerwen LJ, et al. Behavioral and cognitive group treatment for fear of flying. J Behav Ther Exp Psychiatry 2006;37:358–71.

ESSENTIALS OF MARITIME MEDICINE

Jet travel has become standard for rapid long distance travels, but many now select the waterways. Ten million passengers on cruise ships per year represents an increase of over 1,000% the last few decades. The cruising industry has focused on leisure travel, providing visits to various ports in different countries allowing passengers to appreciate different cultural experiences in a relatively short period of time. The average length of a cruise is 7 days, with three to five ports of call. In addition to cruising, a considerable number of travelers are additionally being transported by ferries, with the length of travel from few hours to 3 days. An unknown number of travelers are also exposed to water on the lakes and rivers (eg, rafting, swimming, or diving) and an increasing number of people choose to spend their leisure time sailing or boating at sea—an isolated environment with limited options for medical care. Obviously, health risks will differ according to the type of travel and destination.

The revised International Health Regulations address health requirements for ship operations and construction. There are global standards regarding ship and port sanitation, disease surveillance, as well as response to infectious diseases. Guidance is given for provision of safe water, food, vector and rodent control, and waste disposal. According to Article 8 ILO Convention (No. 164) Concerning Health Protection and Medical Care for Seafarers, 1987, vessels carrying more than 100 crew members on an international voyage of 3 days or longer must provide a physician for care of the crew. Unfortunately, these regulations do not apply to passenger vessels and ferries sailing less than 3 days from shore, although the number of crew and passengers can be more than 1,000. Sailing boats shorter than 12 m, with less than 15 tons gross registered tonnage and fewer than 12 persons aboard are not under the obligations of international conventions but are under the jurisdiction of national laws. The contents of the ship's medical chest must comply with the international agreements for oceangoing trade vessels, but there are no special requirements for supplemental drugs for passenger ships.

A cruise line, as with any other shipping line, may choose to flag its ships overseas, the operational procedures, crew qualifications, as well as policies depending consequently on the country chosen. The flagging nation may also require that health care providers on the ship have certain qualifications and, typically, they must be fluent in the official language of the cruise line. Some countries that flag the ships set standards and health care guidelines for cruise ships and any vessels carrying more than a certain number of passengers or crew. They may regulate the medical facilities available, the staff qualifications, and the medical equipment carried. As cruising has become more popular, other guidelines have come into use, and are usually based on the total number of crew and passengers. Additional organizations of cruise lines may assist in the policy development and promote issues such as safety, prevention of crime, and environmental health.

Medical Problems Aboard Cruise Ships

In general, the kinds of diseases seen aboard ships mirror those on land. The differences are high density of population on the ship and the large number of countries from which the crew originates. These two issues are significant in the transmission of certain diseases on cruise ships. Because cruises attract senior travelers, and because there are now special cruises for groups such as kidney dialysis and cancer patients, above-average incidence rates of health problems may result.

Communicable Diseases

A cruise ship's population is ever–changing, and its stores are constantly being replenished with local food and water. If the passengers and crew who join are infected, or the food and water supplies are contaminated, an infection can spread rapidly throughout the entire community.

Repeated gastrointestinal and respiratory tract outbreaks on board cruise ships have resulted in programs to improve detection and control and to improve and maintain a high level of sanitation. Passengers may also expose themselves on shore through interpersonal interactions, which may result in a variety of outbreaks aboard. The public health impact may not only be the transmission of diseases to the cruise ship passengers, but from crew and passengers to those on land at the ports of call. In addition, crew infected with vaccine-preventable diseases have been responsible for transmitting illness not only to passengers on one cruise, but to passengers on consecutive cruises.

Cruise ship passengers may develop gastroenteritis; the number of outbreaks is increasing in parallel with the increase in, for example, norovirus infections on land. This virus is highly transmissible from person to person through contaminated food and water or by contact with fomites. Hand washing frequently with soap and water or with alcohol-based gels is strongly recommended for cruise passengers.

Outbreaks of other illnesses are not uncommon aboard cruise ships. These include other causes of diarrheal disease, such as salmonella, and respiratory illnesses, such as influenza and legionnaires' disease. Interestingly, outbreaks of influenza may occur in the absence of seasonal disease in the cruising geographic region or regions. Legionella infections have been linked to water sources such as spas. Measles, varicella, and rubella are also diseases that have caused outbreaks aboard ship and are often traced to crew members who come from countries where vaccinations to prevent such diseases are not routinely administered.

Non-infectious Health Problems

Environmental exposure to sun, unusual temperatures, rough weather (see "Motion Sickness" in Part 3, "Noninfectious Health Risks and Their Prevention") or changes in diet may lead to sunburn or exacerbation of preexisting illness. Patients with chronic health conditions should consult their physicians before deciding to embark on a cruise. Cardiovascular events in those with underlying cardiac disease remain a major problem for cruise lines; they are the major cause of mortality and the major cause for discharge of passengers in the midst of a cruise at one of the ports of call.

Being Sick on Board

A ship is basically an isolated international community, and one should not expect the same level of medical service as on shore. Cruise ships doctors found one potential dangerous medical situation in 900 passenger days or six serious incidents in 1,000 passenger months. There are no internationally accepted standards of care for cruise ships, but fortunately, a large number of them have medical facilities staffed and equipped in accordance with the guidance provided by the American College of Emergency Physicians (ACEP) or the International Council of Cruise Lines. They are capable of providing reasonable emergency care on board, serving passengers 24 hours a day. Most large ships now have excellent facilities, but a ship's medical centre has no operating rooms, computed tomography or magnetic resonance imaging scanners, or blood banks. It is usually staffed with one or two doctors and –two to four nurses. It has a couple of consulting rooms, radiography equipment, and a simple laboratory. ACEP guidelines recommend that the ship's medical center should be equipped with defibrillators, external pacemakers, cardiac monitors, infusion pumps, respirators, pulse oximeters and a comprehensive range of medications. The on-board staff can treat attacks, strokes, and chest infections in the intensive care ward and, if necessary, will obtain advice via fax, telephone or, on newer ships, real-time video consultation. They can facilitate the evacuation of a seriously ill or injured person to the nearest appropriate shore medical facility. In some ports, shore facilities are of a much lower level than medical facilities on board; evacuation to a higher level of medical help might be necessary.

Cruise ships are not staffed with obstetricians, and most cruise companies will not accept passengers who will reach the third trimester of pregnancy by the end of the cruise. Complications, including miscarriage or premature labor, will normally require evacuation and treatment on shore.

Prevention

For most passengers, cruising possesses few health risks, which can be minimized by sensible planning and a few precautions before, during, and after the voyage. By buying a ticket for the cruise, passengers enter a contract with the cruise company with the distinct obligation to notify the cruise company of any medical condition that can impact the health and safety of the passenger, or make him or her unfit to travel. Those travelers should be advised to carry a summary of medical records with them on board. Most cruise lines have the ability to accommodate a large number of special requests. Any medical, physical, or dietary condition—including but not limited to the following—should be reported at the time of booking:

- mobility impairment,
- pregnancy,
- allergies,
- diabetes,

- dialysis,
- oxygen use,
- bleeding disorders,
- injectable medication,
- prescription medications, and
- digestive disorders.

Most illnesses and injuries can be treated on board, but patients with serious problems must disembark for specialist care. Treatment on board normally carries a cost: all travelers, and especially those with preexisting medical conditions, should ensure that they purchase an insurance policy that provides timely medical assistance and covers the treatment and evacuation costs of an illness or injury.

Most cruise ships do not carry dentists, so travelers with any dental problem should solve the problem prior to departure.

Although most cruise companies advise passengers on vaccinations requested by the International Health Regulations (IHR), they do not routinely provide information on recommended immunizations or prophylactic medications. A valid international certificate of vaccination (for yellow fever) is required for entry in some ports, and passengers lacking it will not be allowed ashore. Cruise ships are not designated yellow fever vaccination centers and are not authorized to issue proper certificates. Although not based on the IHR, a few still request cholera vaccination.

Eating and drinking on shore increases the risk of gastrointestinal disease, so advice on food and hygiene precautions should be provided. Quarantine regulations require all cases of gastrointestinal disease and all on-board sales of antidiarrheal medications to be documented. To prevent or reduce outbreaks of gastroenteritis caused by the very contagious norovirus, those who present with symptoms at the medical centers are put in isolation in their cabins for at least 24 hours after the last symptom. Some ships also isolate asymptomatic contacts for 24 hours. To ensure full compliance, most cruise lines do not permit the sale of antidiarrheal medications without medical consultation. Passengers may take their own antidiarrheal/antibiotic medications on board but should report that immediately to medical service staff because such self-treatment may reflect an epidemic in the closed, isolated community of the cruise.

Outbreaks of influenza may occur in the absence of seasonal disease, thus anyone traveling to regions where influenza is prevalent should be vaccinated; sometimes the use of standby antiviral treatment should be discussed. Female passengers of childbearing age who do not have documented immunity should be informed on rubella occurrence risk on board.

As stays in port are short and usually only during the day, even if visiting a malarial zone, antimalarial medications may not be necessary. Decisions about the use of protective clothing, insect repellents, and antimalarial medication should be based on general recommendations for short-term stays.

▍ Medical Problems Aboard Ferries and Passenger Ships

Beside cruise ships, passenger transport at sea includes domestic ferries that sail for just a few hours at a time and international passenger ships that travel more than 30 hours, some of them even offering vacations and amusement on board, similar to those on board cruise ships. Only passenger ferries at sea for more than 72 hours with more than 100 passengers are considered cruise ships; they are required to have a medical doctor on board. Shorter range ferries and similar ships, besides having no doctor on board, often do not even have an emergency room.

While on a cruise ship, every passenger will have his own cabin and is likely to stay there if she of he falls ill; on ferries, many of the passengers will have no cabin of their own. Large numbers of them, young and old, will sleep on the deck or dance all night in the bar. On the majority of ferries, there is only basic resuscitation equipment and no defibrillators, so an attempt to bring the passenger or crew member who had a sudden cardiac arrest back to life would presumably be useless. Some tragic accidents caused by human error or overloaded ships have highlighted worldwide problems with ferries. Some simple precautions should be taken: when a ferry is full or obviously overloaded, wait and catch the next one; passengers should be advised to make sure, immediately after boarding, that they know where the life vests and other safety devices are located and how to use them. On cruise ships, passengers are drilled as to emergency safety procedures, while on ferries, as a rule, nobody will spontaneously give such information. Passengers should be familiar with the signals that are going to be used in the case of emergency, and should know the position of their muster station for the life boats.

On ships where there is no medical doctor present, as on ferries or passenger ships, the captain or the deck officer who is properly trained, equipped, and assisted by telemedical (Radio medico) provides medical help. According to the Article 8 ILO Convention (No. 164) Concerning Health Protection and Medical Care for seafarers, 1987, the competent authority shall ensure by a prearranged system that medical advice by radio or satellite communication to ships at sea, including specialist advice, is available at any hour of the day or night. Radio medico is the only possibility the ship's officer has to ask for medical help in the event of disease or accident. Today, there are more than 300 radio stations engaged in radio medico advice all over the world, and mostly free of charge. Modern satellite communications (INMARSAT-International Maritime Satellite Organization) make it accessible (from 70° N latitude to 70° S latitude) in virtually every corner of the world where people travel by sea.

The officers undergo a basic paramedic training and are capable of observing, reporting, and carrying out treatment based on the RM advice but they do not diagnose and treat independently. They are supposed to be the "physicians' eyes, ears and hands." Thus, medical advice can quickly be obtained and proper measures taken in emergencies at sea. The potential of radio-medico advice is, however, overestimated. In many cases, it is a great help but its possibilities are still rather limited.

Sailing

Sailing has become a popular way of spending summer holidays. The problem of an isolated environment can be vital in offshore "blue water" sailing, but even in coastal sailing, it is of major importance. Even in ideal conditions of coastal sailing, it usually takes more than a few hours to reach the nearest medical facility ashore. Weather conditions and distances can limit air rescue by helicopter. One also has to know that not all countries have efficient search and rescue systems.

The range of health care that should be provided for the conditions of sailing tourism exceeds the scope of simple first aid. It can only be realized by means of Radio Medical Advice, the corresponding handbook, the proper education, and the corresponding medicine chest aboard. The aim of this health care is to enable a sailor to perform the tasks necessary to stabilize an injured or ill person until professional help is reached on shore or is able to come from the coast. In "blue water" sailing this aim is higher, and a sailor has to be capable of treating an injured or sick person for longer periods of time.

The boat and crew have to be in the best possible condition. The first responsibility of every skipper should be to determine the risk of the trip, taking into account sailing competence and experience of the crew, current health of each member of the crew, length of time before embarkation, destination, itinerary, length of stay, purpose (cruise or race), food, and water sources. Any member of the crew that regularly takes any medications should take a sufficient supply aboard and notify the skipper about it.

Additional Reading

Committee to Advise on Tropical Medicine and Travel (CATMAT). Statement on motion sickness. Canada Communicable Disease Report 2003;29(ACS11):1–12.

Dahl E. Medical practice during a world cruise. Int Marit Health 2005;56:115–28.

Flemmer M, Oldfield EC 3rd. The agony and the ecstasy. Am J Gastroenterol 2003;98:2098–9.

Golding JF, Gresty MA. Motion sickness. Curr Opinion Neurology 2005;18:29–34.

Miller JM, et al. Cruise ships: high-risk passengers and the global spread of new influenza viruses. Clin Infect Dis 2000;31:433–8.

Schwartz E, et al. Schistosome infection among river rafters on Omo River, Ethiopia. J Travel Med 2005;12:3–8.

Sherman CR. Motion sickness: review of causes and preventive strategies. J Travel Med 2002;9:251–6.

Smith A. Cruise ship medicine. In: Dawood R, editor. Travellers' health. Oxford, UK: Oxford University Press; 2002. p. 277.

http://www.acep.org/webportal/membercenter/sections/cruise/

http://www.iccl.org/policies/medical.cfm

http://www.imha.net/

THE HAJJ: PILGRIMAGE TO SAUDI ARABIA

The pilgrimage to Mecca and Medina in Saudi Arabia, called hajj, is one of the five pillars of Islam. More than 2 million Muslims from more than 140 countries all over the world congregate to perform religious rituals there yearly. This nearly one-month pilgrimage is scheduled according to the lunar calendar and moves 11 days forward in the Gregorian calendar yearly. There are various health risks associated with the hajj (Table 9).

Overcrowding contributes to the rapid dissemination of airborne diseases. Upper respiratory symptoms are the most frequently reported complaints among pilgrims. Influenza vaccination has recently been documented to reduce influenza-like illness among pilgrims. In extreme risk, consider neuraminidase inhibitor prophylaxis. Pneumococcal vaccination is mandatory for those above age 65. Close proximity of pilgrims also facilitates person-to-person transmission of meningococci, and meningococcal outbreaks have been associated with the hajj. The largest meningococcal outbreak occurred in 1987 and was caused by serogroup A. Subsequently, vaccination against serogroup A became compulsory for all hajj pilgrims. In the years 2000 and 2001, other meningococcal disease outbreaks occurred among pilgrims and subsequent transmission to household contacts upon return to their countries of origin has been documented. This generated particular interest, since it was caused by a previously rare serogroup, W135. In 2002, quadrivalent meningococcal vaccine against A/C/Y/W135 became a hajj visa requirement. From 2004, no more meningococcal outbreaks related to hajj were reported

Table 9.   Muslim Calendar — travel related holidays

Year, Gregorian	Year, Islamic	Ramadan starts	Eid Ul-Fitr (end of Ramadan)	Hajj starts	Hajj ends
2007	1428	13 September	13 October	19 December	31 December
2008	1429	02 September	01 October	08 December	20 December
2009	1430	22 August	21 September	28 November	10 December
2010	1431	12 August	11 September	18 November	30 November

from anywhere. Because many Muslim pilgrims come from developing countries where tuberculosis is highly endemic, the health authorities of the Kingdom of Saudi Arabia have implemented prevention measures (such as surgical masks). A pre- and post-hajj purified protein derivative (PPD) status may help to identify latent tuberculosis infection.

Overcrowding has also been associated with stampede. Stampede has most commonly been reported during the ritualistic stoning of the pillars and during the circumambulation of the Kaaba, the center of the Holy Mosque. Heatstroke and severe dehydration have been described in hajj pilgrims. The health authorities now provide clean water at all holy sites.

Inadequate storage and cooking, lack of refrigeration, and improper food handling may contribute to food and waterborne diseases. Diarrhea occurs frequently, and, under the circumstances, proper rehydration is paramount. An antibiotic for self-treatment, the first choice being a quinolone, plus loperamide in the travel kit are indicated. Hepatitis A is endemic in Saudi Arabia; thus, clinicians strongly recommend vaccination.

Most male pilgrims shave their heads upon completion of the rites, which may result in blood-borne diseases and the risk of various infections. Barbers have a high rate of hepatitis B infection. For this reason, hepatitis B vaccination may benefit pilgrims.

In summary, immunize hajj pilgrims with quadrivalent meningococcal vaccine at least 2 weeks, and no longer than 3 years, prior to arrival in the Kingdom (see Part 2). In children under 2 years of age, give two doses of monovalent A meningococcal vaccine, 3 months apart. Likewise, give antimicrobial prophylaxis to pilgrims arriving from high risk areas, such as the Sahel countries, and recommend that pilgrims use ciprofloxacin before leaving Mecca to avoid carrying *Neisseria meningitidis* back to their families. In addition, recommend hepatitis A and B, influenza, and pneumococcal vaccination to hajjis, the last of which is strongly recommended for the usual specific risk groups and, in fact, has recently become mandatory for those over 65 years of age. Additionally, pilgrims below the age of 15 years and all residing in Nigeria now are immunized upon arrival against poliomyelitis; for these groups it is recommended to obtain a documented dose of polio vaccine six weeks prior to applying for a visa. Advise pilgrims to stay in groups but to avoid crowds, to wear masks when crowding occurs, to seek shade as often as possible, and to perform rituals during cooler parts of the day, to maintain adequate hydration, and to protect themselves against the sun.

Additional Readings

Ahmed QAA, et al. Health risks at the hajj. Lancet 2006;367:1008–15.

Shafi S. Hajj 2006: communicable disease and other health risks and current official guidance for pilgrims. Euro Surveill 2005;10:E051215.2

Wilder-Smith A, et al. Acquisition of meningococcal carriage in Hajj pilgrims and transmission to their household contacts: prospective study. BMJ 2002;325:365–6.

General Strategies in Host-Related Special Risks

PRINCIPLES OF MIGRATION MEDICINE

Migrants total 2 to 4 million yearly, compared with 1 billion travelers. Immigrants, refugees, asylum seekers, and illegal immigrants are essentially on a one-way ticket. They move mostly from a poor to a richer or more peaceful country, searching for a better life or to escape war, human rights violations, and poverty or environmental disasters. They often suffer restrictions when accessing health care at their destination.

First, the predeparture phase influences migration health. In addition to socioeconomic conditions, endemicity of diseases and nutrition in the country of origin play primary roles. Lack of hygiene and medical supplies, as well as violence, will hinder future health. Religion and culture influence future health-seeking behavior. Past experiences with the medical infrastructure at the origin will guide expectations at the destination.

Migration itself may be short and uneventful or long and full of deadly risks. The strain suffered may result in post-traumatic stress disorder and will have an impact on adaptation in the post-migration environment. This may greatly differ, depending on the legal status of a person. Access to health services may be restricted to illegal immigrants. Overcrowding may enhance disease transmission. Infections such as human immunodeficiency virus, tuberculosis, and hepatitis B are not properly assessed and treated and therefore further spread occurs. Isolation may perpetuate the psychological stress, resulting in depression and a multitude of psychosomatic symptoms. Owing to cross-cultural differences and language barriers, these problems are often difficult to understand for medical professionals who lack special training.

Mandatory medical screening at the point of entry, with the primary aim of protecting the host population, has been implemented in most countries. This followed the occurrence of a broad variety of unusual infections that were imported to destination countries. (This will be further described in Part 4). Many question the epidemiologic rationale of a non–patient-centered medical act and suggest that immigrants and refugees have health needs to be fulfilled by a regular medical interview and examination.

Improved hygiene at the country of destination may often lead to reduced transmission.

With global mobility, differentiation between travelers and migrants often becomes arbitrary. We must understand that both groups leave a specific biologic environment to be exposed to different biologic characteristics in the new environment, which is a stressful process that results in potential health consequences. This goes far beyond communicable diseases, affecting physical and mental health. Health care professionals must be able to cope with this challenge when in charge of a broad palette of cultures. Also politicians must acknowledge that this population is in urgent need of measures, such as diagnostics and vaccines.

Additional Readings

Barnett ED. Infectious disease screening for refugees resettled in the United States. Clin Infect Dis 2004;39:833–41.

Bischoff A. Language barriers between nurses and asylum seekers: their impact on symptom reporting and referral. Soc Sci Med 2003;57:503–12.

Gushulak BD, MacPherson D. Globalization of infectious diseases: the impact of migration. Clin Infect Dis 2004;38:1742–8.

Loutan L. The health of migrants and refugees. In: Zuckerman J, editor. Principles and practice of travel medicine. John Wiley & Sons; 2001.

FEMALE AND PREGNANT TRAVELERS

Female Travelers

For women who plan to travel alone on a long trip abroad, we recommend a gynecologic checkup before departure to avoid possibly inconvenient or embarrassing experiences.

They should carry a sufficient supply of tampons, sanitary napkins, or pads; remote areas may not carry quality products. Women who prefer not to menstruate while abroad can take oral contraceptives continuously—without interruption between packs. Such a solution can help divers and swimmers avoid attracting sharks and, for visitors to game parks, to avoid attracting animals. Contraception is highly recommended for women of childbearing age who plan to dive because of possible complications in pregnancy. In some eastern countries, for menstruating women, entry is prohibited into some temples.

Women must know that the effect of hormonal contraceptives may be reduced by interaction with antibiotics, laxatives, or charcoal, and the same may occur in diarrhea. Pharmacokinetic properties of some contraceptives do not allow intervals exceeding 27 hours; thus, women using low-dose products must be advised accordingly when they cross more time zones westbound.

If casual sex is a possibility, women should include condoms (or femidoms) in their travel medical kit.

Emergency contraception may often be difficult to implement within 72 hours as needed. It consists of levonorgestrel alone (0.75 mg twice, 12 hours apart) or the Yuzpe regimen (two tablets of medium-dose contraceptive taken with two more 12 hours later).

Pregnant Women

Should pregnancy occur, medical establishments in many developing countries do not have all the facilities to treat complications. For travel during pregnancy, consider specific problems. Preferably, pregnant women should abandon their travel plans whenever they have obstetric or general medical risk factors. In the pretravel assessment of pregnant travelers, the travel medicine advisor should work closely with the obstetrician. Serology for hepatitis B, human immunodeficiency virus, cytomegalovirus, rubella, measles, chickenpox and toxoplasmosis should be carried out. Pregnant travelers should carry a copy of their medical records (including blood type and Rh). Prenatal vitamins, which may be difficult to obtain overseas, should be prescribed in sufficient quantities. Many insurance plans do not cover pregnancy and delivery overseas.

Malaria infection during pregnancy carries a bad prognosis and may be associated with maternal anemia, preterm delivery, low birth weight, intrauterine growth retardation, and fetal death. Therefore, there is universal consensus with the World Health Organization statement, which "advises pregnant women not to travel on vacation to areas where transmission of chloroquine-resistant (*Plasmodium falciparum*) occurs." Pregnant women should avoid other destinations that are far from competent medical facilities. If a pregnant woman decides to travel, the second trimester (weeks 18 to 24) is the safest period; at this time, there is lower risk of spontaneous abortion or premature labor. Travel health professionals should strongly recommend that pregnant women use malaria chemoprophylaxis if they need to, or elect to, travel to high-risk areas. The use of chloroquine, proguanil, and mefloquine (at least during the second and third trimester) is not contraindicated in pregnancy and thus has no reason for interrupting a pregnancy.

In the event of traveler's diarrhea, doxycycline, bismuth subsalicylate, and quinolones are contraindicated; however, azithromycin may be used if necessary, together with loperamide. No prophylactic medication can be recommended, but the usual measures to reduce exposure apply. Pregnant women can tolerate water purification with iodine tablets for a few weeks, but prolonged prevention may result in adverse effects on the fetal thyroid gland.

Various relative contraindications exist for vaccines (see Part 2 for details). Table 7 provides other contraindications. Inactivated vaccines, in general, can be safely administered to pregnant women if their administration is not associated with severe febrile reactions. The Advisory Committee on Immunization Practices endorses tetanus toxoid administration during pregnancy. The manufacturers recommend that nonimmunized or incompletely immunized pregnant women and those immunized more than 10 years previously who may deliver a child under unhygienic circumstances or surroundings should receive one or two properly

---

Table 10 Relative Contraindications to International Travel During Pregnancy

Patients with obstetric risk factors

- History of miscarriage
- Incompetent cervix
- History of ectopic pregnancy (ectopic gestation in present pregnancy should be ruled out prior to travel)
- History of premature labor or premature rupture of membranes
- History of past or present placental abnormalities
- Threatened abortion or vaginal bleeding during present pregnancy
- Multiple gestation in present pregnancy
- History of toxemia, hypertension, or diabetes with any pregnancy
- History of infertility or difficulty becoming pregnant
- Primigravida age > 35 years or < 15 years

Patients with general medical risk factors

- Valvular heart disease or congestive heart failure
- History of thromboembolic disease
- Severe anemia
- Chronic organ system dysfunction that requires frequent medical interventions

Patients contemplating travel to destinations that may be hazardous

- High altitudes
- Areas endemic for or where there are epidemics of life-threatening food or insect-borne infections
- Areas where chloroquine-resistant *Plasmodium falciparum* is endemic
- Areas where live virus vaccines are required and recommended

---

Adapted from: Lee RV. The pregnant traveler. Travel Med Int 1989;7:51–58.

spaced doses of combined tetanus-diphtheria vaccine (Td, adult use dosage), preferably during the last two trimesters, to prevent neonatal tetanus. Live vaccines (such as measles, mumps, rubella, and yellow fever) are contraindicated. Replace oral polio (a live vaccine) with enhanced potency inactivated poliovirus vaccine. The safety of Japanese encephalitis vaccine in pregnancy has not been established and therefore should only be offered to pregnant women after weighing the risks versus benefits. Bacterial polysaccharide vaccines, meningococcal vaccine, and pneumococcal vaccine are listed as Food and Drug Administration (FDA) pregnancy category C. Hepatitis A virus (HAV) infection of the pregnant traveler is not associated with perinatal transmission; however, placental abruption and premature delivery has been reported during acute infection. For pregnant women, the risk of acquiring HAV is the same as for other travelers. Inactivated hepatitis A vaccines belong to FDA pregnancy category C, and, according to the package inserts, the main concern is the possible febrile response associated with vaccination. Passive immunization with human immunoglobulin was the mainstay of prophylaxis for HAV infection for the short-term pregnant traveler, but in view of problems associated herewith (see Part 2, page 213), the travel health professional should discuss inactivated hepatitis A vaccine and weigh risks and benefits in any nonimmune pregnant women traveling to a developing country. Hepatitis B virus (HBV) infection is a risk for travelers exposed to blood or body fluids, especially in countries with high HBV endemicity. Recombinant hepatitis B vaccine series can be administered to pregnant women who are at high risk and are negative by serology for past HBV infection. Hepatitis E virus infection has a particularly high fatality rate during pregnancy (15 to 20%). Food and water precautions are currently the mainstay of hepatitis E virus infection prevention in a traveler, because no vaccine is available yet.

While abroad, fatigue, heartburn, gastrointestinal problems and discomfort, vaginal discharge, leg cramps, increased urination, varicose veins, and hemorrhoids may occur in pregnant women but with a similar frequency to that at home.

In road and air travel, seat belts should be fastened low over the pelvis. Air travel late in pregnancy might precipitate labor; therefore, most airlines have set (varying) limitations, depending on the duration of the flight, with the most frequent cut-off being at 35 weeks. The increased level of clotting factors and the progesterone effect of venous dilatation result in an increased risk of thromboembolic disease. In all prolonged travels, pregnant women should move around every 1 to 2 hours to reduce the risk of thrombosis, and they should wear elastic support stockings or hose. Heparin prophylaxis may be indicated and should be discussed with the obstetrician. Because of the low humidity of flights, hydration is crucial for the pregnant traveler, particularly for placental flow. The fetus is considered safe from desaturation during routine commercial airline flights.

We do not advise travel to destinations at altitudes of 2,500 m and above (except for short excursions), diving, horse riding, safaris, and other expeditions to remote areas during pregnancy.

Diving during pregnancy has been associated with an approximate 15-fold increase in risk of malformation of the fetus and is, consequently, contraindicated during pregnancy.

Nursing mothers serve their infants well in nutritional and anti-infective aspects. To find a place for nursing may be a challenge; in fact, in some societies nursing in public is unacceptable. Fluid intake, eating and sleeping patterns, and stress invariably do affect lactation.

Breast milk will contain small amounts of antimalarial drugs. However, there is no indication that this could harm the infant. The quantity transferred is too small to grant adequate protection against malaria; thus, nursing infants should receive the chemoprophylaxis dosage as recommended (see Part 2). In addition, antibiotics are excreted in the breast milk.

Lactating women should keep in mind that nursing does not grant complete protection against pregnancy, even if menstruation has not yet resumed.

Additional Readings

Kingman CE, Economides DL. Travel in pregnancy: pregnant women's experiences and knowledge of health issues. J Travel Med 2003;10:330–3.

Kozarsky PE, van Gompel A. Pregnancy, nursing, contraception, and travel. In: DuPont HL, Steffen R, editors. Textbook of travel medicine and health. 2nd ed. Hamilton (ON): BC Decker Inc; 2001.

Patton PG. Emergency contraception in a travel context. J Travel Med 1999;6:24–6.

MALE TRAVELERS: CORPORATE TRAVELERS

In pretravel health advice for male travelers, keep in mind three aspects: (1) a considerable proportion traveling alone will have casual sex, some unprotected, (2) men abuse alcohol more often, and (3) they are more accident prone because they take greater risks. Men above age 40 who have urinary system problems should consult a urologist before long-term travel to assess the condition of the prostate.

Corporate travelers are usually men, particularly when the destination is in a developing country. They may have extremely short-, intermediate-, and long-duration travel patterns. Usually, the standard of hygiene is relatively good, but nevertheless various problems may occur, similar to those in short-duration travelers (eg, crews) or in tourists. Under all circumstances, employers should ensure corporate travelers obtain travel health advice and take appropriate measures, even when departure is on short notice, which is often the case. Travel health professionals must emphasize that many vaccines may offer benefits within hours, and it is never too late to start malaria chemoprophylaxis.

In general, the usual travel health rules apply. Again, because many corporate travelers may be unable to refuse the food and beverages that their hosts offer, chemoprophylaxis of traveler's diarrhea may be more appropriate in short-term missions. Rapidly effective medication to treat traveler's diarrhea is a must in travel medical kits. Further, remind this group to avoid unprotected casual sex.

Additional Reading

Kemmerer TP, et al. Health problems of corporate travelers: risk factors and management. J Travel Med 1998;5:184–7.

Prince TS. Corporate travel medicine: benefit analysis of on-site services. J Travel Med 2001;8:163–7.

Rogers HL, Reilly SM. Health problems associated with international business travel. AAOHN J 2000;48:376–84.

INFANTS AND CHILDREN

It is estimated that 4% of overseas travelers are infants and children, and that children account for 25% of travel-related hospitalizations. In the United Kingdom, imported infections have been reported to account for 2% of pediatric hospitalizations. Accidents are the leading cause of mortality in pediatric travelers. Infants and small children are more susceptible to accidents and also to infections than are adults, and they have more serious complications. Malaria is associated with higher mortality in children than in adults. Children are at closer contact with stray animals and therefore have the highest incidence of rabies.

Pretravel pediatric counseling should include the same topics as those for adults as well as the following:

- Water safety and food hygiene
- Oral rehydration and additional strategies in case of diarrhea
- Car safety: seats, seat belts
- Personal protection against mosquito bites
- Malaria chemoprophylaxis (particularly dosage), possibly preparation of capsules by pharmacist, and how to ingest
- Sun: hazards and screen
- Petting of any animals, even if they appear well
- Procedures in case of animal bites, envenomous bites
- Medical insurance, evacuation coverage
- As appropriate: high altitude illness; for adolescents, also consider risks of sexually transmitted diseases

There are some infants who must not travel. Ensure that air travel is avoided with infants under age 2 weeks. Some extend this recommendation to the age of 6 weeks. Travel health professionals should advise parents with very young children against vacationing in countries with high endemicity of tropical or infectious diseases. The World Health Organization strongly discourages traveling with children to malarious areas. Even greater contraindications against travel to developing countries exist for infants and children with immune deficiency, cystic fibrosis, diabetes, serious handicaps, and conditions that require repeated blood transfusions.

Other contraindications to flying are acute middle ear infections and recent ear, nose, and throat surgeries (ie, tympanomastoidectomy, labyrinthectomy). Air travel should be avoided for 2 weeks after surgery and with a history of spontaneous pneumothoraces as is the case for adult air passengers (see "Essentials of Aviation Medicine"). Complete effusions and pneumonostomy tubes protect against middle ear barotraumas by minimizing pressure changes and are not contraindications to flying. About 15% of children experience ear pain during descent. As the process of swallowing decompresses the eustachian tubes, encourage bottle- or breast-feeding infants during descent, and have older children suck on something or chew gum. There are indications that, at altitudes exceeding 2,500 m, children have a greater risk of high-altitude illness compared to adults.

To reduce the impact of jet lag, it may help to begin to shift the sleep schedule a few days prior to travel. Advice on jet lag prevention is similar to that for adults, but children usually get over it much faster than adults because of their adherence to natural circadian rhythms. For a quiet flight, sedation with promethacin syrup may be considered. However, avoid medications such as benzodiazepines. There are no data on melatonin in the pediatric age group.

Compared to adults, motion sickness occurs more often in children. Commonly used therapies for motion sickness in children includes diphenhydramine and dimenhydrinate. Avoid using scopolamine in children under age 12 years, owing to the increased risk of side effects. In the same way, anti-dopaminergics, such as metoclopramide hydrochloride, are more frequently associated with side effects such as extrapyramidal symptoms.

Enhance the safety of children by having parents carry a car seat for any child under age 4. Encourage parents to have seat belts inspected for integrity before accepting a rental vehicle. Traffic patterns vary from country to country, and children unfamiliar to these different regulations are at high risk and, therefore, need constant supervision. Survey hotel rooms for potential hazards; specifically, open electrical wiring and sockets, paint chips, pest poisons or traps, and low or unstable balcony railings. An identification card attached to the child can be simple, but helpful, in the event the child gets lost. Take along a first aid kit. Brief parents about crisis management in case of illness acquired abroad.

Drowning is the second leading cause of death in pediatric travelers. At all times, provide supervision during swimming, and pay special attention to tides, currents, and warnings. Swimming pools in developing countries with hot climates pose a higher risk of ear infections because of bacterial and fungal contamination. Excessive chlorination of water may cause conjunctivitis. Children who stay in the pool for prolonged periods of time should wear protective goggles and earplugs. Cutaneous larva migrans is a risk due to frequent contact with sand. Children should wear protective footwear, as well as place a barrier (ie, towel or sheet) between themselves and the ground.

To prevent heat injuries, children must maintain hydration, wear loose-fitting and light clothing, limit physically demanding midday activities, and avoid direct sun. The risk of melanoma is now more than double in individuals who have had one or more severe sunburns in childhood. Advise the child to wear protective clothing and to use sunscreen. To prevent cold injuries, wear layered clothing, gloves, and woolen socks. The layers should include an underwear layer that takes away moisture, an insulating layer (ie, wool or fleece), and an outside shell (ie, nylon).

If parents still opt to travel to countries with vector-borne diseases, such as malaria, personal protection against mosquito bites is paramount. This can be achieved, to some extent, by wearing light-colored clothes, long sleeves, and full-length pants, and by treating uncovered skin with DEET, EBAAP, or Bayrepel.

It is better to avoid DEET concentrations of > 10%; they may be neurotoxic for smaller children. To avoid contact with eyes and mouth, the agent should not be applied on children's hands. Many consider DEET contraindicated for children under 1 year of age. Repellent cream on skin should be washed off following return to a protected indoor area. Malaria chemoprophylaxis for children follows the same basic rules as for adults, with doses determined according to body weight (see "Malaria" in Part 2, "Infectious Health Risks and Their Prevention").

Traveler's diarrhea in children leads to more rapid dehydration than in adults, often resulting in visits to a physician and, occasionally, hospitalization. Preventive measures and food hygiene, as we describe in Part 2, should be strictly adhered to. Children are more likely to become infected with helminths (Ascaris, Trichuris, hookworm, Strongyloides, and tungiasis) because of more intimate contact with the soil and lack of hygiene. Rapid use of oral rehydration solutions is essential in the event of diarrhea, and professional help is often necessary.

**Table 11 Minimum Ages for Vaccines in Infants
and Minimum Intervals between Doses**

Vaccine	Age of Child	Minimum Interval Between Doses
Diphtheria/tetanus/polio (OPV)	4 wk	4 wk
Diphtheria-tetanus-polio- *Haemophilus influenzae* B (DTP-Hib) combined	6 wk	4 wk
Polio (poliovirus vaccine live oral [OPV])	4 wk	6 wk
Polio (poliovirus inactivated [IPV])	6 wk	4 wk to 6 mo
Measles, mumps, and rubella	6 mo	2nd dose: 12 to 15 mo
Hepatitis B	at birth	1 mo to 2 mo
Varicella	12 mo	4 wk

Appropriate footwear should be worn at all times.

Infants and small children need routine vaccinations. For under age 1 year, certain travel vaccinations are contraindicated (see Part 2, "Infectious Health Risks and Their Prevention"), mainly because vaccines are inactivated by maternal antibodies. Table 11 shows the minimum ages for the first doses and the minimum interval between doses.

Except for the lower age limits, essentially, the travel-related vaccinations that are recommended for infants and children are the same for adults. It is wise, however, to be more generous with hepatitis B and rabies vaccinations for the reasons already described. Rarely, bacille Calmette-Guérin immunization may be indicated. Part 2 provides details.

Additional Readings

Albright TA, et al. Side effects of and compliance with malaria prophylaxis in children. J Travel Med 2002;9:289–92.

Balkhy HH. Traveling with children—the pre-travel health assessment. Int J Antmicrob Agents 2003;21:193–9.

Stauffer WM, et al. Traveling with infants and young children. Part I: Anticipatory guidance: travel preparation and preventive health advice. J Travel Med 2001;8:254–9.

PARENTS PLANNING INTERNATIONAL ADOPTION

International adoption is becoming more frequent. If children are adopted from developing countries, parents and health care providers need to take certain precautions. Although some disease screening is done at the country of origin, serious deficiencies have been identified. Children offered for adoption show frequent growth and developmental delays, and abnormal thyroid function tests exist in 10%. For this reason, all children require complete physical and mental examinations and developmental screening. Standard developmental screening guidelines, however, may not be culturally appropriate for some ethnic groups.

Fever of unknown origin can be a symptom of malaria or tuberculosis in children arriving from tropical or subtropical areas. Health care providers need to be informed about the country of origin of these children to alert them to the possibility of tropical diseases. Perform a tuberculin skin test, as well as serologic studies for hepatitis B and sexually transmitted diseases, including human immunodeficiency virus. Intestinal parasites such as Ascaris, Trichuris, Clonorchis, and Giardia can pose problems in children and be spread to others. Routinely take a blood film and stool samples.

Assess the immunization status. Immunization schedules may vary, and vaccines may differ from those available in the industrialized world. Immunization documentation may be in a language other than English, and always consider self-reported immunization histories as inadequate. If no documentation exists, it is safest to assume that no vaccinations have been given, and a primary series as recommended in the country of residence should be started. International adoption programs cause pediatric populations from endemic countries to increase in low endemic areas, possibly spreading infections to close contacts. Therefore, parents of adopted children from developing countries should take precautions themselves by being immunized against hepatitis A and B, measles, mumps, and rubella.

Additional Readings

Miller LC. International adoption: infectious disease issues. Clin Infect Dis 2005;40:286–93.

The main aim is to help athletes compete at full strength at their destination. Studies have shown that mood state, anaerobic power and capacity, and dynamic strength were affected by rapid trans-meridional travel, and that even highly trained athletes suffer from jet lag. Competitive athletes are also exposed to the additional negative consequences of a shift from the optimal circadian window of performance. Heavy, particularly prolonged, exertion has acute and chronic adverse influences on systemic immunity. Changes occur in several compartments of the immune system and body (eg, the skin, upper respiratory tract mucosal tissue, lung, blood, and muscle). Although still open to interpretation, most exercise immunologists believe that, during this "open window" of impaired immunity (which may last between 3 and 72 hours, depending on the parameters measured) viruses and bacteria may gain a foothold, increasing the risk of subclinical and clinical infection. The infection risk may be amplified when other factors related to immune function are present, including exposure to novel pathogens during travel, lack of sleep, severe mental stress, and malnutrition or weight loss.

Prior planning is therefore the key to optimal performance. The goal is primarily to minimize jet lag and the risk of infections. Strongly advise arrival long before the competition to allow time for acclimatization and adjustment to the new time zone. Melatonin has no adverse effects on athletic performance and may be given against jet lag. Complete the vaccination of athletes well in advance of the planned travel, including hepatitis A, hepatitis B, influenza, as well as updating routine vaccinations such as tetanus with diphtheria. The indication of other vaccinations, such as typhoid fever, yellow fever, Japanese encephalitis, etc., will depend on the destination of the sports event. Chemoprophylaxis for malaria, and even leptospirosis, may be indicated. For example, during the Eco Challenge in Sabah 2000, multiple participants of this expedition race were exposed to Leptospira-containing water and developed leptospirosis. Those on doxycycline malaria prophylaxis were not affected.

To prevent traveler's diarrhea, advise individuals to avoid eating out, and restrict the team to food imported from their home country and prepared by an experienced cooking team in clean facilities. Prophylactic antidiarrheal medication is usually not recommended owing to the fear of side effects that can thus reduce strength, but a non-absorbed agent, such as rifaximin could be considered. Team medical staff should become familiar with the major medical and injury concerns of athletes, and a comprehensive team medical kit should be organized. In addition, all team medical staff should be made aware of the current list of banned substances, and seek to minimize medication use by their athletes. There should be enough time offered for appropriate rest and balanced nutrition. After the event, the team medical staff should hold an appropriate debriefing session with a view to planning improvements for the future.

Additional Readings

Hill DW, et al. Effects of jet lag on factors related to sport performance. Can J Appl Physiol 1993;18:91–103.

Milne C, et al. Medical issues relating to the Sydney Olympic Games. Sports Med 1999;28:287–98.

Nieman DC. Special feature for the Olympics: effects of exercise on the immune system: exercise effects on systemic immunity. Immunol Cell Biol 2000;78:496–501.

Turbeville SD, et al. Infectious disease outbreaks in competitive sports: a review of the literature. Am J Sports Med 2006; [Epub ahead of print]

PREEXISTING HEALTH CONDITIONS AND ELDERLY TRAVELERS

General Notes On Preexisting Health Conditions

Preexisting illness may be improved or aggravated during stays in tropical or subtropical climates. The health care provider must evaluate each patient on the basis of the existing condition and of the travel characteristics, particularly the planned duration of the stay. Remind such travelers to check whether their insurance policy covers both hospitalization abroad and repatriation if their health condition deteriorates while abroad. If a patient has a particularly complicated medical problem, provide the individual with the name and telephone number of a specialist at the destination, if possible. Besides illness, some conditions also need to be considered, be they congenital or postoperative—an example being asplenia.

Travelers on medication should carry enough to last the entire trip, plus a few days extra. Equivalent medications may not be available in other countries, dosage and strength are frequently different, and conversion factors are not readily discernable. Most medication should be carried on the person or in the hand luggage to ensure a supply of medication in case of lost or stolen luggage. Because hand luggage may also be stolen, in the event of serious medical disorders, it would be wise to have complete duplicate supplies of medication in hand luggage and checked-in luggage.

Travelers with preexisting medical conditions should carry their physician's office and emergency telephone and fax numbers, as well as a copy of all pertinent medical records. When appropriate, the physician should also provide a copy of the most recent electrocardiogram and any significant test results. An official document detailing the necessary medical supply is advisable for patients carrying syringes or medications that are likely to be questioned by customs officials (see Figure 16).

The following is a general discussion of major conditions in the context of travel; the guidelines for each need to be tailored on an individual basis.

Additional Reading

Ericsson CD. Travellers with pre-existing medical conditions. Internat J Antimicrob Agents 2003;21:181–8.

Watson DAR. Pretravel health advice for asplenic individuals. J Travel Med 2003;10:117–21.

▌Cardiovascular Disease

Cardiovascular conditions do not necessarily preclude travel. Persons who are able to tolerate vigorous exercise at home will usually manage well during travel and at the destination, unless this is at an exceptionally high altitude (eg, Altiplano in South America). Unstable coronary artery disease and recent myocardial infarction, however, are often a reason against travel, due to the stress of travel, the exertion of carrying heavy luggage, and abrupt changes in climate that may aggravate the condition. Pretravel cardiology consultation, possibly with coronary angiography and 24-hour electrocardiography, may be considered in doubtful cases, particularly for prolonged stays abroad (see "Fitness to Fly" in "Essentials of Aviation Medicine"). Stable coronary heart disease is no contraindication for travel.

Advise patients with arrhythmias requiring medication, conditions requiring anticoagulation, or a risk of endocarditis against prolonged stays in developing countries. In contrast, those with stable hypertension can tolerate a prolonged stay abroad or altitude exposure. If necessary, a patient can be instructed to self-check the blood pressure. Some antihypertensive medications such as β-blockers may interfere with a compensatory increase in the heart rate at high elevations. This may result in shortness of breath and symptoms that mimic acute mountain sickness.

Low blood pressure can be aggravated in zones with a hot climate, and antihypertensive or diuretic medication may result in low blood pressure symptoms in any person.

Mild to moderate congestive heart failure usually causes no problems during air travel but may result in progressive problems upon arrival. Patients on diuretics are particularly prone to suffer electrolyte imbalance during bouts of travelers' diarrhea (or due to excessive perspiration), and in such cases, prophylactic antibiotics may be considered. Altitudes above 2,400 m (8,000 ft) can also compromise cardiopulmonary function in travelers with pre-existing heart or lung disease or severe anemia.

Long flights or bus, car, and train rides may present a risk of venous (and rarely arterial) thrombosis for patients with varicose veins and similar risk factors, particularly if they have cramped, uncomfortable seats and are unable to move their legs for a long time. Advise these patients to request well in advance (possibly with a medical certificate) seats next to the aisle or in the first row, if there is ample space there. They must be reminded to maintain adequate fluid intake during the flight, to walk around periodically, and to avoid in-flight sleeping medication. In selected cases, pressure stockings, low-dose preflight heparin, or low-molecular-weight heparin may be considered; aspirin probably gives insufficient protection. Part 3 discusses this in more detail (see "Deep Vein Thrombosis and Pulmonary Embolism").

Ensure that travelers with cardiovascular conditions have a cardiology consultation before travel, in the event they have any concerns. They should always take care to minimize stress by allowing themselves ample time, by getting assistance in carrying heavy luggage, and, if necessary, asking for a wheelchair. Patients with pacemakers or implanted defibrillators should get clearance from security staff and avoid passing through metal detectors. Theoretically, the metal detectors should not induce magnetic interference that results in deprogramming of such instruments, but this possibility cannot be ruled out, particularly in developing countries where the machines may be faulty.

Additional Reading

Leon MN. Cardiology and travel (part 1): risk assessment prior to travel. J Travel Med 1996;3:168–71.

Pulmonary Disease

Chronic respiratory insufficiency in patients with low arterial oxygen saturation and low forced expiratory volume who need oxygen supplementation for long periods on a daily basis are certainly unfit for pleasure travel but, if necessary, may be transported by air. Patients with chronic obstructive pulmonary disease with acceptable levels of arterial blood gases on the ground may well require oxygen during the flight, because oxygen saturation will drop. Similarly, chronic obstructive pulmonary disease may be aggravated by high altitude, and these patients often suffer from increased dyspnea. In contrast, patients with asthma may experience easier breathing. During a flight, gases in the gastrointestinal tract will expand, and this may impair respiration to a critical point in some patients with more severe pulmonary disease.

According to statistics from British Airways, among all in-flight emergencies due to respiratory disorders, asthma (5.6%), dyspnea (3.3%), hyperventilation (1.6%), and hypoxia (1.3%) were the most frequent ones encountered. Rarely, a pneumothorax may occur or recur. Dry cabin air has been associated with a flare-up of bronchial irritation and asthma. The incidence of pulmonary embolism following venous thrombosis (as already described) during a flight is probably underreported. Aggravation of sleep apnea syndrome after long flights has been described anecdotally.

Bronchopulmonary disease may be exacerbated, particularly in cities with smog, whereas chronic bronchitis may improve in a humid, warm climate. Advise patients with chronic obstructive airway disease to take ample medication to cope with episodes of aggravation, as required.

Additional Reading

Coker RK. Managing passengers with respiratory disease planning air travel: British Thoracic Society recommendations. Thorax 2002;57:289–304.

▌ Metabolic and Endocrinologic Disease

The most frequent problem among this group of disorders is insulin-dependent diabetes. These patients should avoid travel unless they are stable, able to assess their blood sugar, and can adapt the insulin dose. All long-term travelers should ensure they are free of comorbid complications. There are potential problems of hypo- and hyperglycemia that may be caused by the disruption of daily routine and the stresses of travel. The tropics are associated with additional health risks for patients with diabetes. Diabetic patients should plan for increased monitoring of blood glucose during travel.

Before travel, patients with diabetes must make sure they have in their hand luggage sufficient stock of the following:

- Insulin, as usually used (plus some extra)
- Insulin (regular)
- Injection material

- Blood glucose meters (with extra batteries) and blood glucose testing strips
- Urine ketone and glucose testing strips
- Sugar and snacks for treating hypoglycemic episodes and in case of meal delays
- Sugar substitutes
- Glucagon emergency kit for use in case of hypoglycemia resulting in unconsciousness (prior to travel, patients should instruct a travel companion both in the signs of hypoglycemia and in the use of the kit)
- First aid kit
- Diabetes log book
- Medical certificate, stating that the patient is diabetic
- Insurance certificate that guarantees coverage for hospitalization and/or evacuation

Diabetic travelers should request special diets for the flight at least 24 to 48 hours in advance. They should take appropriate preventive measures against motion sickness, which may result in hypoglycemia caused by decreased caloric intake. Selecting appropriate seats in the bus (the front), plane (over the wing), and on a boat (low, in the center [see Part 3, "Noninfectious Health Risks and Their Prevention"]) may be beneficial. Patients with insulin pumps should inform security staff that they should avoid passing through metal detectors. Although, theoretically, these should not induce magnetic interference resulting in deprogramming of an insulin pump, this cannot be ruled out, particularly in developing countries where the machines may be faulty.

Flights crossing no more than three time zones represent no problem to insulin-dependent diabetics, but in further westbound flights with prolongation of the day, additional doses of regular insulin may be necessary. In contrast, for eastbound flights with shorter days, reducing the insulin dose or regular insulin rather than prolonged action insulin may be indicated. When administering insulin during the flight, put one-half as much air in the bottle as normal, due to decreased air pressure at high altitude. Dehydration because of prolonged flights may make glucose control more difficult; therefore, the individual should consume plenty of nonalcoholic fluids and should frequently monitor blood sugar. Patients should consult their endocrinologist or another competent medical professional for detailed and personalized pretravel advice. Oral hypoglycemics for patients with non–insulin-dependent diabetes (type 2) can be taken as prescribed without any adjustments for time zone changes.

In hot climates, during travel and at the destination, insulin should ideally be refrigerated, although it will keep for at least 1 month unrefrigerated if protected from freezing or temperatures above 30 °C (86 °F). If insulin is likely to be exposed to heat above 50 °C (approximately 120 °F), protect with a wide-mouthed thermos or insulated bottle. For trips exceeding 1 month in duration, patients with diabetes should check in advance the local availability and equivalent brand names of their usual form of insulin.

Diabetes increases susceptibility to heat-related problems. Symptoms of hypo- or hyperglycemia may mimic some of the symptoms of heat exposure, such as weakness, dizziness, headache, and confusion. Increased perspiration may result in an increased risk of cutaneous infection; therefore, measures of hygiene should be strictly followed. Diabetic patients with autonomic neuropathy, a condition that interferes with sweating, should avoid hot climates, or ensure air-conditioned environments are available. Remind patients with diabetes to drink lots of fluids. This is particularly important in senior travelers with type 2 diabetes to avoid dehydration and hyperosmolar coma. Before vigorous exercise, it may be necessary to slightly reduce the dose of insulin. Traveler's diarrhea may be prevented with chemoprophylaxis in an individual with diabetes.

Diabetic patients must rigorously carry out diabetic foot care and obey common sense rules. In addition, they must avoid going barefoot and must frequently change their socks to keep the feet dry and comfortable. They must inspect their feet carefully each day and seek immediate medical attention if they detect a foot infection or non-healing cut or puncture wound. If staying in humid climates, an antifungal powder is a useful addition to the first aid kit.

If vomiting occurs, and individuals with type 1 diabetes are unable to eat, patients should use insulin (preferably regular insulin) at a reduced dose regularly. During any illness, carefully monitor blood sugar levels to accurately determine insulin requirements.

Obtain the names and addresses of local diabetes associations by consulting appropriate Web sites (see Appendix B, page 550). Local diabetes associations can provide information about physicians specializing in diabetes in many parts of the world, as well as restaurants offering special diets, pharmacies open 24 hours, and other useful information. The American Diabetes Association provides a wallet-size "Diabetic Alert Card" with emergency information in 13 languages.

Hyperuricemia may become a problem if recurrent bouts of gout occur. Hyperlipidemia is of comparatively little relevance with respect to travel.

Additional Reading

Brubaker PL. Adventure travel and type 1 diabetes: the complicating effects of high altitude. Diabetes Care 2005;28:2563–72.

Burnett JCD. Long- and short-haul travel by air: issues for people with diabetes on insulin. J Travel Med 2006;13:255–260.

Driessen SO, et al. Travel-related morbidity in travelers with insulin dependent diabetes mellitus. J Travel Med 1999;6:12–5.

Suh KN, Mileno MD. Challenging scenarios in a travel clinic: advising the complex traveler. Infect Dis Clin North Am 2005;19:15–47.

Renal and Urinary Tract Disorders

Renal insufficiency may be complicated during long-term travel by dehydration because of excessive perspiration or diarrhea. In addition, serious metabolic problems may occur following dietetic errors or diarrhea, resulting in hyperkalemia, hyponatremia, or metabolic acidosis. Finally, azotemia may increase the risk of infection through various mechanisms that decrease immunocompetence. Again, this may result in reduced efficacy of inactivated vaccines. For long-term travelers, renal insufficiency may be tolerated, if slight. If severe, however, we advise avoiding extensive travel or prolonged stay in a developing country.

Whenever a patient on hemodialysis wishes to travel, it is initially necessary to organize dialysis at the destination, indicating the characteristics of the patient and of the dialysis. Various tour operators specialize in tours and cruises for patients on dialysis and kidney-transplant patients, with necessary access to medical resources. The patient may, however, need to be adequately equipped with all the required materials (eg, erythropoietin), particularly for prolonged stays. The patient must take particular care to avoid infections, through immunization or chemoprophylaxis. Remind patients to drink enough fluids to avoid thrombosis of the arteriovenous fistula. They must also obtain insurance coverage for medical expenses.

Patients with urolithiasis may have an increased risk of recurrence, especially during the first months of stay in a warm climate, thus the need for them to drink plenty of fluids. A predeparture ultrasonic evaluation may occasionally be indicated. Prostatic hypertrophy and other reasons for urgency to urinate may be a disturbing handicap, particularly in planes and buses.

Gastrointestinal Disorders

Chronic inflammatory bowel disease may predispose travelers to enteric complications if they are staying in areas with high risk of gastrointestinal infection. Chronic hepatitis is a serious concern because of the risk of additional liver infections, which may lead to deterioration of the condition. Patients with chronic hepatitis should therefore decide against traveling to those countries where other types of hepatitis are hyperendemic.

Patients on acetylsalicylic acid (eg, aspirin) or those using non-steroidal anti-inflammatory products must be aware of the risk of gastric mucosal injury and the risk of bleeding. Even though there are theoretic concerns that agents reducing gastric acidity may increase the risk of traveler's diarrhea, this has only been demonstrated in gastrectomy. There is some evidence that the proton pump inhibitors may be a risk factor for acquiring diarrhea, whereas antacids and other H2 blockers do not seem to cause an increased incidence of gastrointestinal infections. Patients with diverticulosis should carry antibiotics, such as a quinolone, and metronidazole to treat a bout of diverticulitis; such patients should abstain from antimotility agents in the event of diarrhea; subsequent constipation may result in aggravation of diverticulosis or diverticulitis. Hemorrhoids may flare up after prolonged sitting, alcohol abuse (both risk factors of long flights), and after consumption of spicy food. In these patients, the travel medical kit must contain the necessary medications.

In expedition participants traveling to remote areas, elective surgical care to prevent potential problems (eg, of appendicitis) may be considered.

Dermatological Disorders

Sunlight, heat, moisture, cold dry climate, and positive or negative emotions may aggravate or alleviate some skin diseases. A few people have a genetically determined higher susceptibility to photosensitivity.

Psoriasis is usually improved by ultraviolet light, but sunburn of the untanned skin may cause Koebner phenomenon and lead to exacerbation. Ultraviolet light induces peeling of the skin and thus improves acne vulgaris, although few patients report an aggravation. Patients with atopic dermatitis usually observe a reduction of their skin lesions in summer, but perspiration can aggravate the disease. Ultraviolet light improves T-cell lymphomas of the skin when used therapeutically. Vegetative disorders, such as some forms of urticaria, may improve during a vacation with greater exposure to sunlight.

Sunlight may provoke symptomatic herpes simplex infection. This often occurs in people skiing in the sun (herpes solaris). Sunlight, or more specifically ultraviolet light, may also aggravate seborrheic dermatitis, rosacea, Mallorca acne (acne estivalis), and transient acantholytic dermatosis. Photosensitivity and sunlight can provoke discoid and systemic lupus erythematosus, respectively. Generally, sunlight aggravates other serious dermatoses such as erythema multiforme, bullous pemphigoid, and pemphigus vulgaris. Porphyria cutanea tarda is a photosensitive disease with bullae formation on the light-exposed areas. Psoriasis is only rarely aggravated. The same applies for chronic venous insufficiency, tinea pedis (athlete's foot), tinea versicolor (liver spots), and disseminated superficial actinic porokeratosis. Inform patients who take oral retinoids that they would easily get a sunburn in the mountains, because of the higher amount of UV radiation at a higher altitude.

Heat plays a prominent role in intertrigo and hyperhidrosis. Persons with anhidrotic ectodermal dysplasia have no eccrine sweat glands and experience heat congestion when they are exposed to sun and heat. Travel to tropical countries may be life-threatening in such cases.

A dry climate may unfavorably influence ichthyosis vulgaris and atopic dermatitis. Persons with dry skin should use a body lotion after a shower, take brief showers, and use soap only on the intertriginous areas.

Cold will aggravate Raynaud's disease and syndrome, peripheral vascular malperfusion, vasculitis due to cryoglobulins and cryofibrinogens, erythrocyanosis crurum, acrocyanosis, and cold panniculitis.

The recommended vaccinations generally given to potential travelers are usually well tolerated. In the past, the smallpox and bacille Calmette-Guérin vaccines (rarely indicated now) had created problems.

In contrast, all agents used for malaria prophylaxis (chloroquine, amodiaquine, mefloquine, proguanil, doxycycline, and sulfadoxine/pyrimethamine) may be associated with exacerbation of psoriasis or may result in phototoxicity.

Allergies

Travelers prone to allergies may be able to avoid during their travel the usual allergens they encounter at home, but they face the risk of being exposed to new ones, and avoidance of allergens is more difficult in a foreign environment.

House dust mites thrive in tropical conditions and can be particularly sensitizing. The risk of seasonal reactions to pollens varies region by region. Food allergies are a constant threat due to unknown ingredients in exotic dishes. Various insect bites may result in anaphylaxis. Some medications recommended for use during travel in tropical areas may trigger hypersensitivity reactions.

Travelers with allergies should carry identification cards that include a list of substances they are allergic to and should take a travel medical kit containing antihistamines or corticosteroids with them.

Degenerative rheumatologic disease is often improved during a stay in a warm climate. Depending on the type of aircraft seat, low back pain could often be aggravated during and after a long flight; thus, arranging for stopovers during long journeys and spending a night in bed may help.

Neurologic Diseases

Among neurologic diseases, epilepsy is of particular relevance to travelers; mefloquine and, to a lesser extent, chloroquine may lead to a recurrence of seizures and are therefore contraindicated. Headaches may improve while abroad; tension headaches, in particular, may disappear, because during travel, the person is removed from the usual factors causing stress.

Psychiatric and Psychological Disease

Psychological and psychiatric diseases play an important role, particularly in the case of long-term residents in a foreign country. They are among the most frequent reasons for turning down an applicant who wishes to move to another country. Patients with, or with a history of, substance abuse and persons who cannot easily adapt to new conditions are not good candidates for a prolonged stay abroad (see Part 3, "Noninfectious Health Risks and Their Prevention").

Transplantation Patients

Transplantation patients, particularly in an initial phase, are under immunosuppressive medication. This increases the risk of infection and results in a contraindication to live vaccines. Inactivated vaccines are usually not contraindicated, but immunogenicity may be diminished due to medication. For this reason, when possible, perform all immunization pre-transplantation; however, this, by far, is not always feasible.

Additional Readings

Boggild AK, et al. Travel patterns and risk behavior in solid organ transplant recipients. J Travel Med 2004;11:37–43.

Kofidis T, et al. Traveling after heart transplantation. Clin Transplant 2002;16:280–4.

Stark K, et al. Immunizations in solid-organ transplant recipients. Lancet 2002;359:957–65.

Senior Travelers

The past few years have seen a clear increase in the proportion of senior travelers, even for adventure tours in remote parts of the world.

With age, various physiologic changes occur. There is a decrease in muscle tone and strength, joint flexibility, and pulmonary and cardiovascular performance. Elderly travelers are less tolerant of hot climates, because of the reduced ability of peripheral blood vessels to dilate and the skin to perspire. Senior travelers are less sensitive to thirst. Because of decreased kidney function, they are more susceptible to fluid and electrolyte disturbances from diarrhea. Jet lag and the adverse side effects of sedatives prescribed to counter jet lag are both seen more frequently in the older population. With increasing age, there is a decline in sharpness of vision and hearing, impairment of night vision, difficulty in turning the head sideways, and longer reaction times. Impaired hearing and sight may cause failure to detect approaching vehicles, and therefore, elderly travelers driving cars are prone to greater accident risks. Poorer balance and postural instability results in an increased risk of falling and fractures, especially hip fractures. The course of many infections bears a higher rate of complications or death, such as hepatitis A, hepatitis B, or malaria. On the other hand, senior persons are less likely to get chronic hepatitis B or to suffer from motion sickness. Psychological reaction times are slower, and possible short-term memory loss may result in more stress and increased difficulty to adapt to changes. This may ultimately result in confusion.

A medical checkup before the journey is wise, particularly if one suffers from a chronic disease. A way to overcome the limitations of age and infirmity is to take advantage of organized tours that cater to the elderly. A leisurely cruise is another alternative that allows travelers to set their own pace. Luggage with wheels or a collapsible luggage cart is useful for all travelers. Encourage travelers with hearing loss to ensure that they have a hearing aid and to take along extra batteries.

Immunization requirements for the elderly traveler are no different from other adults, except that they also require pneumococcal vaccination and annual influenza vaccine administration. Many senior travelers may already be immune against hepatitis A by infection; serologic pre-vaccination screening may be cost-effective in this group. Seroconversion rates may decrease with age, and post-vaccination verification may be indicated (see Part 2, "Infectious Health Risks and Their Prevention"). Yellow fever vaccination has been associated with an increased rate of fatal adverse events in senior travelers.

Malaria prophylaxis is essential for the older traveler at risk of exposure. Persons age 60 years and older tend to have fewer adverse events to chemoprophylaxis, despite the frequent use of co-medication. However, use mefloquine cautiously in patients with bifascicular block.

Denture adhesive is often difficult to find in many countries; thus, advise travelers to take along enough for the entire trip. Encourage patients to soak dentures overnight in purified water; stains are unlikely to occur from water treated with iodine. If a pure water source is unavailable, use beer, soft drinks, or bottled mineral water for a period of up to 4 weeks.

While abroad, elderly travelers are less likely to be affected by travelers' diarrhea, but are more likely to suffer fluid and electrolyte imbalances. Prompt therapy that includes oral rehydration solutions is essential. Beware of potential drug interactions (eg, trimethoprim and sulfamethoxazole combinations) that may potentiate oral hypoglycemics, and some quinolones prolong the half-life of theophyllines.

Additional Readings

Leder K et al. Travel vaccines and elderly persons. Clin Infect Dis 2001;33:1553–66.

Linton C, Warner NJ. Travel-induced psychosis in the elderly. Int J Geriatr Psychiatry 2000;15:1070–2.

HIV INFECTION AND OTHER IMMUNODEFICIENCIES

Most immunodeficient travelers now encountered in travel medicine are infected by human immunodeficiency virus (HIV). However, principles important to this group also pertain to travelers with immunodeficiency of a different origin.

Overall, the increased risk of infection in developing countries results in increased risks of diseases, particularly when the CD4 count (the number of helper T cells per cubic millimeter of blood) is low. Recommend that persons with a CD4 count of < 200/mm^3 cancel their travel plans to destinations with a high risk of infections. In addition, medical facilities in many developing countries may not be sufficiently equipped to assess and treat such patients.

When a known HIV-infected individual travels to a developing country, include the following in the pretravel evaluation: (1) perform medical history, (2) find out travel plans (for recommended restrictions, see above), (3) conduct laboratory evaluation of hematologic parameters, including CD4 levels prior to departure, and consider tuberculin skin testing.

In addition to the advice given to all travelers, instruct the HIV-infected traveler extensively as follows:

1. Avoid unsafe sexual practices or sharing of needles.
2. Avoid gastrointestinal infection by refusing potentially contaminated food and beverages and carrying medication for rapid self-treatment. In AIDS patients, gastric secretory failure is common. This allows a larger number of viable pathogens to enter the small bowel. There may also be a depletion of CD4-positive T cells in the intestinal tissues, and impaired mucosal immune function may exist. Thus, HIV-infected travelers may be more susceptible to diseases transmitted via the oral-fecal route.
3. There is an increased risk for developing respiratory infections during travel. In HIV-infected patients, there may be a risk of dissemination of disease or secondary complications; in those with tuberculosis, there is risk of the disease becoming active. Thus, self-treatment of sinusitis with decongestants, antihistamines, and antibiotics is important, especially before air travel.

4. Avoid sunlight, because HIV-infected persons on various medications are more prone to hypersensitivity reactions. In these patients, the sun may also reactivate herpes simplex infection.

5. Personal protective measures against mosquito bites are particularly important in this population to avoid vector-borne infections such as malaria or dengue fever.

6. To seek immediate evaluation and to receive prompt medical treatment if illness occurs is vital. If possible, before travel begins, identify a physician at the destination who is informed about HIV infection.

With respect to immunizations, evaluate the potential benefit and harm with particular care; the benefit of immunization may be reduced due to an impaired antibody response resulting in decreased protective efficacy. Those with CD4 counts > 300/mm^3 usually develop antibodies, but this does not necessarily mean they will be clinically protected; those with CD4 counts < 100/mm^3 will not form antibodies. The potential harm may be increased when using live vaccines as dissemination or increased reactions may occur. With the use of inactivated or toxoid vaccines (influenza, tetanus, hepatitis B), clinicians have observed a small increase in the expression of HIV-1, but nevertheless, they are considered safe. Multiple concomitant immunizations may accelerate the progression of HIV disease.

Generally, HIV-infected persons should be immunized or have protective antibodies against the following:

- Pneumococcal pneumonia (booster every 5 years until age 65)
- Influenza (yearly or at six-month intervals; if the other hemisphere is visited, use appropriate vaccine for that hemisphere)
- *Haemophilus influenzae* B (single dose, no booster)
- Hepatitis B (check serum antibodies to make certain that they are not already immune)
- Tetanus and diphtheria (booster every 10 years)
- Measles (check antibodies to see if immune)
- Hepatitis A (note impaired immune response, especially in patients with clinical signs of acquired immunodeficiency syndrome; in advanced disease, immune globulin may be considered)

Depending on the destination and travel characteristics, consider the following:

- Poliomyelitis (use inactivated vaccine)
- Yellow fever (protective and safe in those with CD4 count > 500/mm^3; seroconversion limited to 85% and safe when CD4 count is 200 to 500/mm^3; contraindicated if CD4 count < 200/mm^3)
- Typhoid (use inactivated vaccine)
- Meningococcal disease
- Rabies (in view of impaired immunogenicity, check antibody response)
- Japanese encephalitis

Part 2 provides details on vaccines.

With respect to malaria chemoprophylaxis, there are no special recommendations, but a few travel medicine experts prefer to use doxycycline chemoprophylaxis for the additional benefit in preventing traveler's diarrhea in HIV patients.

The travel medical kit should contain sufficient antimicrobial agents (eg, rather than a short course, a seven-day course against traveler's diarrhea is preferred in patients with HIV infection). There should be enough medication for the entire trip, plus at least an extra week's supply. Labeling of medications to distinguish medicines such as cotrimoxazole for diarrhea from that for *Pneumocystis carinii* pneumonia helps avoid possible problems with customs officials.

For long-term travelers with HIV infection, many countries issue restrictions beyond the World Health Organization's International Health Regulations (see Appendix C). Because entry requirements keep changing, it is best to obtain the latest information from the consulate of the host country at the time of booking travel arrangements.

Asymptomatic patients returning from short trips who report having had no health problems during travel most likely need no post-travel screening. Those who report diarrhea, respiratory problems, or other disease symptoms require appropriate evaluation.

For asymptomatic patients on extended trips, for routine post-trip testing, include a complete blood count with differential, stool examination for ova and parasites, and tuberculin testing with controls, if previously a skin test was negative for tuberculosis.

Additional Readings

Castelli F, Patroni A. The human immunodeficiency virus-infected traveler. Clin Infect Dis 2000;31:1403–8.

Colebunders R, et al. Antiretroviral treatment and travel to developing countries. J Travel Med 1999;6:27–31.

Furrer H, et al. Increased risk of wasting syndrome in HIV-infected travellers: prospective multicentre study. Trans R Soc Trop Med Hyg 2001;95:484–6.

Mahto M, et al. Knowledge, attitudes and health outcomes in HIV-infected travellers to the USA. HIV Med 2006;7:201–4.

Salit IE, et al. Travel patterns and risk behaviour of HIV-positive people traveling internationally. Can Med Assn J 2005;172:884–8.

Simons FMJ, et al. Common health problems in HIV-infected travelers to the (sub)tropics. J Travel Med 1999;6:71–5.

HANDICAPPED TRAVELERS

The benefits of modern travel are increasingly available to people with physical limitations, despite difficulties posed by physical, and sometimes even cultural, barriers. In many areas of the world, there is an increased awareness and support for their needs. Some agencies and tour operators have developed an expertise in dealing with handicapped travelers. Tours are available for people with a wide range of special physical or medical requirements. Information can be obtained from the following organizations.

Wheelchair users are usually advised that a lightweight folding chair or "junior" model is most convenient during travel. It is useful to carry the necessary tools for repairs as well. Most new aircraft are designed for wheelchair access, and some older planes still in service have been retrofitted for wheelchair access. Many cities throughout the world publish accessibility handbooks, and their tourist bureaus will provide information.

Depending on the destination, transport of guide dogs for the blind across international borders can be a major problem. Lengthy quarantines for the animals may be imposed. Check regulations with the embassy or local consulate of the destination country prior to travel and obtain all the necessary medical and legal documents in advance. It is also important to inquire about requirements for reentry into the country of origin.

Hearing-impaired travelers need to inform transportation and hotel staff of their handicap, so they do not miss travel announcements or emergency information and alarms. On airline flights, they should request preloading privileges and should notify flight attendants about their hearing problem. Attendants will show the emergency equipment and exit locations and keep them informed of announcements.

There are no rules restricting travel of the mentally challenged or others with mental disabilities as long as they are self-sufficient. If the need for assistance is anticipated, requests for help en route, at airports, or elsewhere should be made well in advance. Tours and excursions exist in many countries for those with special needs. Some people may become disoriented in a strange town and lose their way. It helps for them to carry a card with the name, address, and telephone number of their hotel or other residence, as well as a card showing their destination in order to obtain directions or assistance if they get lost.

Additional Reading

Jorge A et al. Preflight medical clearance of ill and incapacitated passengers: 3-year retrospective study of experience with a European airline. J Travel Med 2005;12:306–11.

PETS

Travelers should let the international carrier or national airlines know well in advance that they want to carry a pet and the intended destination. Pets should be at least 8 weeks old and fully weaned for eligibility to travel. Depending on the airline, pets up to approximately 5 kg are allowed to travel in the cabin. There are restrictions on importation of exotic pets, particularly when they are on the list of endangered animals. The International Air Transport Association issued regulations that determine the type of transport containers for pets. There are specialized pet transport companies (e.g. www.worldcarepet.com).

Formalities for animals may take a long time. Usually, there are regulations to control specified diseases. If a pet is presented without the necessary documents, it will be quarantined or destroyed at the owner's expense. The most frequent requirement is proof of immunization against rabies if originating from a rabies endemic country (see "Rabies" in Part 2, "Infectious Health Risks and Their Prevention"). For some countries (eg, Australia) importation from a rabies endemic country may also involve a prolonged period of quarantine prior to importation and quarantine after arrival. Dogs may need other vaccines, for example, against distemper, canine viral hepatitis, parvovirus, and leptospirosis. In addition, some countries require proof that pets are free of ectoparasites, resulting in treatment within 48 hours predeparture. Others require a health certificate issued by a veterinarian after a pretravel checkup.

Pets need an identification with a collar and a name tag that includes the full address to prove ownership and to assure return if the pet gets lost. Some now implant a percutaneous information transducer (PIT) microchip subcutaneously, which includes the description, PIT number, and vaccinations.

In some countries, pets must be restrained while traveling in a car, which may be relevant for car rental.

Additional Reading

Leggat PA, Speare R. Traveling with pets. J Travel Med 2000; 7:325–9.

INFECTIOUS HEALTH RISKS AND THEIR PREVENTION

ANGIOSTRONGYLIASIS

Infectious Agent

Two species of *Angiostrongylus* cause two distinct diseases: *Angiostrongylus cantonensis* causes eosinophilic meningitis and is prevalent in Southeast Asia and certain tropical Pacific islands. *Angiostrongylus costaricensis* causes an eosinophilic inflammation of the gastrointestinal tract that can mimic appendicitis and is found mainly in Central and South America. *Angiostrongylus cantonensis*, also known as the rat lungworm, lives as an adult in the pulmonary arteries of the rat.

Transmission

The life cycle involves the rat and mollusks (slugs, snails, etc.), with humans being incidental hosts. Adult worms in rodent pulmonary arteries produce fertilized eggs that develop into first-stage larvae, migrate up the bronchi, are coughed up, swallowed and then passed in the feces. Larvae are consumed by land snails or slugs (in particular *Achatina fulica*). When humans consume a mollusk with viable larvae, the larvae migrate to the central nervous system (CNS).

Global Epidemiology

The spread of this parasite over Southeast Asia, the Pacific Islands and elsewhere is related to infected rats being transported aboard ships, or via importation of mollusks such as the giant African snail (*Achatina fulica*), which is capable of carrying many parasites.

Risk For Travelers

In Thailand, eosinophilic meningitis may be related to the ingestion of sliced, pickled Pila snails, which are eaten as a delicacy.

Clinical Picture

When the larvae migrate through the CNS, they cause an eosinophilic pleocytosis. Typically, the cerebrospinal fluid (CSF) shows 100 to 5,000 leukocytes per microliter, 10 to 90% of which are eosinophils. The CSF protein is usually elevated. Peripheral eosinophilia is not a consistent finding. Patients present with headache, nausea, vomiting, and neck stiffness. Fever may not be a common sign in adults. Paresthesias are a distinctive complaint; they are asymmetrical and usually noted on the extremities. Transient cranial nerve palsies, especially on the facial nerve, can occur, but serious neurologic sequelae are unusual. The duration of illness ranges from 2 to 8 weeks. Most cases resolve spontaneously without sequelae. There is no specific treatment. Anthelmintics and corticosteroids have been tried, but it is difficult to assess efficacy in the absence of controlled studies.

Incubation

2 weeks

Prevention

Prevention is by educating travelers that snails, slugs, freshwater shrimp, and crabs must be cooked, not simply marinated or refrigerated, before they are eaten. Vegetables must be washed if eaten uncooked. Mollusks like the giant African land snail, *Achatina fulica*, should be handled carefully to avoid contamination of the fingers with larvae. Control of mollusks and planarians and reducing the number of rats are important measures.

Additional Reading

Lim JM, et al. Eosinophilic meningitis caused by *Angiostrongylus cantonensis*: a case report and literature review. J Travel Med 2004;11:388–90.

ANTHRAX

Beginning with the mail-related anthrax terrorist attack in the United States in 2001, there has been a heightened concern about the potential for anthrax dissemination in the general public. The organism produces two important toxins, edema toxin and lethal toxin, which explain the clinical expressions of the infection. Anthrax causes cutaneous, inhalational, and gastrointestinal disease, depending on route of spread. Cutaneous and inhalational anthrax are the most frequent manifestations. An edematous and erythematous skin lesion with a necrotic center characterizes cutaneous anthrax. In the inhalational form, the patient presents initially with mediastinitis associated with cough, shortness of breath, and chest pain. Toxemia, the second phase, is generally fatal. Rhinitis (nasal stuffiness) and sore throat suggest a non-anthrax cause of a respiratory disease.

Anthrax outbreaks occur occasionally during the summer in central Asia (Uzbekistan, Russian Federation) among those who have consumed the meat from diseased animals. Several cases of cutaneous anthrax have been documented in travelers returning from Haiti and in personnel working with materials imported from Pakistan. In Germany in the 1970s, four of 29 individuals diagnosed with anthrax had traveled abroad. Particularly at risk were those who had purchased handicrafts made from animal products such as skin, hair, or wool contaminated with *Bacillus anthracis*. An inactivated vaccine, available primarily for armed forces personnel, is administered subcutaneously (SC) in 3 doses at 2-week intervals, with 3 further doses at 6, 12, and 18 months, providing a 93% reduction in disease occurrence. Boosters are required yearly. Mild local reactions to the vaccine occur in 30% of cases (higher rates in females), and systemic reactions are rare ($< 0.2\%$). According to the United States Food and Drug Administration, Biothrax, an anthrax vaccine adsorbed that is produced by BioPort Corp, is licensed and distributed in the United States.

Anthrax is not considered a travel-related disease requiring immunization. Travelers should avoid contact with souvenirs that may be contaminated.

Additional Reading

Inglesby TV, et al. Anthrax as a biological weapon, 2002: updated recommendations for management. JAMA 2002;287:2236–52.

Schumm WR, et al. Comments on the Institute of Medicine's 2002 report on the safety of anthrax vaccine. Psychol Rep 2002;91:187–91.

Van den Enden E. Cutaneous anthrax, Belgian traveler. Emerg Infect Dis 2006;12:523–5.

Arenaviral Hemorrhagic Fevers

Argentine, Bolivian, Venezuelan, and Brazilian hemorrhagic fevers are caused by arenaviruses, as is Lassa fever. Rodents are the hosts. Infection occurs through inhaling or ingesting contaminated excreta or by the etiologic agent entering through the skin or mucous membranes. Most of these infections take their names from the areas where they are prevalent. Lassa fever, named after the town in Nigeria where the fever was first reported, occurs in West and Central Africa (eg, Liberia, Sierra Leone, and Nigeria). The incubation period for Lassa fever is 3 to 16 days; 7 to 14 days for the other hemorrhagic fevers. Illness begins with chills and fevers accompanied by malaise, weakness, headache, myalgia, and upper gastrointestinal symptoms (including anorexia, nausea, and vomiting). Purulent pharyngitis and aphthous ulcers mark Lassa fever. Other early signs of these fevers are conjunctivitis, skin rash, and facial edema. Before the end of the first week, dehydration, hypotension, bradycardia, and hemorrhage may be seen. Bleeding from the nose and gums, gastrointestinal tract, and urinary tract or uterus is particularly common with the hemorrhagic fevers and less frequent in Lassa fever. Neurologic signs are commonly found in the Bolivian form of hemorrhagic fever. Leukopenia and thrombocytopenia are common during the early phase of these fevers. The acute phase lasts between 1 and 2 weeks. In fatal cases, uremia and hypovolemic shock usually occur after the first week of illness.

The diagnosis is by isolating the virus from the blood, cerebrospinal fluid, throat washings, or other body fluids. Serologic approaches (eg, immunofluorescence) are generally employed. Treatment is supportive, involving replacing electrolyte and fluid deficiencies and administering plasma expanders in the early stages of the disease, taking care to avoid pulmonary edema. Specific virus-immune human plasma may be administered to treat Argentine hemorrhagic fever, and a phase-three trial with a live attenuated vaccine was successful. Ribavirin given early in the course of Lassa fever benefits.

Additional Reading

Macher AM, et al. Historical Lassa fever reports and 30-year clinical update. Emerg Infect Dis 2006;12:835–7.

Maiztegui JI, et al. Protective efficacy of a live attenuated vaccine against Argentine hemorrhagic fever. J Infect Dis 1998;177: 277–83.

Tesh RB. Viral hemorrhagic fevers of South America. Biomedica (Bogota) 2002;22:287–95.

AVIAN INFLUENZA

Infectious Agent

Only influenza A viruses infect birds, and all known subtypes of influenza A viruses can infect birds. Avian influenza A H5 and H7 viruses can be distinguished as "low pathogenic" and "high pathogenic" forms on the basis of genetic features of the virus and the severity of the illness they cause in poultry; influenza H9 virus has been identified only in a "low pathogenicity" form. Each of these three avian influenza A viruses (H5, H7, and H9) theoretically can be partnered with any one of nine neuraminidase surface proteins; thus, there are potentially nine different forms of each subtype (eg, H5N1, H5N2, H5N3, H5N9). The current concern is about H5N1 because of its rapid epizootic geographic expansion.

Transmission

Most cases of H5N1 influenza in humans are thought to have occurred from direct contact with infected poultry in affected countries. Transmission of H5N1 viruses to two persons through consumption of uncooked duck blood may also have occurred in Vietnam in 2005. Several clusters of probable person-to-person transmission associated with close contact within a family are thought to have occurred in Thailand and Indonesia.

Global Epidemiology

The avian influenza A (H5N1) epizootic (animal outbreak) first evolved in Asia at the end of 2003 and has since been reported in almost all countries in Asia and parts of Europe, the Near East, and Africa. At the time of writing, more than 300 human cases had been reported. The public health threat of a pandemic arising from novel influenza subtypes, such as influenza A (H5N1), would be greatly increased if the virus gains the ability to easily spread from one human to another. It is of public health concern that H5N1 infections are not only observed in birds but also among pigs in China and in felines. In addition, Germany reported H5N1 infection in a stone marten (a weasel-like mammal).

Risk For Travelers

To date, no case in a traveler has been reported, but a theoretical risk of infection cannot be excluded if travelers make contact with infected animals.

Clinical Picture

Symptoms of avian influenza in humans have ranged from typical human influenza-like symptoms (eg, fever, cough, sore throat, and muscle aches) to eye infections (H7N7), pneumonia, severe respiratory diseases (such as acute respiratory distress in H5N1), and other severe and life-threatening complications. H5N1 is also associated with diarrheal disease. Case fatality rate due to H5N1 is currently about 60%. An atypical fatal case of encephalitis in a child in southern Vietnam in 2004 was identified retrospectively as H5N1 influenza through testing of cerebrospinal fluid, fecal matter, and throat and serum samples.

Incubation

3 to 7 days

Communicability

Person-to-person transmission exceptionally occurred after very close contact.

Susceptibility

There is hardly any natural immunity to H5N1 infection in the human population.

Minimized Exposure In Travelers

Visits to poultry farms and bird markets where live poultry are raised or kept should be avoided, along with contact with poultry as well as surfaces that may have been contaminated by poultry feces or secretions. Uncooked poultry or poultry products, including blood, should not be consumed. All foods from poultry, including eggs and poultry blood, should be cooked thoroughly. Egg yolks should not be runny or liquid. Because influenza viruses are destroyed by heat, the cooking temperature for poultry meat should be 74 °C (165 °F).

Chemoprophylaxis

Neuraminidase inhibitors, such as oseltamivir (Tamiflu) or zanamivir (Relenza) would probably be effective to protect persons who are exposed to H5N1, but this is currently not indicated for any travelers.

Immunoprophylaxis

Several (pre-pandemic) vaccines began testing with mixed success, the first expected to become available in 2007. Several countries bought stocks to be able to offer pre-pandemic priming to subjects at high risk or to the entire population.

Principles of Therapy

The H5N1 viruses are often resistant to amantadine and rimantadine. Most of the H5N1 viruses tested have been susceptible to the neuraminidase inhibitors oseltamivir (Tamiflu) and zanamivir (Relenza), but some resistance to them has been reported. The effectiveness of these drugs when used for treatment of H5N1 virus infection is enhanced when used within 24 (or 48) hours.

Community Control Measures

The World Health Organization and many nations have published pandemic plans to be implemented in the event that H5N1 or any other influenza virus should become more easily transmitted and pose a pandemic threat. Specifically related to travel, health alerts would be issued, deferral of nonessential travelers coming or going to affected areas would be advised, and anyone traveling would be advised to perform daily self-checking for fever, to report symptoms, and would be instructed on how to behave if illness occurs. Entry screening for travelers arriving from affected areas has been demonstrated to be ineffective, but some exit screening procedures may be implemented (eg, by health declarations, thermal scanning). Measures to increase social distance will be recommended, such as closure of schools, cancellation of mass gatherings; on board planes, such travelers would be separated. On flights from affected areas, masks would be offered to all passengers upon boarding, although recommendations with respect to wearing masks (and as to type of mask) are inconsistent.

Additional Reading

Democratis J, et al. Use of neuraminidase inhibitors to combat pandemic influenza. J Antimicrob Chemother 2006;6:1–5.

Tellier R. Review of aerosol transmission of influenza A virus. Emerging Infect Dis 2006;12:1657–62.

Viboud C, et al. Air travel and the spread of influenza: important caveats. Plos Medicine 2006;3:e503.

World Health Organization. Avian influenza fact sheet (April 2006). Wkly Epid Rec 2006;81:129–136.

www.who.int/csr/disease/avian_influenza/en/index.html.

BARTONELLOSIS

Infectious Agent

Bartonella bacilliformis is a facultative intracellular bacillus that attacks erythrocytes.

Transmission

Sandflies (*Lutzomyia verrucarum*)

Global Epidemiology

Narrow river valleys between 500 m and 3,200 m above sea level in Peru, Colombia, and Ecuador. The acute form of the disease gets its name from an outbreak that occurred in 1871 near La Oroya, Peru. More than 7,000 people perished. Some survivors later developed a skin disease, called verruga peruana (Peruvian warts). These skin lesions were observed prior to the 1871 outbreak—perhaps as far back as the pre-Columbian era—but a connection to Oroya fever was unknown. In 1885, a young medical researcher, Daniel Carrion, inoculated himself with blood from a lesion to study the course of the skin disease. When he became ill with Oroya fever, the connection became apparent. Oroya fever is often called Carrion's disease in honor of his fatal experiment. The bacteria, *B. bacilliformis*, was isolated by Alberto Barton in 1909.

Risk for Travelers

There have been a few cases in returning travelers from affected areas in South America

Clinical Picture

Acute bartonellosis (Oroya fever) is an acute anemic febrile disease. Erythrocyte parasitization levels can be as high as 100%. Symptoms are fever, chills, severe anemia, hepatosplenomegaly and jaundice.

With chronic bartonellosis (verruga peruana), 2 to 20 weeks after recovery from Oroya fever (or sometimes without any pre-

ceding illness), fever, arthralgia, and a series of crops of verru-
cae appear as painless, erythematous papules, nodules, or large
angioma-like cutaneous lesions, particularly on the extremities.

Incubation

1 to 30 weeks (mean of 2 months)

Diagnosis

Bartonellosis is identified by symptoms and the patient's history,
such as recent travel in areas where bartonellosis occurs. Isolation
of *B. bacilliformis* from the bloodstream or lesions can confirm
the diagnosis. Serologic diagnosis by enzyme immunoassay is
possible.

Principles of Therapy

Antibiotics have dramatically decreased the fatality associated
with bartonellosis. Prior to the development of antibiotics, the
fever was fatal in 40% of cases. With antibiotic treatment, that
rate has dropped to 8%. The bacteria are susceptible to several
antibiotics, including chloramphenicol, penicillins, and amino-
glycosides. Blood transfusions may be necessary to treat the
anemia caused by bartonellosis. Fatalities can result from complications associated with severe anemia and secondary infections.
Once the infection is halted, an individual can recover fully.

Prevention

Avoiding sandfly bites is the primary means of prevention. Sandfly
eradication programs have been helpful in decreasing the sandfly population, and insect repellant can be effective in preventing
sandfly bites.

Other Bartonella Infections

B. quintana causes trench fever. The clinical manifestations of
B. henselae infections are cat-scratch disease, encephalitis,
meningitis, FUO, endocarditis, bacillary angiomatosis, and
bacillary peliosis.

Additional Readings

Koehler JE, et al. Case records of the Massachusetts General Hospital. Case 30-2005. A 56-year-old man with fever and axillary lymphadenopathy. N Engl J Med 2005;353:1387–94.

Matteelli A, et al. Short report: verruga peruana in an Italian traveler from Peru. Am J Trop Med Hyg 1994;50:143–4.

BOTULISM

Botulism, usually a paralytic disease, results from ingestion of a neurotoxin produced by one of a number of *Clostridium botulinum* types (A, B, E, F, or G). The toxin is destroyed by boiling liquids for 5 to 10 minutes or by heating food for 30 minutes at 80 °C. Travelers usually contract botulism from eating improperly canned foods in which heat-resistant spores of *C. botulinum* have germinated and multiplied. The customary incubation period for botulism is 1 day but may range from a few hours to 1 week or slightly longer. The patient usually experiences nausea, vomiting, and general weakness. Autonomic dysfunction may occur, causing dryness of the mouth, ileus, constipation, diarrhea, urinary retention, and hypotension. The hallmarks of the disease are neurologic impairments, including double or blurred vision, ptosis, dysphonia, dysarthria, and dysphagia in the early stages, and weakness of the peripheral and respiratory muscles as the disease progresses. The patient is usually alert, conscious, and without fever. Dilated pupils in an alert patient suggest botulism, as does generalized muscle weakness without sensory loss. Treatment includes respiratory support, purging the intestine with lavage, purgatives, and saline enemas, and administering a trivalent antitoxin. The latter is an equine-derived material directed against *C. botulinum* types A, B, and E, and is available from the Centers for Disease Control and Prevention (CDC).

One-half of each dose of antitoxin may be given intravenously and one-half intramuscularly or the full dose intravenously. Hypersensitivity to equine-derived antiserum (urticaria or angioedema) occurs in up to one-fifth of patients, and anaphylaxis may occur in a smaller number, mainly after repeat use. Specific human immune globulin may be available in small quantities in some countries. The armed forces of some countries have access to a vaccine.

Additional Reading

Arnon SS, et al. Botulinum toxin as a biological weapon: medical and public health management. JAMA 2001;285:1059–70.

Reller ME. Wound botulism acquired in the Amazonian rain forest of Ecuador. Am J Trop Med Hyg 2006;74:628–31.

Roblot F. Botulism in patients who inhale cocaine: the first cases in France. Clin Infect Dis 2006;43:e51–2.

BRUCELLOSIS

Infectious Agent

The specific microorganism responsible for human infection depends upon its animal host: cattle host, *Brucella abortus*; goats and sheep, *B. melitensis*; pigs, *B. suis*; and dogs, *B. canis*.

Transmission

Brucellosis is a worldwide infection that is most commonly found in the developing regions. The organism passes from its animal host to humans through inhalation of infected aerosols, through direct contact with infected animals, or by ingesting unpasteurized milk or cheese.

Clinical Picture

There are three different clinical manifestations of brucellosis due to *B. melitensis*, the most frequent cause of brucellosis. The acute form is characterized by acute onset of fever, malaise, weight loss, often associated with arthralgias and myalgias. The relapsing form (Malta fever) usually reflects incomplete treatment or failure of treatment and is characterized by hepatic involvement and arthritis, occasionally uveitis and orchidoepididymitis. Chronic brucellosis is characterized by either a cyclic course with back pain, arthralgias, fatigue, and depressive mood, or by a chronic localized form presenting with spondylitis or uveitis. The disease is characterized by fever and systemic signs and symptoms, such as chills, myalgias, and headache, with an insidious onset. Relapse following treatment is common. Diagnosis is usually confirmed in a patient with a compatible illness by demonstrating an elevated titer of specific antibodies in serum samples. Brucellosis should always be considered when diagnosing a patient with febrile illness who has traveled to a developing region (especially South America) or southern Europe, particularly if there has been contact with animals or ingestion of unpasteurized milk or cheese. Clinicians can make a diagnosis by recovering organisms from blood cultures or by performing a serologic study. Brucellosis is treated with an antimicrobial agent, including doxycycline (200 mg/d) plus rifampin (600 to 900 mg/d) (or streptomycin with doxycycline), trimethoprim/sulfamethoxazole (160/800 mg bid) or a fluoroquinolone (eg, ciprofloxacin 500 mg bid, or levofloxacin 500 mg qd PO) for 6 weeks.

Additional Reading

Memish ZA, et al. Brucellosis and international travel. J Travel Med 2004;11:49–55.

Pappas G, et al. The new global map of human brucellosis. Lancet Infect Dis 2006;6:91–9.

CHIKUNGUNYA

Infectious Agent

Chikungunya virus (CHIKV) is a member of the genus *Alphavirus*, in the family Togaviridae.

Transmission

Aedes aegypti (the tiger mosquito) is the main vector.

Global Epidemiology

West, central, and southern Africa and many areas of Asia. The virus circulates throughout much of Africa, with transmission thought to occur mainly between mosquitoes and monkeys.

Risk for Travellers

As demonstrated particularly in 2006, travellers may be infected by CHIKV.

Clinical Picture

Headache, fatigue, nausea, vomiting, muscle pain, rash, and joint pain. The term "chikungunya" is Swahili for "that which bends up." Acute chikungunya fever typically lasts a few days to a couple of weeks, but as with dengue, West Nile fever, and other arboviral fevers, some patients have prolonged fatigue lasting several weeks. Chikungunya is often mistaken for dengue in dengue-endemic areas; the main clinical feature that differentiates chikungunya from dengue is its severe arthralgia, often prolonged. Haemorrhagic manifestations do not occur in chikungunya.

Communicability

The infection is not communicable from person to person.

Incubation Period

2 to 12 days, but is usually 3 to 7 days.

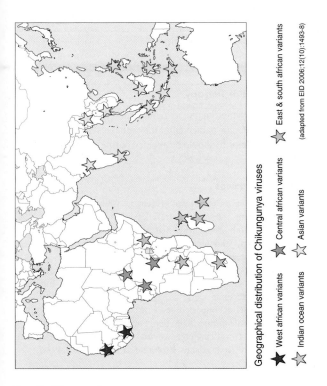

Geographical distribution of Chikungunya viruses

West african variants
Central african variants
East & south african variants

Indian ocean variants
Asian variants

(adapted from EID 2006;12(10):1493-8)

Figure 15   Chikungunya virus

▌ Minimized Exposure in Travelers

Personal protective measures against mosquito bites in daytime

▌ Chemoprophylaxis

Not applicable

▌ Immunoprophylaxis

Not applicable

▌ Principles of Therapy

Treatment is symptomatic; rest, fluids, and ibuprofen, naproxen, acetaminophen, or paracetamol may relieve symptoms of fever and aching. Aspirin should be avoided during the acute stages of the illness.

Additional Readings

Center for Disease Control and Prevention. Chikungunya fever diagnosed among international travellers–United States, 2005–2006. MMWR Morb Mortal Wkly Rep 2006;55:1040–2.

Charrel RN et al. Chikungunya outbreaks — The Globalization of vectorborne diseases. N Engl J Med 2007;356:769-71.

Hochedez P et al. Cases of chikungunya fever imported from the islands of the South West Indian Ocean to Paris, France. Euro Surveill 2007;12:Epub

Krastinova E, et al. Imported cases of chikungunya in metropolitan France: update to June 2006. Euro Surveill 2006;11:E060824.1.

Parola P et al. Novel chikungunya virus variant in travelers returning from Indian Ocoan Islands. Emerg Infect Dis 2006;12:1493-7.

CHOLERA

Infectious Agent

Vibrio cholerae, a motile, curved, gram-negative bacterium of the family Vibrionaceae, has a single polar flagellum. Two serogroups, O1 and O139 ("Bengal") have been implicated in human cholera epidemics. Among serogroup O1, there are the classic and El Tor biotypes and the Inaba and Ogawa serotypes. Strains expressing both Inaba and Ogawa serotypes are classified as serotype Hikojima. The principal virulent component of *V. cholerae* is an enterotoxin composed of a central A subunit and five B subunits arranged in circular form. Nontoxigenic O1 strains and non-O1/O139 strains can cause diarrhea and sepsis but not epidemics.

Most laboratories in the developed nations do not routinely test for *V. cholerae* in diarrheal stool samples, and such a test must be explicitly requested if cholera is suspected.

Cholera infection is spread through oral contact with fecal matter. Humans are the only known natural hosts. For a previously healthy person to become infected, contact with more than 105 cholera bacteria is usually required.

Global Epidemiology

Cholera is linked to poverty. It often occurs when overcrowding is accompanied by poor sanitation and untreated drinking water. Cholera is spread mainly through contaminated drinking water, other beverages, ice, ice cream, locally grown vegetables, raw fish, and shellfish. Food and beverages sold by street vendors are particularly suspect.

Cholera occurs throughout the developing world (Figure 16). In 2005, a total of 52 countries reported 131,943 cases of cholera with 2,272 deaths; the case fatality rate was 1.7%. The World Health Organization (WHO) Weekly Epidemiological Record regularly identifies areas where infections have been documented.

Currently, the eltor biotype predominates, except in Bangladesh, where the classic biotype has reappeared. After its detection in 1992, strain O139 caused major epidemics in both Bangladesh and Calcutta the following year. Although O139 continues to be

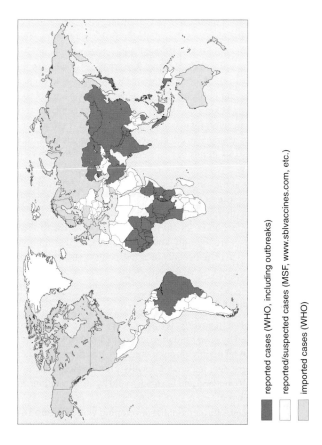

Figure 16   Cholera 2004–2006, summary of outbreaks and imported cases

detected in Southeast Asia, it has not yet resulted in an eighth cholera pandemic, as initially feared.

Risk for Travelers

There are about 100 cases of imported cholera reported to the WHO each year. This figure, however, is deceptive because many travelers are treated and cured while abroad, many are cured without diagnosis, and many are oligosymptomatic or asymptomatic.

Retrospective surveys reviewed cases of cholera imported to the United States from 1961 to 1980 and from 1965 to 1991, and to Europe and North America from 1975 to 1981. All three surveys concluded that the rate of importation of cholera from an endemic to a developed country was usually < 1 case in 100,000 travelers. Many had acquired cholera in North Africa or in Turkey, despite these countries having, at the time, reported no or few cases of cholera to the WHO. Recent data identify Mexico as a country where the infection is frequently acquired. Risk factors for cholera infection in the endemic areas were consumption of seafood (particularly raw), unboiled water, and food and beverages from street vendors. The *V. cholerae* strains are becoming resistant to antimicrobial treatment.

Evidence exists that the incidence of cholera is increasing, at least under specific circumstances. A retrospective analysis of all cases of cholera reported to national surveillance centers in the developed countries in 1991 found an attack rate of 13.1 per 100,000 (mean duration of stay < 2 weeks) in 38 cases of cholera imported from Bali to Japan. According to Japanese quarantine officers and other local experts, this is likely a low estimate; despite tight surveillance at Japanese airports, some returning travelers do not report diarrheal illness. Similarly, the only follow-up study to date observed a rather high incidence of 5 cases per 1,000 US government employees in Lima in the first 3 years of the epidemic (1991 to 1993). More than 90% of cases of cholera imported from Asia were *V. cholerae* Ogawa eltor infections, whereas in most cases, cholera contracted in Latin America was of the Inaba serotype, eltor biotype. Importation of O139 infections to Denmark and the United States have been reported.

Clinical Picture

V. cholerae infections may lead to a broad spectrum of clinical illnesses. In eltor infections, for each symptomatic case, up to 50 asymptomatic or mildly symptomatic cases indistinguishable from other diarrheal causes occur. The proportion of a typical clinical picture in classic biotype infections is one to five.

Severe watery diarrhea is experienced in < 5% of cases, often accompanied by vomiting, due to acidosis, without nausea, abdominal pain, or fever. Up to 1 liter hourly of stool is produced in the first day, becoming colorless, odorless, and flecked with mucus; these are often described as "rice-water stools." Dehydration (cholera gravis) results, leading to a loss of body weight of > 10% within the first 24 hours. Patients may die within 2 hours from circulatory collapse, if no treatment is provided. More commonly, diarrhea from *V. cholerae* infections leads to shock, accompanied by drowsiness or unconsciousness, in 4 to 12 hours and to death in 18 hours to several days. Bicarbonate losses lead to acidosis, as well as hypovolemia. Hypokalemia produces cardiac arrhythmia, renal failure, and leg cramps. Hypoglycemia may cause seizures in children with cholera.

The overall case fatality rate of cholera is currently low. It was 0.9% in the Latin American epidemic of 1991 to 1994. Case fatality rates of 1 to 2% have been noted among surveyed travelers. Untreated severe cases are often fatal.

Incubation

The incubation period in cholera ranges from several hours to 5 to 7 days.

Communicability

Patients may be infective 3 days prior to the onset of symptoms. They are usually noninfective after 2 to 3 weeks but occasionally become persistent carriers. In developed countries, no secondary outbreaks could be attributed to the several hundred patients with imported cholera in 1990 to 1993. The secondary infection rate may reach 17% from household contacts in developing countries.

Susceptibility and Resistance

Adults, particularly those over age 65, are more often affected than children. Persons with the "O" blood group are more likely to develop symptoms and to experience severe illness. Hypochlorhydria apparently also predisposes to developing symptomatic illness whereby an infective dose of 104 organisms causes diarrhea in 90% of such individuals and a dose of 103 causes diarrhea in 50%. Japanese tourists demonstrate an elevated attack rate, possibly because of the prevalence of atrophic gastritis among the population. Atrophic gastritis is also common among Peruvians, particularly young people of the lowest socioeconomic level. This may be partly due to infection with *Helicobacter pylori*. The role of H2-receptor antagonists in predisposition to cholera remains unclear.

Infection with *V. cholerae* results in antibody production to both subunits of the enterotoxin. Resistance to reinfection is limited in duration, lasting longest against the homologous biotype. Infection with the classic biotype confers better protection against eltor biotypes than vice versa.

Minimized Exposure in Travelers

Basic sanitation and public health procedures are essential to fighting cholera. The state of Ceara, Brazil, reduced the number of cholera cases from 20,000 in 1994 to 35 in 1995 by instituting such measures.

Travelers could virtually avoid cholera by being careful about what they eat and drink. Most tourists and business people, however, do not avoid local culinary temptations. Travelers should avoid raw or undercooked seafood and tap water in areas with endemic cholera.

Chemoprophylaxis

Antibiotics for prophylaxis of traveler's diarrhea may provide some protection against cholera. Antimicrobial prophylaxis for cholera has been considered only for closed situations, wherein a group may have had common exposure, such as on board a ship.

Immunoprophylaxis by Cholera Vaccine

Only one cholera vaccine is currently available: Oral Cholera (and enterotoxigenic *Escherichia coli* [ETEC]) Vaccine: Whole Cell, Recombinant B-Subunit (WC/rBS), marketed as Dukoral.

The oral vaccine CVD 103-HgR (Orochol, Mutacol) is no longer produced, and the obsolete parenteral vaccine seems to have disappeared everywhere.

Immunology and Pharmacology

Viability: inactivated

Dosage and antigenic form: 10^{11} whole cell inactivated *V. cholerae* 01 representing the (classic) Inaba and Ogawa serotypes and classical and eltor biotypes, plus 1 mg recombinant B-subunit cholera toxin

Adjuvants: buffer

Preservative: none

Allergens/Excipients: none

Mechanism: induction of specific immunoglobulin (Ig) A and IgG intestinal antibacterial and antitoxin antibodies

Administration

Schedule: two oral doses administered with a 1- to 6-week interval. In children aged 2 to 6 years, 3 doses are required.

Recipients should not eat or drink 1 hour before or 1 hour after ingesting the vaccine.

Booster: although no clinical efficacy data have been generated on repeat booster dosing, a single booster dose is recommended after 2 years for adults and children older than 6 years of age, and after 6 months for children aged 2 to 6 years. However, immunological data suggest that, if up to 2 years have elapsed since the last vaccination, a single booster dose should be given. If more than 2 years have elapsed since the last vaccination, the primary course should be repeated.

Route: oral

Storage: store at 2 to 8 °C (35 to 46 °F). Discard frozen vaccine (air passengers should keep Dukoral in the carry-on luggage!) According to the manufacturer Dukoral can be exposed at least 14, possibly 35, days to room temperature without any effect on its potency.

Availability: registered in more than 50 countries worldwide including the European Union, Canada, Australia, New Zealand, and South Africa (but not in the United States), produced by SBL Vaccin in Stockholm, now a Crucell company.

Protection

Onset: 7 days after the second dose

Efficacy: studies in three different continents (Asia, South America, and Africa) all show a field efficacy of 85% against cholera O1 serogroup. Whether Dukoral has any protective efficacy against *V. cholerae* O139 (Bengal) has not been studied, but that may theoretically be possible because the cholera toxin produced by *V. cholerae* O139 is identical to the cholera toxin produced by *V. cholerae* O1 (eltor). So far not assessed in non-immunes, except for the Peruvian military shortly after the introduction of cholera on the Latin American continent.

Also, 60 to 70% efficacy against LT-producing enterotoxigenic *Escherichia coli* has been documented, since this is structurally, functionally, and immunologically similar to cholera toxin B (CTB). The two toxins cross-react immunologically.

Duration: 78% after 1 year in subjects over 5 years; 60% after 2 years; in children 2 to 5 years 100% protection is seen the first 6 months.

Contraindications

Absolute: none

Relative: previous adverse reactions to the vaccine, any acute illness, diarrhea, or vomiting. In contrast, Dukoral has been given to ulcer and to colonectomized patients, and no side effects other than those reported by healthy volunteers were reported.

Children: safety and immunogenicity has been studied in children from age 1 year, efficacy from 2 years—thus contraindicated at a lower age.

Pregnant women: not contraindicated, based on the nature of the vaccine and the oral route.

Lactating women: according to the manufacturer not contraindicated. It is unknown whether cholera vaccine or corresponding antibodies are present in human breast milk. Dukoral has been given to a large number of breast-feeding women in different studies, and no adverse events in relation to breast-feeding have been reported. Both the pregnant woman and her child in utero may be protected.

Immunodeficient persons: not contraindicated. Persons receiving immunosuppressive therapy or having other immunodeficiencies may experience a diminished antibody response to active immunization. Dukoral has been well tolerated in HIV-infected people.

Adverse Reactions

Few, mainly from buffer (eg, belching, abdominal discomfort, vomiting rarely). No serious adverse reactions have been documented.

Interactions

Food and beverages at 1 hour before and after vaccine ingestion. There is uncertainty about interaction with other oral vaccines. Oral live typhoid vaccine can be given concomitantly with Dukoral. Immunosuppressant drugs and radiation therapy may result in an insufficient response to immunization.

Recommendations for Vaccine Use

Persons following the usual tourist routes are at virtually no risk of *V. cholerae* O1 infection, unless they break the most fundamental rules of food and beverage hygiene.

Vaccination against cholera cannot prevent importation of the disease. For this reason, the World Health Assembly amended the International Health Regulations in 1973, so cholera vaccination is no longer required of any traveler. Currently, no country requires proof of cholera vaccination from travelers arriving from nonendemic countries. Several rarely visited countries and local authorities in some countries, however, still request proof of vaccination from travelers who have passed through endemic areas in the previous 5 days. In these cases, give cholera vaccination at least 6 days prior to entry, and record it in the International Certificate of Vaccinations.

In view of the minimal risk of cholera to prudent travelers, immunization is of questionable benefit and, according to the CDC, "almost never recommended." Immunization against cholera is suggested only for special high-risk individuals who live and work in highly endemic areas under inadequate sanitary conditions, such as refugee camps.

Self-Treatment Abroad

Not applicable, as travelers will not know their precise diagnosis.

Principles of Therapy

Cholera patients require immediate therapy. Rapid rehydration is crucial to prevent death and should never be withheld until laboratory confirmation is obtained. Depending on the degree of dehydration, oral rehydration with WHO oral rehydration solutions may be sufficient. For patients who have lost more than 10% of their body weight or are experiencing severe vomiting, lethargy, or an inability to drink, treat them with intravenous fluid and electrolyte replacement until the oral medication can be taken.

Antibiotics will decrease the duration of illness. Tetracycline and doxycycline are recommended. If the strains are resistant, erythromycin, co-trimoxazole, quinolones, etc, may be used. Oral administration is usually feasible; vomiting subsides soon after initiation of rehydration.

Community Control Measures

Current International Health Regulations (Appendix A) require reports on any case of cholera. Isolation of patients is unnecessary, but cleanliness (enteric precautions) should be practiced around the patient, whether or not they are hospitalized. Feces can be directly discharged in sewers without preliminary disinfection.

Some countries trace contacts of imported cholera. Observing persons who shared food and beverages with a cholera patient is recommended for 5 days from last exposure. Give household members chemoprophylaxis for 3 days with doxycycline or tetracycline if there is likelihood of secondary transmission.

Additional Readings

CATMAT. Statement on new oral cholera and travellers' diarrhea vaccination. Can Commun Dis Rep 2005;31:1–11.

Hill DR, et al. Oral cholera vaccines: use in clinical practice. Lancet Infect Dis 2006;6:361–73.

Steffen R, et al. Cholera: assessing the risk to travellers and identifying methods of protection. Travel Med Infect Dis 2003;1:80–88.

Tarantola A. Current cholera epidemics in west Africa and risks of imported cases in European countries. Euro Surveill 2005;10:E050901.2.

World Health Organization. Oral cholera vaccine use in complex emergencies: what next. Report of a WHO meeting; Cairo 2005 [PDF]. Available at: http://www.who.int/topics/cholera/publications/cholera_vaccines_emergencies_2005.pdf (accessed Jan. 14, 2007).

World Health Organization. Cholera 2005. Wkly epid Rec 2006; 81:297–307.

DENGUE

Infectious Agent

The causative agents of dengue fever are four serotypes of the dengue fever virus, belonging to the Flaviviridae family (single-stranded, non-segmented RNA viruses). Dengue virus serotypes are distinguishable by complement fixation and neutralization tests.

Transmission

The infection is spread through the bite of the *Aedes aegypti* mosquito (tiger mosquito) and others of the same genus. *A. aegypti* is an efficient vector for several reasons: it is highly susceptible to dengue virus, feeds preferentially on human blood, is a daytime feeder, has an almost imperceptible bite, and is capable of biting several people in a short period for one blood meal. As a peridomiciliary mosquito, it is well adapted to urban life as it typically breeds in stagnant water in a wide variety of man-made containers that collect rainwater (such as tires, tin cans, pots, and buckets). Viremic humans represent the reservoir of infection. In Africa and Southeast Asia, there is a jungle cycle of dengue, with monkeys serving as a reservoir.

Global Epidemiology

Dengue viruses are now the most common cause of arboviral disease in the world, with an estimated annual 100 million cases of dengue fever (DF), 250,000 cases of dengue hemorrhagic fever (DHF) and an annual mortality rate of 25,000. Dengue viruses are spread throughout the regions where *A. aegypti* are found—tropic and subtropical areas between 30° north and 20° south latitude. The principal geographic urban and rural areas include the Caribbean, Latin America (including Mexico), Northern Australia, the South Pacific, Southeast Asia, and Hawaii (Figure 17). Transmission occurs at altitudes below 2,000 feet, predominantly during the rainy seasons. Sustained cold weather will interrupt transmission by destroying the mosquito vector.

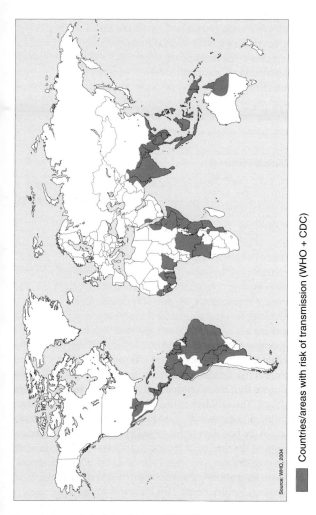

Countries/areas with risk of transmission (WHO + CDC)

Source: WHO, 2004

Figure 17   Geographic distribution of dengue, 2003–2005.

Risk for Travelers

Attack rates of dengue among travelers visiting endemic areas depend on the intensity of local prevalence. Prospective studies on seroconversion rates based on dengue immunoglobulin (Ig) M in travelers (which include asymptomatic and symptomatic cases) revealed an incidence of dengue of 2.9% (in those traveling for a mean of one month) and 6.7% (in those traveling for a mean of 6 months). Risk factors for acquiring dengue depend on duration of travel, season, and destination. The majority of dengue virus infections in travelers are acquired in Asia (followed by the Americas) and only a small proportion in Africa.

Clinical Picture

Dengue (breakbone fever) typically begins with fever lasting 1 to 5 days. Most cases are characterized by mild muscle aches, back pain, frontal or retro-orbital headache, pharyngitis, arthralgia, and cough. Bradycardia may occur. Scleral and pharyngeal redness is commonly found. Transient generalized macular rash that blanches under pressure is common early in the illness; petechiae may be seen later. Thrombocytopenia below 100,000/mm^3 is commonly found. Biphasic febrile illness is common. On resolution, the rash may desquamate.

Although the mechanisms for developing severe hemorrhagic disease are not fully understood, the main risk factor for developing dengue hemorrhagic syndrome and dengue shock syndrome is thought to be secondary infection with another serotype. Children are more at risk than adults, females more than males, well nourished more than malnourished, and Asian and Caucasians more than black. The hallmark of this syndrome is a capillary leakage syndrome, accompanied by hemorrhagic manifestations. Patients present in the first days similarly to DF, but then plasma leakage develops at the time of defervescence around 4 to 7 days after the onset of disease. Abdominal pain and vomiting, restlessness, change in level of consciousness, and a sudden change from fever to hypothermia may be the first clinical warning signs, associated with a significant decrease in platelets and rise in hematocrit. The diagnosis of DHF is made based on the combination of hemorrhagic manifestations, platelet count < 100,000/mm^3, and objective evidence of plasma leakage shown by either fluctuation of packed cell volume > 20% during the course of illness or clinical signs of plasma leakage, such as pleural effusion, ascites, or hypoproteinemia. Hemorrhagic manifestations without capillary leakage do not constitute DHF. A positive tourniquet test is incorporated in the World Health Organization clinical case definition of DHF, but differentiates poorly between dengue and DHF and seems to be not very specific. Mortality of DHF can be up to 10 to 20%, but it is as low as 0.2% in hospitals with staff experienced in the management of the disease.

Dengue shock syndrome (DSS) is DHF plus narrow pulse pressure, hypotension, and shock. It is often associated with a case fatality rate exceeding 40%.

Incubation Period

The incubation period for dengue usually ranges from 4 to 7 days (minimum 3 days to maximum 14 days) after being bitten by a mosquito harboring the virus.

Communicability

The infection is spread from viremic local persons to susceptible individuals through the bite of an *Aedes* mosquito. Mother to child (vertical) transmission has been described, as well as non-vector transmission via needle stick injury.

Susceptibility and Resistance

Most travelers visiting endemic areas are susceptible to dengue. Prior infection with one serotype confers immunity to that serotype but not cross protectivity to others. There is some evidence that a second infection with a heterologous dengue virus serotype carries a significantly higher risk of developing dengue hemorrhagic fever, although other factors such as genetic disposition and degree of viremia may also play a role.

Minimizing Exposure

The single most effective dengue preventive measure for travelers to endemic areas is taking precautions to avoid mosquito bites, such as using mosquito repellents (based on deet [diethyltoluamide]), protective clothing (the best being permethrin-impregnated), and insecticides. *Aedes* are daytime biting mosquitoes, hence these measures have to be taken during the day (in particular in the morning and late afternoon), and the utility of insecticide treated bed nets at night is therefore limited. *Aedes* are also indoor feeders and are often found in dark areas (ie, inside closets and bathrooms, behind curtains, and under beds), and it is advisable to spray these areas with insecticides. Care should be taken not to leave out trash, pots, or any other containers that could potentially fill with rainwater and become breeding grounds.

Chemoprophylaxis

None available

Immunoprophylaxis

Various inactivated, live vector subunit, and attenuated dengue vaccines are under development. None are available as of this writing.

Diagnosis

At the point of care, the diagnosis of dengue is often clinical and potentially life-threatening, and treatable causes of fever need to be excluded first, such as malaria or typhoid fever. Laboratory results will take some time. Figure provides an algorithm. The most commonly used test for dengue is the IgM capture enzyme-linked immunosorbent assay, but this test is negative early in the illness, should only be done at least 4 to 5 days after the onset of symptoms, and only gives a probable diagnosis. A confirmed diagnosis is established by virus culture, polymerase chain reaction (PCR) or serologic assays. All these tests have their limitations. PCR is not available in many settings, and is only sensitive very early in the disease. A four-fold or greater rise in dengue IgG titers as a confirmatory test requires a convalescent serum. Cross-reactions with other flaviviruses interfere with serologic testing, in particular the enzyme-linked immunosorbent assay IgG, and this has a bearing on interpreting results in travelers exposed to other flavivirus infections (including previous vaccinations against flavivirus infections such yellow fever and Japanese encephalitis). Self diagnosis kits are marketed in some countries.

Principles of Therapy

Treatment is symptomatic and supportive, with the primary aim to prevent mortality from severe DHF/DSS. Mild or classic dengue is treated with antipyretics (ie, paracetamol [acetaminophen]), bed rest, and oral (rarely parenteral) fluid replacement; most cases can be managed on an outpatient basis. Aspirin, non-steroidal anti-inflammatory drugs, and intramuscular injections are best avoided because of bleeding tendencies. For this reason, the use of bismuth subsalicylate is, on theoretical grounds, not indicated in dengue endemic areas. Platelet and hematocrit determinations should be repeated at least every 24 hours in order to promptly recognize the development of DHF and institute fluid replacement.

Other Arboviral Diseases

Four agents produce illness similar to dengue but often without skin rash: sandfly fever, Rift Valley fever, Ross River fever, and Colorado tick fever. Sandfly fever occurs in the Mediterranean area, in the Middle East, in Russia, and in India. Ross River fever occurs in eastern Australia and the South Pacific. Colorado tick fever is seen among campers or hunters in the western United States.

Additional Readings

Cobelens FG, et al. Incidence and risk factors of probable dengue virus infection among Dutch travellers to Asia. Trop Med Int Health 2002;7:331–8.

Halstead SB, Deen J. The future of dengue vaccines. Lancet 2002;360:1243–5.

Jelinek T, et al. Epidemiology and clinical features of imported dengue fever in Europe. Clin Infect Dis 2002;35:1047–52.

Wilder-Smith A, et al. Dengue in travelers. N Engl J Med 2005;353:924–3.

DERMATOLOGIC INFECTIONS

Common dermatologic bacterial infections include impetigo, furunculosis, erysipelas, ecthymata, cellulitis, tropical ulcer, erythrasma, intertrigo, pitted keratolysis, cat-scratch disease, and borreliosis. Atypical mycobacterioses such as aquarium granuloma or mycobacterial ulcus (Buruli ulcer) can occur. Among the viral infections, herpes, condylomata acuminata, and common warts are the most important. Fungi and yeasts include tinea of the type corporis, faciei, barbae, cruris, pedis, manuum, nigra, and unguium; perleche, *Candida intertrigo, C. paronychia,* and pityriasis versicolor. Various parasitic diseases are frequently transmitted, including trichomoniasis, cutaneous leishmaniasis, and creeping eruption. Epizootic infestation is possible through pediculosis (see also Part 3).

Additional Readings

James WD. Imported skin diseases in dermatology. J Dermatol 2001;28:663–6.

Lupi O, et al. Tropical dermatology: bacterial tropical diseases. J Am Acad Dermatol 2006;54:559–78.

DIPHTHERIA

Infectious Agent

Corynebacterium diphtheriae strains are classified based on severity of illness produced: gravis (serious), mitis (mild), or intermedius biotype. All may produce toxins, but it is mostly the toxigenic strains that produce lesions. Non-toxigenic strains have been associated with infective endocarditis.

Transmission

Diphtheria is transmitted through contact with a patient, by an asymptomatic carrier, or occasionally by contaminated materials or raw milk.

Global Epidemiology

Although it can occur throughout the world, immunization programs have, to a large extent, eliminated diphtheria. It should be noted, however, that in many countries more than 40% of adults lack protective levels of circulating antitoxin. In temperate zones, the disease most often occurs in the colder months among non-immunized children but may also appear in adults who have not received booster doses of vaccine. From 1992 to 1997, there was an epidemic of diphtheria throughout the New Independent States of the former Soviet Union.

Risk for Travelers

Several cases have been reported of travelers importing the infection from the New Independent States of the former Soviet Union to Northern and Western Europe, and at least one died in Russia. Cutaneous diphtheria may be imported after visits to tropical regions. Of 23 cases diagnosed in Switzerland from 1990 to 1994, 11 were imported, mainly from Southeast Asia, India, and East Africa. Many of these patients were intravenous drug users with poor personal hygiene.

Clinical Picture

Diphtheria is an acute bacterial disease characterized by pseudomembranous pharyngitis (patches of gray-white membrane), often accompanied by lymphadenopathy, a bull neck, and serosanguineous nasal discharge. The infection may involve the tonsils, pharynx, larynx, nose, and occasionally, other mucous membranes or the skin. Complications after 1 to 6 weeks include neurologic problems and myocarditis. The case fatality rate is 5 to 10%.

Cutaneous diphtheria with open sores may occur as a primary or secondary infection in the tropics. There is usually no systemic toxicity, and post-diphtheric complications, such as myocarditis or polyneuritis, are rare.

Incubation

The incubation period is 2 to 5 days, occasionally longer.

Communicability

Communicability extends usually no longer than 2 weeks, but chronic carriers may shed the agent for more than 6 months. Effective antibiotic therapy promptly terminates organism shedding.

Susceptibility and Resistance

The toxoid can induce prolonged active immunity to classic diphtheria, but immunized persons may still contract cutaneous diphtheria. Recovery from a clinical attack does not always result in lasting immunity. Inapparent infection, however, often results in immunity.

Chemoprophylaxis

Penicillin given intramuscularly (IM) as a single dose or erythromycin for 10 days is recommended for contacts, regardless of their immune status.

Immunoprophylaxis by Diphtheria Vaccine

Immunology and Pharmacology

Viability: inactivated

Dosage and antigenic form: 6 to 25 international units (IU) (pediatric doses depending on product) or 2 IU (adult dose) toxoid made from *Clostridium diphtheriae* toxin

Adjuvants: aluminum phosphate, hydroxide, or potassium sulfate

Preservative: 0.01% thimerosal

Allergens/Excipiens: not > 0.02% residual-free formaldehyde

Mechanism: induction of protective antitoxin antibodies against diphtheria toxin

Administration

Schedule: for primary immunizing series, three 0.5 mL doses are given 6 to 8 weeks apart at ages 2, 4, and 6 months, a fourth dose at age 15 to 24 months, and a fifth at age 4 to 7 years. There are slight differences in the various national immunization schedules. Combined vaccines are usually used (with tetanus, pertussis Hib, HBV, IPV, etc.). Note that, in older children (age limit 7 to 12 years, depending on the product) and in adults, a vaccine containing less IU is used.

Booster: after 5 years (but in practice after 10 years, as given with tetanus vaccine)

Route: deeply IM

Site: deltoid

Storage: store at 2 to 8 °C (35 to 46 °F). Discard frozen vaccine.

Availability: worldwide.

Protection

Onset: immunity begins to develop several weeks after second dose. Total immunity develops after completing the basic series.

Efficacy: > 95%.

Duration: 5 to 10 years

Protective level: anti-diphtheria antitoxin levels of 0.01 antitoxin units per mL are generally considered protective, although 0.1 units per mL are optimal.

Adverse Reactions

Redness, tenderness, and induration surround the injection site; transient fever, malaise, generalized aches and pains;

(rarely) flushing, generalized urticaria or pruritus, tachycardia, hypotension.

Contraindications

Absolute: persons with a previous hypersensitivity reaction to diphtheria vaccine doses, particularly thrombocytopenia or neurologic symptoms, or with known hypersensitivity to any component of the vaccine

Relative: any serious acute illness

Children: Defer first dose to age 2 months

Pregnant women: category C. Use only if clearly indicated.

Lactating women: it is unknown whether diphtheria toxoid or corresponding antibodies are excreted in breast milk. Problems in humans have not been documented. Use if clearly needed.

Immunodeficient persons: persons receiving immunosuppressive therapy or having other immunodeficiencies may experience diminished antibody response to active immunization. Defer primary diphtheria immunization until treatment is discontinued. An additional dose may be injected at least 1 month after immunosuppressive treatment has ceased. Nonetheless, routine immunization of symptomatic and asymptomatic human immunodeficiency virus-infected persons is recommended.

Interactions

Immunosuppressant drugs and radiation therapy may result in an insufficient response to immunization. In patients receiving anticoagulants, administer subcutaneously.

Recommendations for Vaccine Use

Immunization against diphtheria is routine worldwide. After completing a primary series, administer a booster dose every 10 years for life, usually in conjunction with tetanus immunization.

Since the occurrence of the diphtheria epidemic in the New Independent States of the former Soviet Union, pilgrims to Mecca in Saudi Arabia from these areas have been required to show proof of diphtheria vaccination.

Self-Treatment Abroad

None. Medical consultation is required.

Principles of Therapy

Patients: administer the antitoxin as soon as possible if diphtheria is suspected, even before microbiologic confirmation. Prescribe erythromycin or penicillin. (In some countries only the equine antitoxin is available.)

Carriers: single-dose penicillin IM

Community Control Measures

In most countries, notifying public health authorities is mandatory. Strict isolation is indicated for pharyngeal diphtheria and contact isolation for cutaneous diphtheria. Adults in contact with the disease whose occupation involves handling food, especially milk, should abstain from work until bacteriologic examination establishes they are not carriers.

Additional Readings

Center for Disease Control and Prevention. Fatal respiratory diphtheria in a U.S. traveler to Haiti—Pennsylvania, 2003. MMWR Morb Mortal Wkly Rep 2004;52:1285–6.

Lumio J, et al. Epidemiology of three cases of severe diphtheria in Finnish patients with low antitoxin antibody levels. Eur J Clin Microbiol Infect Dis 2001;20:705–10.

Sing A, et al. Imported cutaneous diphtheria, Germany, 1997–2003. Emerg Infect Dis 2005;11:343–4.

DRACUNCULIASIS

Dracunculiasis (guinea worm, dragon worm, Medina worm, serpent worm) is a tissue nematode infection caused by *Dracunculus medinensis*. The disease is widely distributed in West Africa, from Mauritania to Cameroon, in the Nile Valley and eastern equatorial Africa, and the Arabian Peninsula. The infection is acquired when copepods containing the larvae in drinking water are ingested. The larvae develop into adult worms within 12 months; then, the fertilized adult females migrate to form a superficial cutaneous blister. Symptoms relate to the local ulcer that forms or to immunologic reactions such as urticaria. Chronic complications may include contracture of extremities. Treatment involves manual extraction of the worm by winding it on a stick, using gentle traction. Patients should also receive tetanus toxoid. Simple prevention measures such as filtering drinking water through a mesh fiber or boiling it before drinking should be followed (Figure 18).

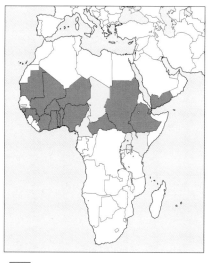

■ endemic countries

□ countries under pre-certification surveillance

Figure 18   Geographic distribution of guinea worm (WHO 2005, many other countries of Africa not yet certified as free)

In 1986, an estimated 3.5 million cases of dracunculiasis occurred in 20 countries, and 120 million persons were at risk for the disease. That year, the World Health Assembly adopted a resolution calling for the eradication of dracunculiasis. This report describes the status of the global dracunculiasis eradication program as of July 2005, indicating that, during January to July 2005, a total of 8,191 indigenous cases of dracunculiasis were reported from nine countries, with at least 150 million persons at risk. Despite the substantial reductions in dracunculiasis cases since 1986, eradication of dracunculiasis will require international commitment, ongoing surveillance, and intensified interventions at national, state, and local levels.

Additional Readings

Center for Disease Control and Prevention. Progress toward global eradication of dracunculiasis, January 2004-July 2005. MMWR 2005;54:1075–7.

Ebola Fever

Risk For Travelers

There have been few anecdotal cases imported to industrialized nations.

Abrupt onset with fever, malaise, myalgia, conjunctival injection, sore throat, headache and abdominal pain, diarrhea. The pharynx is often inflamed with herpetic lesions. A maculopapular rash may occur, followed by widespread hemorrhagic disease. The case fatality rate is 50 to 90%.

Incubation

2 to 21 days

Communicability

As long as blood and secretions contain virus (in semen up to 2 months), there is frequent nosocomial spread.

Global Epidemiology

Tropical Africa, most likely from the Ivory Coast to Kenya and Congo (ex-Zaire)

Minimized Exposure in Travelers

Avoid contacts with Ebola patients in hospitals.

Chemoprophylaxis

Not applicable

Immunoprophylaxis

None available

Self-Treatment Abroad

None. A physician should treat the patient.

No sexual intercourse until semen is demonstrated to be free of the virus.

Additional Readings

Freedman DO, et al. Emerging infectious diseases and risk to the traveler. Med Clin North Am 1999;83:865–83.

Isaacson M. Viral hemorrhagic fever hazards for travelers in Africa. Clin Infect Dis 2001;33:1707–12.

Jeffs B. A clinical guide to viral haemorrhagic fevers: Ebola, Marburg and Lassa. Trop Doct 2006;36:1–4.

Weber DJ, et al. Risks and prevention of nosocomial transmission of rare zoonotic diseases. Clin Infect Dis 2001;32:446–56.

ECHINOCOCCOSIS

Infectious Agent

Echinococcus granulosas, E. multilocularis, and *E. vogelii* are tapeworms (found primarily in dogs, but also wolves, foxes, sheep, goats, and camels).

Transmission

Transmitted through direct contact with infected feces and ingesting viable parasite eggs with food. Eggs remain viable in the feces of tapeworm-infected canines for weeks, allowing transmission to individuals with no direct contact with the vector animal.

Global Epidemiology

Most of the world; endemic in South America, North Africa, the Middle East, the United States (especially the lower Mississippi Valley and Alaska), northern and Western Canada, India, Southern Europe, Australia, and New Zealand (especially in areas where sheep are raised).

Risk for Travelers

Minimal, unless exposed to infected dogs or living among populations involved with sheep raising in endemic areas.

Clinical Picture

Most people with *Echinococcus* infections are asymptomatic, especially in the lengthy early stages. Most patients have one such cyst. The hydatid cysts form in the liver in 50 to 79% of patients, or in the lung in 20%, and the remaining 10% may be found in the brain, heart, or the bones. Hepatic cysts may exist as long as 20 years before becoming large enough to be visible or to cause pressure-related problems, such as pain, nausea, cirrhosis, and other manifestations of liver disease. Pulmonary cysts may also grow for many years before causing dyspnea, cough, or hemoptysis. Cysts in the brain produce problems consistent with a slow-growing, space-occupying lesion. Rupture of the cyst or other means of cyst spillage produces infection, occasional obstruction, or allergic reaction in the affected organ. In severe cases, the allergic reaction can lead to anaphylactic shock.

Incubation

Usually years, and can take decades

Chemoprophylaxis

In endemic areas, prevention is primarily via prophylactic treatment of dogs with praziquantel 5mg/kg on a monthly basis to remove the adult tapeworms. Ranchers should be educated to not feed their dogs scraps from butchered animals. Prolonged freezing of meat or through cooking of meat kills cysts in the tissue.

Vaccination

None available.

Diagnosis

Ultrasonography, computed tomography (CT), or magnetic resonance imaging are commonly used. Immunoblot (Western blot) and enzyme-linked immunosorbent assay are 80 to 100% sensitive for liver cysts but only 50 to 56% for lungs and other organs. If the CT shows a cyst, regardless of confirmation by serology, the diagnosis should be made.

Principles of Therapy

Surgical excision of the cyst remains the treatment of choice for symptomatic cysts. Albendazole is the drug of choice in treatment because it is absorbed best. Albendazole is given orally at 10 to 15 mg/kg/d or fixed doses of 400 mg bid (with meals) in adults cycled for at least 3 months. Percutaenous aspiration, injection, respiration can be done for solitary and easily accessible hepatic cyst without biliary communication.

Additional Reading

Bell C, et al. Management of hepatic and intracardiac echinococcal cysts. Surg Infect 2006;7:309–13.

FASCIOLA HEPATICA

Infectious Agent

Fasciola hepatica is a liver and bile duct parasite. It is a large fluke (30 mm by 15 mm), flat and leaflike. Adult liver flukes produce fertile eggs, which are passed through the bile ducts to the small intestine. The eggs are shed in the feces and, if conditions are adequate, a ciliated miracidium will penetrate the snail, develop through one generation as a sporocyst and two generations of rediae. Finally, a free living cercariae is produced, which leaves the snail. These encyst as metacercariae on submerged objects such as plant material. If they are ingested by herbivorous animals feeding on the plants, they penetrate the gut and migrate through the peritoneal cavity to the liver. They undergo extensive migrations through the liver; this migration may take 6 to 8 weeks. From the liver, the adults can enter the bile ducts and shed eggs into the intestine.

Global Epidemiology

They are found in herbivorous mammals and man. *F. hepatica* has been reported worldwide, especially in sheep-raising areas. Over 2 million people are infected. In the United States, *F. hepatica* is found mostly in the Gulf Coast states and Pacific Northwest.

Risk for Travelers

A variety of freshwater plants upon which metacercariae encyst, such as watercress, water lettuce, mint, and parsley are important sources of human infection because they are often eaten raw in salads. Snails are the first intermediate host. The major natural reservoirs are sheep, cattle, goats, buffalo, etc. *F. hepatica* has been described mainly in immigrants.

Clinical Manifestations

Acute Hepatic (Invasive) Stage

Within 6 to 12 weeks of ingestion of metacercariae, symptoms occur that reflect larval migration through the small intestinal wall, the peritoneal cavity, and liver capsule. Abdominal pain, eosinophilia, intermittent fever, malaise and weight loss, sometimes urticaria, and chest pain are predominant features. Computed tomography scans frequently reveal single or, more frequently, multiple small, hypodense lesions. In addition, tunnel-like, branching hypodense lesions may be observed peripherally in the liver, representing the pathologic changes created by the migration of the immature fluke through the liver.

Chronic Biliary (Obstructive) Stage

Once *F. hepatica* has migrated through the liver, it arrives at the common bile duct, where it reaches maturity and produces eggs. Fever, anorexia, and abdominal pain resolve and the patient may become asymptomatic. Eosinophilia is infrequent. Some develop intermittent biliary obstruction mimicking biliary colic or acute cholecystitis, or even ascending cholangitis with fever, jaundice, and upper abdominal pain.

Diagnosis:

An enzyme-linked immunosorbent assay antigen capture technique has a sensitivity of 100% and specificity of 98%. In the biliary stage, eggs of *F. hepatica* can be found in stool specimens; during the acute hepatic stage, usually not.

Treatment

Triclabendazole 10 mg/kg with one or two single daily doses

Additional Reading

Jensenius M, et al. Fascioliasis imported to Norway. Scand J Infect Dis 2006;57:326–30.

FILARIASIS

Eight human filarial parasites are transmitted through arthropod bites. They include lymphatic filariasis caused by *Wuchereria bancrofti*, *Brugia malayi*, and *Brugia timori*; *Onchocerca volvulus*, *Loa loa*, *Mansonella perstans*, *Mansonella streptocerca*, and *Mansonella ozzardi*. We discuss the more important filarial parasites further.

▌ Lymphatic Filariae

The lymphatic filarial parasite *W. bancrofti* is endemic in Haiti, South America, Africa, the South Pacific, and Southeast Asia (including India and Indonesia). *B. malayi* occurs in India, the Philippines, Malaysia, Indonesia, and China. *B. timori* is found in Indonesia. Fever is the first clinical manifestation of symptomatic lymphatic filariasis. Asymptomatic infection is common in local populations. In travelers, expatriates, and military personnel, localized inflammatory reactions and lymphangitis of the lower extremities or genitalia more commonly occur, with or without immediate hypersensitivity reactions such as urticaria and eosinophilia. Filarial fever is often associated with localized reactions in episodic fashion. With chronic infection, refractory edema and elephantiasis may occur. Biopsy of affected lymph nodes reveals eosinophils surrounding adult worms and sexually immature parasites. Signs and symptoms do not recur if afflicted individuals leave the endemic area. The presence of microfilariae in the blood or new rapid tests provide the diagnosis. Lymphatic filariasis is treated with drug combinations consisting of ivermectin and diethylcarbamazine (DEC) or albendazole.

Tropical eosinophilia is seen mainly in persons living in an area in which lymphatic filariae are endemic. The clinical manifestations of infection relate to pulmonary reactions to microfilariae such as nocturnal coughing and wheezing. Since the parasites are nocturnal, obtain the blood between midnight and 4 a.m. to increase the chances of detection. Antifilarial immunoglobulin E antibodies may be sought in travelers with a compatible illness. Treatment is with a 2-week course of DEC (Figure 19).

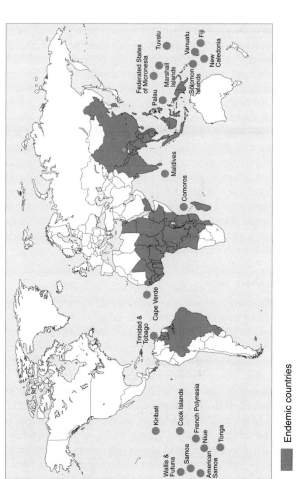

Figure 19   Geographic distribution of human lymphatic filariasis (WHO 2005)

Loiasis

Loa loa infection is seen in Central and West Africa. The insect vector is the deerfly, which deposits larvae in the skin. Adult worms later migrate throughout the subcutaneous tissue, including the conjunctivae. Microfilariae can be found in the blood, with a diurnal variation peaking at approximately noon. Migratory angioedema and egg-like swellings over bony prominences (Calabar swellings) may be found. Immune reactions to antigens released by the migrating worms account for the angioedema accompanying the disease. Swellings resolve over several days but typically recur. Adult worms may be visible during migration through the ocular conjunctivae. Demonstrating the presence of microfilariae in blood obtained at midday results in diagnosis. Administering DEC for 3 weeks is the appropriate therapy. Corticosteroids are given for the first 3 days in the presence of neurologic symptoms on initiation of DEC (Figure 20). Initial treatment with albendazole may be indicated in cases with high microfilaremia to prevent encephalopathy.

Onchocerciasis

Onchocerciasis (river blindness) is caused by chronic infection by the filarial parasite *O. volvulus*. The infection is transmitted by bites of blackflies and typically occurs in West and Central Africa, Guatemala, southern Mexico, Venezuela, northwest Brazil, Colombia, Ecuador, Yemen, and Saudi Arabia near the Red Sea. Cutaneous and ocular-tissue inflammatory reactions occur in response to the microfilariae. Infiltrates of lymphocytes, histiocytes, eosinophils, and plasma cells are found on biopsy of the involved tissue. Microfilariae are not prevalent in the blood of persons with the infection. Scarring of the cornea from inflammation may lead to blindness. Mobile skin nodules are often found. Travelers tend to experience less severe infections than permanent residents in endemic areas. Infected travelers characteristically present with pruritus and an intermittent papular rash, erythema, and edema or thickened skin. Nodules occur occasionally in travelers with onchocerciasis. Demonstrating microfilariae in skin biopsies results in diagnosis. Typically, multiple skin snips are examined for microfilariae. Ivermectin is given in a single oral dose (150 µg/kg). The drug has no effect on adult worms, and further treatment may be required (Figure 21).

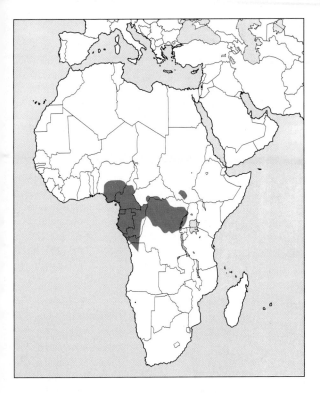

Figure 20   Geographic distribution of *L. loa* (WHO 1989, adapted 2000)

Additional Readings

Ezedine K, et al. Onchocerciasis-associated limb swelling in a traveler returning from Cameroon. J Travel Med 2006;13:50–3.

Leggat PA. Could it be lymphatic filariasis? J Travel Med 2004;11:56–60.

Nguyen JC, et al. Cutaneous onchocerciasis in an American traveler. Int J Dermatol 2005;44:125–8.

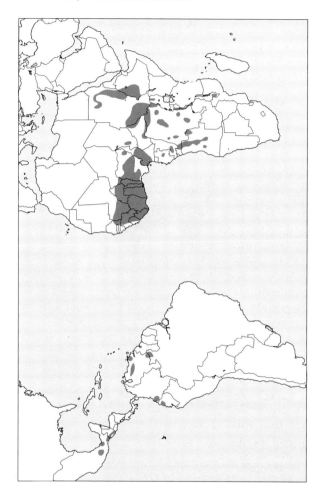

Figure 21   Geographic distribution of onchocerciasis. The Filarial Genome Network. Adapted 2006

FILOVIRUS INFECTIONS

Marburg and Ebola viruses, members of the family Filoviridae, are capable of causing the highly fatal African hemorrhagic fever in humans and primates. Marburg virus infection was first identified in Germany and Yugoslavia among handlers of tissue from Ugandan monkeys and primates. Both infections are endemic in Africa. Ebola virus infection has been reported in Zaire, Sudan, Kenya, and the Ivory Coast. So far one veterinary pathologist has imported Ebola from the Ivory Coast to Switzerland (none of the staff got infected), while Marburg fever occurred in 25 laboratory staff (7 died) after the importation of African green monkeys from Uganda to Yugoslavia and Germany. Secondary infections occurred in 6 hospital staff, all survived. Also three travelers died from Marburg after stays in Zimbabwe (one infected nurse survived), and Kenya 1975 to 1987.

Following an incubation period of 3 to 18 days, patients experience headache, myalgias, back pain, and, occasionally, abdominal discomfort. Nausea, vomiting, and diarrhea (accompanied by passage of mucus and blood) commonly develop followed by the appearance of a maculopapular rash on the trunk, which then spreads to the extremities. Mental function is compromised, followed by spontaneous bleeding from multiple body sites. Death occurs from the end of the first week through to the second week of illness. Clinicians diagnose by identifying the virus in body tissue or by serologic studies. There is no specific treatment. Supportive treatment consists of administering fluid and electrolytes, blood, platelets, or fresh, frozen plasma to control the hemorrhage, and dialysis for renal failure. Heparin has been used against disseminated intravascular coagulation, although its value has not been established. Control measures are unavailable, because the spread mechanism is unconfirmed. Nosocomial spread may be prevented by standard infection control measures.

Additional Readings

Isaacson M. Viral hemorrhagic fever hazards for travelers in Africa. Clin Infect Dis 2001;33:1707–12.

Zeller H, et al. Infections by viruses of the families Bunyaviridae and Filoviridae. Rev Sci Tech 2000;19:79–91.

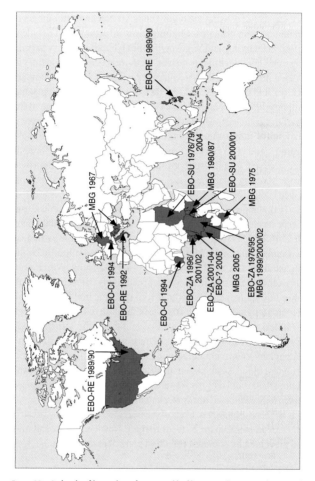

Figure 22 Outbreaks of hemorrhagic fever caused by filoviruses. All important documented episodes are shown with the year of emergence and/or re-emergence. *EBO-CI* Ebola subtype (?) Côte d'Ivoire; *EBO-RE* Ebola subtype Reston; *EBO-SU* Ebola subtype Sudan; *EBO-ZA* Ebola subtype Zaire; *EBO-?* Ebola subtype unknown; *MBG* Marburg

GNATHOSTOMIASIS

Infectious Agent

Gnathostoma spinigerum. Because the larva cannot mature into the adult form in humans, the third-stage larva can only wander within the body of the host; clinical symptoms of gnathostomiasis then occur because of the inflammatory reaction provoked by these migrating larvae.

Global Epidemiology

Human gnathostomiasis is found mainly in Thailand, India, Japan, China, Malaysia, the Philippines, India, and Vietnam. Increasingly, cases are being reported in Central and South America, possibly related to eating ceviche.

Risk to Travelers

G. spinigerum is acquired by eating uncooked food infected with the larval third stage of the helminth; such foods typically include fish, shrimp, crab, crayfish, or frog.

Clinical Picture

There are four distinct clinical manifestations: cutaneous, visceral, ocular, and cerebral gnathostomiasis.

Cutaneous Gnathostomiasis

After ingestion of larvae, epigastric pain, nausea, and vomiting may last for 2 to 3 weeks, consistent with penetration of the intestinal wall and migration of the worm. A larva located in the subcutaneous tissues produces edema and inflammation and is felt as an indurated, pruritic, erythematous lesion. The swelling may resolve, but it will reappear later in another location because of the proclivity of the larva for migration in the tissues. If the larva reaches the superficial epithelium, it manifests as cutaneous larva migrans.

Eosinophilic Meningitis

When migrating through the central nervous system, radiculomyelitis with marked radicular pain is a common symptom. The pain lasts 1 to 5 days and is often accompanied by paralysis of one or more extremities; paraplegia is common, sometimes followed by triplegia and quadriplegia. The main clinical characteristic of *Gnathostoma* encephalitis is the migratory nature of the neurologic symptoms. Cerebrospinal fluid eosinophilia is prominent.

Diagnosis

A diagnosis of gnathostomiasis should be considered for patients with a history of transient, migratory cutaneous or subcutaneous swellings, or nonspecific gastrointestinal symptoms for which a potential epidemiologic exposure is identified. Management of the disease thereafter is usually relatively straightforward, although more than one course of treatment may be required to effect a cure. In cases of eosinophilic meningitis plus an appropriate travel or food history, serology for gnathostomiasis should be taken. Serologic testing for gnathostomiasis can be performed, for example, in the Department of Helminthology of the Faculty of Tropical Medicine at Mahidol University in Bangkok, Thailand. Clinical diagnosis of cutaneous gnathostomiasis is confirmed by recovery of the larva and study of its morphologic characteristics. Larvae recovered from humans have measured from 2.5 to 12.5 mm in length by 0.4 to 1.2 mm in width.

Treatment

The reported efficacy of albendazole in the treatment of gnathostomiasis is > 90%.

Prevention

Avoid uncooked or undercooked fish, shrimp, crab, crayfish, or frog.

Additional Readings

Gorgolas M. Cutaneous and medullar gnathostomiasis in travelers to Mexico and Thailand. J Travel Med 2003;10:358–61.

Hennies F, et al. Gnathostomiasis: import from Laos. J Dtsch Dermatol Ges 2006;4:414–6.

Hantavirus

Hantaviruses, belonging to the Bunyaviridae family, chronically infect various rodents throughout the world. Transmission to humans results from contact with excretion (eg, urine) from an infected rodent. Different hantaviruses are found in Asia, eastern and western Europe, and North America. In the Asian and European forms, hemorrhagic fever with renal disease or nephropathia epidemica, a milder form of renal disease, are the common manifestations. In North America, hantavirus pulmonary syndrome is found without a significant renal component. Diagnosis is made by detecting a virus-specific antibody, particularly immunoglobulin (Ig) M, or by direct virus isolation. The customary procedure for documenting serologic response to infection is by enzyme-linked immunosorbent assay testing. An elevated IgM titer with a compatible clinical illness establishes the diagnosis. The IgG antibodies persist for decades at high titers. Intravenous ribavirin administered for 10 days may have some treatment value, if given early in the disease (up to the fourth day of illness). Supportive treatment is important (Figure 23). In South Korea, an inactivated vaccine (Hantavex) is available.

Additional Readings

Caramelo P, et al. Puumala virus pulmonary syndrome in a Romanian immigrant. J Travel Med 2002;9:326–9.

Dos Santos MC, et al. Human hantavirus infection, Brazilian Amazon. Emerg Infect Dis 2006;12:1165–7.

Mailles A, et al. Larger than usual increase in cases of hantavirus infections in Belgium, France and Germany, June 2005. Euro Surveill 2005;10:E050721.4.

Murgue B, et al. First reported case of imported hantavirus pulmonary syndrome in Europe. Emerg Infect Dis 2002;8:106–7.

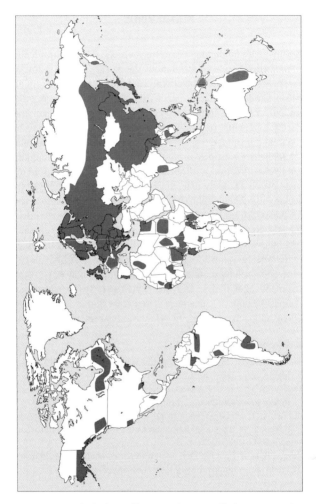

Figure 23   Geographic distribution of hantavirus infections. Strickland. Hunter's Tropical Medicine and Emerging Infectious Disease. 8th ed. 2000, adapted.

HEPATITIS

Several distinct hepatic infections are grouped as hepatitides due to their similar clinical presentations and because, prior to the 1970s, it was impossible to differentiate the various etiologies, most of them viruses. These include the hepatotrophic viruses hepatitis—A, B, C, D (delta), E, and G—and members of the herpes virus group, coxsackievirus, dengue, yellow fever, and other agents. Hepatitis can also be a manifestation of Leptospira, Mycobacterium, Rickettsia, hantavirus, and of bacteremia. Mixed infection is possible.

In all infections, there is a similar acute illness; prodromal symptoms include malaise, fever, headache, and, later, anorexia, nausea, vomiting, and right upper quadrant pain. Dark urine, light-colored stools, and jaundice may follow. Subclinical forms are common in infants and children, whereas in adults, the prognosis gets worse with increasing age. Jaundice can be prolonged, and hepatic coma and death may occur. Chronic illness may be a result of hepatitis B and hepatitis C infections.

HEPATITIS A

Infectious Agent

Hepatitis A virus (HAV), a picornavirus.

Transmission

Person-to-person transmission usually occurs as a result of fecal-oral contact and occasionally by way of contaminated needles. Outbreaks may be related to contaminated water or ice cubes or foods such as shellfish, lettuce, and strawberries, or other foods that become contaminated during handling.

Global Epidemiology

Crowded living conditions and poor sanitation result in hepatitis A (HA) being highly endemic throughout the developing world. Most infections occur at an early age, and almost all children acquire protective immunity, which probably lasts for life. Outbreaks of clinical HA are rare; children usually experience asymptomatic or mild infection. As economic and hygienic conditions improve, exposure gradually shifts to older age groups, in which the proportion of clinical infection increases. In the developed countries, a large proportion of the population remains susceptible to HA because of low endemicity and, as a result, may acquire it at any age during travel. Figure 25 illustrates the public health impact on various industrialized communities in the time before hepatitis A vaccines were introduced on the market. The incidence of hepatitis A in Southern Europe has drastically decreased: for instance, in Italy in 1998, a rate of 6 (in southern Italy, 19) per 100,000 was recorded, which can be compared to rates of 20 to 48 per 100,000 in eight states in the western United States.

Risk for Travelers

In nonimmune travelers, the average incidence of HA for each month staying in a high-risk area is 30 per 100,000, increasing to 2,000 per 100,000 for those facing unfavorable hygienic conditions (eg, backpackers, aid workers in remote areas, missionaries). Recent data suggest that tourists no longer have an increased risk of hepatitis A in southern Europe, whereas evidence exists that risk is increased for workers who originated in those areas when they return to visit their families.

Clinical Picture

Fulminant, fatal HA rarely occurs, but chronic infection has not been reported. The case fatality rate is < 0.1% in children but exceeds 2% in those older than age 40.

Incubation

The incubation period is 15 to 50 days.

Communicability

Excretion of the virus in the stool, hence communicability, is highest in the latter half of the incubation period, continuing for several days after the onset of jaundice. Prolonged viral excretion has been documented in infants. Boiling contaminated water or cooking contaminated food at 85 °C for at least 1 minute inactivates the virus. Drinking water is also made safe by chlorination.

Susceptibility and Resistance

Susceptibility is general for all nonimmune persons. Lifelong homologous immunity results after infection. Higher proportions of asymptomatic to symptomatic cases are seen at younger ages (see "Global Epidemiology").

Minimized Exposure in Travelers

Travelers can avoid hepatitis A by being careful about what they eat and drink. Most tourists and business people, however, do not avoid local culinary temptations.

Chemoprophylaxis

None available.

█ **Immunoprophylaxis**

Hepatitis A Vaccines

Various hepatitis A vaccines exist in the developed countries:

- Avaxim (Sanofi Pasteur Mérieux Connaught) a Crucell company, 160 U
- Epaxal 24 IU (Berna Biotech Ltd., formerly Swiss Serum and Vaccine Institute)
- Havrix 720 EL U (pediatric) and 1440 EL U (adult) (SmithKline Beecham Biologicals)
- Vaqta 25 U (pediatric) and 50 U (adult) (Merck and Co.)

The various types of units are not comparable, but all vaccines have a similar profile and are therefore described under a single heading. There is a live attenuated hepatitis A vaccine available in China, which is not discussed here.

Immunology and Pharmacology

Viability: inactivated

Antigenic form: whole virus, strains GBM (Avaxim), RG-SB (Epaxal), HM-175 (Havrix), CR326F (Vaqta), all cultivated on human MRC-5 diploid cells

Adjuvants: aluminum hydroxide, except in the virosome formulated vaccine Epaxal: 10 µg influenza-hemagglutinin, phospholipids

Preservative: Avaxim and Havrix: 100 µg 2-phenoxyethanol; Epaxal: none; Vaqta: none

Allergens: none

Excipiens: various (eg, formalin traces, proteins)

Mechanism: neutralizing anti-HAV antibodies protect against infection

Application

Primary schedules and initial booster:

Pediatric:

Epaxal	0, 6 to 12 months, all ages ≥ 1 year (a few countries ≥ 5 years)
Havrix 720 EL U	0, 6 to 12 months, ages 1 to 18 years
Vaqta 25 µg	0, 6 to 18 months, ages 2 to 17 years

Adult:

Avaxim	0, 6 to 12 months, all ages ≥ 16 years
Epaxal	0, 6 to 12 months, all ages

Havrix 1440 EL U   0, 6 to 12 months, ages $\geq$ 19 years

Vaqta 50 µg   0, 6 to 18 months, ages $\geq$ 18 years

Subsequent boosters: probably none needed, lifelong protection

Route: IM

Site: deltoid, except in infants, mid-lateral muscles of the thigh. No gluteal application to avoid suboptimal immune response

Storage: store at 2 to 8 °C (35 to 46 °F). Discard frozen vaccine.

Availability: worldwide there is at least one vaccine available, except in some developing countries. Twinrix, a combination of Havrix 720 EL U and Engerix-B 20 µg, is also widely available. The application is as with Engerix-B.

Protection

Onset: protective antibodies can be demonstrated within 2 weeks in most recipients (80 to 98%). In view of the prolonged incubation time of natural infection, immediate protection may result from immunization after a single dose of any hepatitis A vaccine, except for Twinrix in adults, because the content herein is only 720 EL U.

Efficacy: close to 100%, very few anecdotal reports on vaccine failures

Duration: approximately 3 to 5 years after initial dose, lifelong after initial booster, according to consent conference statement. Currently, the package inserts still consider protection after two doses to be limited to 25 to 30 years, depending on the vaccine used. If the booster is given "late" there is no need to restart the series.

Protective level: anti-HAV-concentration exceeding 10 to 20 IU/mL. It is not necessary to test anti-HAV after immunization, as vaccine efficacy is close to 100%; additionally, most commercially available anti-HAV tests do not detect the low levels obtained after immunization.

Adverse Reactions

Local reactions occasionally occur, consisting of pain, swelling, or erythema at the injection site. These reactions may persist for several days. Epaxal produces fewer local reactions because of lack of aluminum.

Recipients occasionally develop mild temperature, malaise, or fatigue. These reactions may persist for a few days.

No life-threatening adverse reaction to hepatitis A vaccines has been documented.

Contraindications

Absolute: persons with previous hypersensitivity reaction to hepatitis A vaccine doses or with known hypersensitivity to any component of the vaccine

Relative: any serious acute illness

Children: safety and efficacy in infants aged under 1 year has not been established.

Pregnant women: category C. Hepatitis A vaccine and corresponding antibodies cross the placenta. Generally, most IgG passage across the placenta occurs during the third trimester. Problems have not been documented and are unlikely. Use if clearly needed.

Lactating women: it is unknown if hepatitis A vaccine or corresponding antibodies are excreted in breast milk. Problems in humans have not been documented and are unlikely. Use if clearly needed.

Immunodeficient persons: persons receiving immunosuppressive therapy or having other immunodeficiencies may experience diminished antibody response.

Table 10 Protecting travelers simultaneously against hepatitis A and hepatitis B.

Immunization schedules for adults depending on the departure date.

Departure in days	Dose #1 Day 0	Dose #2	Dose #3	Dose #4
0 – 6	Hepatitis A (full dose*) plus Hepatitis B	Hepatitis B ≥ 28 days	Hep A+B (Twinrix) ≥ 180 days	–
7 – 27	Hep A+B (Twinrix)	Hep A+B (Twinrix) ≥ 7 days	Hepatitis B ≥ 14 days after dose 2	Hep A+B (Twinrix) ≥ 11 months after dose 2
≥ 28	Hep A+B (Twinrix)	Hep A+B (Twinrix) ≥ 28 days	Hep A+B (Twinrix) ≥ 150 days after dose 2	

* Twinrix contains only 720 EL U (= half dose) and that would not assure immediate protection against hepatitis A after a single vaccine dose; protection against hepatitis B will occur only in part of the vaccinees some 2 weeks after the second vaccine dose.

Interactions

Immune globulins reduce the antibody titer obtained from vaccination, compared to vaccine alone. Similarly, maternal antibodies may interfere, but there is still sufficient priming.

Immune response of hepatitis A vaccine given with other vaccines is not compromised and does not compromise the immune response of the other vaccines.

Immunosuppressant drugs and radiation therapy may compromise the effectiveness of the vaccine.

In patients receiving anticoagulants, give subcutaneously.

Immune Globulin

Most experts consider immune globulin (IG) obsolete for prevention of hepatitis A, but this chapter is still included because the US Center for Disease Control and Prevention (CDC) still considers this an option. For susceptible persons, hepatitis A vaccine is mostly preferable to immune globulin; it grants specific protection for longer duration. In many countries, there is mounting concern that decreasing anti-HAV prevalence may result in an insufficient content of antibodies in immune globulins. There is no indication that immune globulins may transmit hepatitis B virus, hepatitis C virus, human immunodeficiency virus (HIV), or as yet undetectable infective agents. Consider immune globulin for travelers who plan only one trip, lasting no longer than 5 months, because of cost benefits—but in most industrialized nations, none is available. Giving IG alone in a young person who is likely to travel again is not recommended because it does not provide long-term protection and does not guarantee protection against fatal, fulminant hepatitis A.

Immunology and Pharmacology

Viability: inactive

Antigenic form: human immune globulin, unmodified, with varying content of antibodies reflecting the antibody diversity of the donor population

Adjuvants: none

Preservative: usually none, occasionally thimerosal

Allergens/Excipients: none

Mechanism: induction of passive immunity

Application

Schedule: single dose 1 to 14 days before potential exposure to hepatitis A

Dosage: for travel < 3 months, 0.02 mL/kg body weight (usually 2 mL in adults); for travel > 3 months, 0.06 mL/kg. Post-exposure prophylaxis is also possible within 14 days maximum: 0.02 mL/kg body weight.

Booster: none. If no active hepatitis A vaccine was administered, give same dose every 4 to 6 months

Route: IM, not IV. Use different injection site than for hepatitis A vaccine

Site: preferably in the upper outer quadrant of the gluteus muscle, maximum 5 to 10 mL per site to limit pain and discomfort

Storage: store at 2 to 8 °C (35 to 46 °F)

Availability: in some countries—in industrialized countries, however, there is concern about low anti-HAV content. Products with guaranteed titers are sometimes imported from developing countries. Some products have guaranteed titers of 100 IU/mL.

Protection

Onset: immediate

Efficacy: approximately 85%. At least one case of fulminant, fatal hepatitis A has been described, despite adequate pretravel IG application.

Duration: 3 to 5 months, depending on dosage

Adverse Reactions

Local pain and tenderness are frequent. Persons having received IG tend to faint more often afterward than do active vaccine recipients. Urticaria and angioedema may occur in rare instances.

Contraindications

Absolute: patients with isolated IgA deficiency, because of the risk of an anaphylactoid reaction. Patients with a history of systemic allergic reactions following the administration of human IG.

Relative: patients with thrombocytopenia and coagulation disorders, considering the IM route and considerable volume injected. Patients receiving anticoagulants may have extensive hematomas after an IG injection.

Children: not contraindicated

Pregnant women: not contraindicated

Lactating women: not contraindicated

Immunodeficient persons: not contraindicated

Interactions

Immunoglobulin may diminish the antibody response to various live vaccines (except yellow fever and oral poliomyelitis vaccines)

and to hepatitis A vaccine. Live vaccines should therefore be administered > 14 days before, or > 6 weeks after, IG application.

Recommendations for Vaccine Use

In view of the considerable risk of hepatitis infection in the developing world, the World Health Organization and most experts agree that all travelers visiting the following regions should be immunized: Africa; Asia, except Japan and Singapore; Latin America; the Caribbean; and remote parts of Eastern Europe (Figure 24). This recommendation is based on the observation that many cases of hepatitis A have been contracted in these regions by travelers with standard tourist itineraries, accommodation (even in luxury hotels!), and food-consumption behaviors. The risk is higher for travelers off the beaten track. Often, it is wise to consider simultaneous immunization against hepatitis A and hepatitis B with the combined vaccine, Twinrix, particularly in young travelers and others who potentially will stay over 1 month (cumulative in their lifetime) in developing countries. The schedule is the same as for the hepatitis B vaccine Engerix-B (see below). For adult travelers leaving within less than 7 days, it is a mistake to give only a single dose of Twinrix as they will be insufficiently protected against hepatitis A (see above, Protection, Onset). In such customers one must give a full first adult dose of hepatitis A vaccine plus a first dose of hepatitis B vaccine. When departure is after a week or longer, two doses of Twinrix at least 7 days apart will protect against hepatitis A. There is no way to offer protection against hepatitis B to a majority of travelers within less than 4 weeks.

To eliminate unnecessary immunization, test for antibodies for hepatitis A virus (anti-HAV IgG) in travelers who may have developed lifelong immunity previously by natural infection. This is most likely among those who

- have a history of undetermined hepatitis
- were raised in a developing country or who lived there for at least 1 year
- were born before 1945 in countries of very low endemicity, such as northern and western Europe, or before 1960 in countries of low endemicity (Figure 25)

Such testing may provide benefits only if the cost of screening (laboratory and consultation fee) is considerably less than the

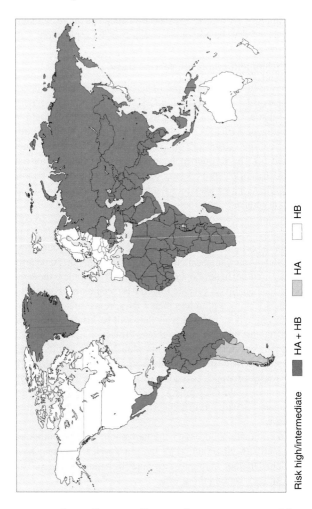

Figure 24   Risk areas of hepatitis A and hepatitis B where vaccine use is recommended (WHO 2006)

cost of immunization and if testing does not interfere with subsequent receipt of vaccine or immune globulin.

In most countries, IG with a sufficient content of anti-HAV antibodies is no longer available. Although there is no indication that immune globulins may transmit hepatitis B virus, hepatitis C virus, or HIV, there is some unsubstantiated concern about yet undetectable infective agents. Only the CDC publication "Health Information for International Travel" in 2005 to 2006 still recommends IG for "travelers who are < 2 years of age, are allergic to a vaccine component, or otherwise elect not to receive vaccine." The same source also advises that "in case of travel within 4 weeks of vaccine administration, a dose of IG (0.02 mL/kg) may be given alone or in addition to hepatitis A vaccine, at a different site, for optimal protection." Most travel health professionals worldwide only give the vaccine without IG, even if departure is imminent. Although anti-HAV antibodies can serologically be demonstrated only (10 to)14 days after immunization, fast protection seems to occur, and no documented case of vaccine failure resulted from this pragmatic approach. This strategy is also supported by studies in primates where post-exposure vaccine doses gave good protection. The immediate efficacy of the booster vaccine dose is undisputed. Even if given later than 8 years after the initial dose, a rapid rise of antibodies from the booster grants immediate protection; thus it is not indicated to restart a hepatitis A vaccination series.

Community Control Measures

Notification of authorities is required in most countries, as isenteric precautions during the first 2 weeks of illness, such as sanitary

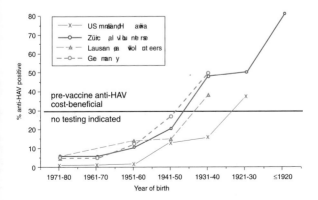

Figure 25 Seroprevalence of anti-HAV in American, German, and Swiss travelers

disposal of feces, urine, and blood. No quarantine is needed, but provide passive immunization of contacts through IG (0.02 mL/kg of body weight) as soon as possible for all household and sexual contacts. Consider active immunization of population at risk.

Additional Readings

Connor BA. Hepatitis A vaccine in the last-minute traveler. Am J Med 2005;118 Suppl 10A:58–62.

Iwarson S, et al. Excellent booster response 4–6 yr after a single primary dose of an inactivated hepatitis A vaccine. Scand J Infect Dis 2002;34:110–1.

Junge U, et al. Acute hepatitis A despite regular vaccination against hepatitis A and B. Dtsch Med Wochenschr 2002;127:1581–3.

Mutsch M, et al. Hepatitis A virus infection in travelers, 1988-2004. Clin Infect Dis 2006;42:490–7.

Steffen R. Changing travel-related global epidemiology of hepatitis A. Am J Med 2005;118:46S-49S.

Van Damme PA, et al. Do we need hepatitis A booster vaccinations? J Travel Med 2004;11:179–80.

Wallace MR et al. Safety and immunogenicity of an inactivated hepatitis A vaccine among HIV-infected subjects. Clin Infect Dis 2004;39:1207-13.

HEPATITIS B

Infectious Agent

Hepatitis B virus (HBV), a hepadnavirus, is the infectious agent for hepatitis B (HB). It consists of a core antigen (HBcAg), surrounded by a surface antigen (HBsAg). The HBsAg is antigenetically heterogenous with four major subtypes: adw, ayw, adr, and ayr. The third antigen, (HBeAg), is a soluble part of the core and an indirect marker of infectivity. The respective antibodies are anti-HBc, anti-HBs, and anti-HBe.

Transmission

Transmission is parenteral. The HBV is transmitted by percutaneous and permucosal exposure to infective body fluids, with minute doses being sufficient for infection. Razors and toothbrushes have been implicated as occasional vehicles of transmission. Perinatal transmission occurs mainly in hyperendemic areas.

Global Epidemiology

Close to 40% of the world's population has experienced infection with HBV, and there are an estimated 20 million new infections yearly worldwide. The highest HBsAg seroprevalence rates, reaching 15%, are found in Asia. There are 350 million people worldwide positive for HBsAg and, thus, potentially infectious (Figure 24).

In areas of high endemicity, infection often occurs in infancy and childhood, often causing chronic rather than apparent infection. In low-endemicity countries, exposure to HBV may be common in groups with high-risk behavior, such as intravenous drug users, heterosexuals with multiple partners, homosexual men, and medical personnel.

Risk for Travelers

Data show that the risk of HB is low in tourists whose stay in an endemic area is of short duration. This may not be so if they break fundamental rules of hygiene (see "Minimized Exposure in Travelers" below) or receive blood transfusions in countries where donated blood is not routinely screened for HBsAg. Among long-term residents of endemic areas, the incidence rate of symptomatic HB ranges from 0.2 per 1,000 per month (Africa, Latin America) to 0.6 per 1,000 per month (Asia). The rates of seroconversion, including asymptomatic infection, are 0.8 and 2.4 per 1,000 per month, respectively. However, surveys in Canada and Europe have demonstrated that 10 to 15% of all travelers to developing countries are at risk of contracting HB, some unintentionally (eg, when medical treatment becomes necessary), some carelessly (eg, piercing, tattooing, casual sex).

Clinical Picture

See the introduction to the hepatitis section (page 61). Fulminant fatal cases with hepatic necrosis and chronic forms potentially leading to cirrhosis or primary hepatocellular carcinoma result in a cumulative case fatality rate of 2%.

Incubation

The incubation period for HB ranges from 45 to 180 days, with 60 to 90 days being most common.

Communicability

All people who are HBsAg-positive are potentially infectious. Communicability may commence many weeks before the onset of symptoms and persist throughout the acute clinical course. In patients with chronic infection, infectivity persists, particularly in HBeAg-positive persons and, to a lesser extent, in anti-HBe positive patients. The virus may remain stable on environmental surfaces for more than 7 days.

Susceptibility is general. As described above, the younger the patient, the milder the clinical course. Protective immunity against all subtypes follows infection if anti-HBs develops and HBsAg is negative. Individuals with Down syndrome, lymphoproliferative disease, human immunodeficiency virus (HIV) infection, and those on hemodialysis are more likely to develop chronic infection.

Minimized Exposure in Travelers

Travelers are advised to abstain from unprotected sex, intravenous drug use, tattooing, piercing, acupuncture, and unnecessary dental or medical treatment where proper sterilization of equipment is suspect. Give unscreened whole blood or potentially hazardous blood products only to patients in dire need.

Chemoprophylaxis

None available.

Immunoprophylaxis

Hepatitis B Vaccines

Various hepatitis B vaccines exist in the developed countries:

- Engerix-B (SmithKline Beecham Biologicals)
- GenHevac B (Pasteur Merieux Connaught)
- Recombivax HB (Merck and Co), other brand names locally

The vaccines have a similar profile and are therefore described under a single heading. Additional vaccines are available, particularly in Asia, such as Heprecomb in Japan, or Hepavac Gene (Berna Biotech Ltd, a Crucell company, formerly Swiss Serum and Vaccine Institute) in South Korea and Poland. Others are used by UNICEF.

Immunology and Pharmacology

Viability: inactivated

Antigenic form: recombinant purified antigen of hepatitis B virus surface-coat (HBs) protein

Adjuvants: aluminum hydroxide

Preservative: 0.005 to 0.01% thimerosal, increasingly vaccines are free from thimerosal

Allergens/Excipiens: less than 5% yeast protein or plasmid DNA

Mechanism: induction of specific antibodies against hepatitis B virus surface antigen

Application

Schedule: three doses, with the second dose after 1 month and the third after 6 to 12 months. For travelers, accelerated schedules have been shown to be effective with doses of 20 µg given at 0, 7, and 21 days or 0, 14, and 28 days, but a fourth dose is then required at 12 months (Figure 27).

Dosage: Engerix-B for adults and adolescents age > 15 years—20 µg in 1 mL

Engerix-B junior for newborns and children up to age 15 years—10 µg in 0.5 mL

GenHevac B for all age groups—20 µg in 0.5 mL

Recombivax HB for adults and adolescents age > 15 years—10 µg in 1 mL

Recombivax HB for newborns and children up to age 15 years—5 µg in 0.5 mL

Recombivax HB for dialysis patients—40 µg in 1 mL

(Note: The age cut-off at 15 years applies to European countries. In some countries, two-dose regimens with adult doses are licensed for children for some vaccines. Consult the package inserts. Other parts of the world may have other cut-offs.)

Control of antibody response: Testing to determine antibody responses is not necessary after routine vaccination, e.g. in young travelers. Knowledge of response to vaccination is, however, important in the following groups:

- persons at risk of occupationally acquired infection
- infants born to HBs-Ag positive mothers
- immunocompromized persons
- sexual partners of HBs-Ag positive persons Assessment 1-2 months after administration of the last dose of the primary vaccination series (in infants at 8-15 months of age) is considered a reliable marker of immediate and long-term (probably lifelong) protection. Protective antibody levels of " 10 (in some countries 100) mIU/ml will be detected in > 95% of infants, children and young adults, after the age of 40 years that rate drops to below 90% and by 60 years protective antibody levels are achieved by 65-75% of vaccinees. If measurement is indicated after a longer delay, it may be recommended to first give an booster dose of hepatitis B vaccine as antibodies may have dropped below the 10 mIU/ml. Those with no or low response will require additional doses every 6

to 12 months. Some individuals are known to have seroconverted after more than 10 doses, it may be beneficial to use double-strength vaccines (as for dialysis patients) and to switch from one product to another.

Booster: although in most countries boosters are now considered unnecessary (see above), some still recommend a booster after 5 to 10 years.

Route: intramuscularly. Intradermal injections of a one-tenth dose results in suboptimal antibody titers, probably due to inadequate technique.

Site: deltoid. Infants, anterolateral thigh.

Storage: store at 2 to 8 °C (35 to 46 °F). Discard frozen vaccine.

Availability: worldwide, there is at least one product available. Plasma-derived vaccines are predominant in the developing countries and recombinant vaccines in the developed countries. In many countries, the combined hepatitis A and hepatitis B vaccine Twinrix is available (see Hepatitis A and "Protection" below).

Protection

Onset: if an accelerated regimen is used, 40 to 85% have seroconverted by days 21 and 28, respectively (Figure 26); over 95% are protected with all regimens approximately 7 to 8 months after starting immunization.

Efficacy: 96 to 99% seroconversion among infants, children, and adolescents; 94 to 98% seroconversion among adults aged 20 to 39 years; 89% seroconversion in adults aged > 40 years 1 to 2 months after third dose.

Duration: lifelong for symptomatic infection in responders. Booster vaccinations would be warranted in certain situations, such as in immunocompromised hosts.

Protective level: anti-HBs titer of ≥ 10 mlU/ml is considered protective.

Adverse Reactions

Adverse reactions are similar for the various hepatitis B vaccines. Local reactions (17 to 22%) may involve pain, swelling, tenderness, pruritus, induration, ecchymosis, warmth, nodule formation, or erythema at the injection site.

Systemic complaints (10 to 15%) include fatigue, weakness, headache, fever > 37.5 °C (100 °F), malaise, nausea, diarrhea, and dizziness. Fewer than 1% of recipients may experience sweat-

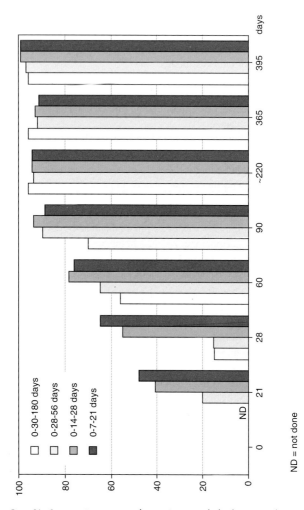

Figure 26 Seroprotection rates against hepatitis B using standard and various rapid immunization schedules.

ing, aches, chills, tingling, pharyngitis, upper respiratory tract infection, abnormal liver function, thrombocytopenia, eczema, purpura, tachycardia or palpitations, erythema multiforme by temporal association, hypertension, anorexia, abdominal pain or cramps, constipation, flushing, vomiting, paresthesia, rash, angioedema, urticaria, arthralgia, arthritis, myalgia, back pain, lymphadenopathy, hypotension, anaphylaxis, bronchospasm, or Guillain-Barré syndrome. Many of these events may simply have been temporally associated with immunization. A slight, but not significant, increase in the relative risk of first attacks or relapse of demyelating diseases, mainly multiple sclerosis, has been discussed. The illness must, however, have been preexisting as it takes years for clinical features to develop.

Transient positive HBsAg reactions have been described (Abbott's enzyme-linked immunosorbent assay and neutralization tests) after administration of Engerix B.

Contraindications

Absolute: persons with a previous hypersensitivity reaction to hepatitis B vaccine doses

Relative: persons with a history of hypersensitivity to yeast or other vaccine components, or any serious acute illness

Children: not contraindicated. Hepatitis B vaccine is tolerated well and highly immunogenic in newborns, infants, and children. Maternal antibodies do not interfere with pediatric immunogenicity.

Pregnant women: category C. It is unknown whether hepatitis B vaccine or corresponding antibodies cross the placenta. Generally, most IgG passage across the placenta occurs during the third trimester. Use if clearly needed.

Lactating women: it is unknown whether hepatitis B vaccine or corresponding antibodies are excreted in breast milk. Problems in humans have not been documented. Use if clearly needed.

Immunodeficient persons: persons receiving immunosuppressive therapy or having other immunodeficiencies may experience a diminished antibody response. Response may be impaired in HIV-positive persons. Dialysis patients and other immunocompromised persons should receive 40 ju g doses.

Interactions

Immune response of hepatitis B vaccines given with other vaccines is not compromised and does not compromise immune responses of other vaccines. In one study, the concomitant application of yellow fever vaccine resulted in a lower antibody titer than expected for yellow fever. It should not be concluded from this that the vaccines should be separated by at least 1 month.

Immunosuppressant drugs and radiation therapy may produce an insufficient response to immunization.

Recommendations for Vaccine Use

Hepatitis B immunization has recently become routine in many countries, so most infants or adolescents are immunized. Planned travel is an opportunity to vaccinate those not vaccinated previously.

The risk of hepatitis B transmission in the average tourist is low. Only a minority of travelers are clearly at risk because of their planned activities, such as those who expose themselves to potentially infected blood and blood-derived fluids (including those from instruments that have not been properly sterilized) and those travelers who have unprotected sexual contact. Any traveler, however, may be involved in an accident or medical emergency that requires surgery. According to the World Health Organization, the vaccine should be considered for virtually all travelers to high and intermediate endemic areas (see Figure 24).

Some travel health professionals recommend immunization for those whose behavior places them at risk (see "Minimized Exposure in Travelers" page 218). Although protection against hepatitis B is indicated in such circumstances, immunization may give a false sense of security against other infections, including HIV.

Self-Treatment Abroad

None. Medical consultation is required and consider passive-active immunization in case of exposure. Give hepatitis B immune globulin (HBIG, 0.06 mL/kg body weight) as soon as possible, but within 24 hours after exposure.

Principles of Therapy

Usually none. Provide α-interferon in some patients with chronic hepatitis B. Lamivudine and adenofovir are also established in therapy. There are newer antivirals being evaluated on clinical trials.

Community Control Measures

Notification is mandatory in many countries. Universal precautions should be taken to prevent exposure to contaminated blood and body fluids. No quarantine is needed. Contacts should be immunized with hepatitis B immunoglobulin and/or hepatitis B vaccine.

Additional Readings

Connor B et al. Hepatitis B risks and immunization coverage among American travelers. J Travel Med 2006;13:273-80.

Keystone JC. Travel-related hepatitis B: risk factors and prevention using an accelerated vaccination schedule. Am J Med 2005;118:63S–68S.

Nothdurft HD, et al. A new accelerated vaccination schedule for rapid protection against hepatitis A and B. Vaccine 2002;20:1157–62.

Zuckerman JN, et al. Hepatitis A and B booster recommendations: implications for travelers. Clin Infect Dis 2005;41:1020–6.

WHO. Hepatitis B vaccines. Wkly epid Rec 2004;79:255-63.

Hepatitis C

Hepatitis C (HC) is a parenterally transmitted infection, with hepacavirus as the infectious agent. It has historically been associated with transfusion but may also be transmitted by exposure to contaminated needles or syringes. It occurs worldwide, with prevalence rates of 0.5 to > 10% (Figure 27). Like hepatitis B, the infection may progress to chronic hepatitis, cirrhosis, and hepatocellular carcinoma. Transmission from mother to child is uncommon, and the chance of spreading through sexual or household contact is low. Immune globulin from unscreened donors may reduce the risk of sexually transmitted HC infection.

Hepatitis C has not been associated with travel. There is no vaccine commercially available. Patients with chronic hepatitis C who acquire hepatitis A infection have a substantial risk of fulminant hepatitis (41%) and death (35%). Hepatitis A vaccination is strongly recommended for chronic HC patients traveling to high- or intermediate-risk areas; it should, in fact, be considered for all HC patients.

Additional Readings

Andenaes S, et al. Prevalence of hepatitis A, B, C, and E antibody in flying airline personnel. Aviat Space Environ Med 2000;71:1178–80.

Coward RA, et al. Hepatitis C and holiday dialysis. Nephrol Dial Transplant 2000;15:1715.

Jaureguiberry S. Acute hepatitis C virus infection after a travel in India. J Travel Med 2005;12:55–6.

Miller LC, Hendrie NW. Health of children adopted from China. Pediatrics 2000;105:E76.

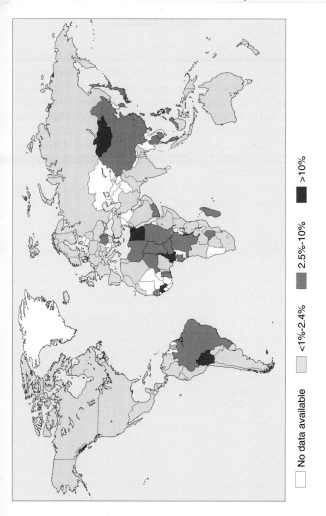

Figure 27   Global prevalence of hepatitis C (WHO 2001)

DELTA HEPATITIS

Delta hepatitis (HD) is caused by a defective RNA virus that can only replicate in the presence of the HB virus. It occurs most often in the Mediterranean region and South America and may result in a more serious clinical course for those with acute or chronic HB infection. Hepatitis D has not been identified as a pathogen associated with travel.

Immunization against HB will protect against viral hepatitis D.

Additional Readings

Rizzetto M. Hepatitis D. Virology, clinical and epidemiological aspects. Acta Gastroenterol Belg 2000;63:221–4.

HEPATITIS E

Infectious Agent

The hepatitis E virus (HEV) has not been conclusively classified. It is most likely either a calicivirus or related to a rubella virus.

Transmission

As with hepatitis A, outbreaks are related to contaminated water. Transmission through fecal-oral contact is less likely as secondary household cases are uncommon. Sexual transmission is possible as there is a high incidence among young adults. Hepatitis E (HE) may be a zoonosis since it can often be linked to swine HEV.

Global Epidemiology

Hepatitis E has been associated with waterborne epidemics, mainly in Asia and specifically in India and Nepal, but has been detected in all regions with inadequate sanitation. The attack rate is highest among young adults.

Risk for Travelers

Many cases of HE have been associated with travel, particularly to Nepal, but the mechanism remains to be determined by further study of HE among travelers and immigrants.

Clinical Picture

The clinical course resembles that of HA, with a large proportion of anicteric infections and their severity increasing with age. There is no evidence of a chronic form. Case fatality rate is usually 3%, but a rate of 20% has been noted in pregnant women.

Susceptibility and Resistance

Susceptibility is unknown. More icteric cases occur with increasing age.

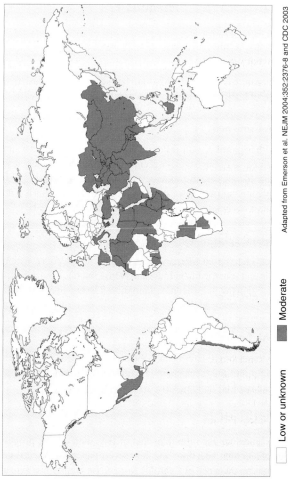

Adapted from Emerson et al. NEJM 2004;352:2376-8 and CDC 2003

Moderate

Low or unknown

Figure 28   Geographical distribution of Hepatitis E

Minimized Exposure in Travelers

Travelers should avoid drinking tap water. Like all enterically transmitted infections, travelers can minimize risk by avoiding potentially contaminated food and liquids.

Chemoprophylaxis

None available.

Immunoprophylaxis

None commercially available, although several candidates were tested. The immune globulin (IG) prepared from plasma collected in non–HE-endemic areas does not grant protection, whereas IG rich in hepatitis E antibodies may possibly offer protection.

Self-Treatment Abroad

None. Medical consultation is required.

Communicability

The period of communicability is unknown but persists for at least 2 weeks after the onset of jaundice.

Additional Readings

Aggarwal R, et al. Role of travel as a risk factor for hepatitis E virus infection in a disease-endemic area. Indian J Gastroenterol 2002; 21:14–8.

He J, et al. Evidence that rodents are a reservoir of hepatitis E virus for humans in Nepal. J Clin Microbiol 2002;40:4493–8.

Hyams KC. New perspectives on hepatitis E. Curr Gastroenterol Rep 2002;4:302–7.

Potasman I, et al. Lack of hepatitis E infection among backpackers to tropical countries. J Travel Med 2000;7:208–10.

Sadler GJ. UK acquired hepatitis E—an emerging problem? J Med Virol 2006;78:473–5.

Hepatitis G

The hepatitis G (HG) virus, a flavi-like virus, is transmitted parenterally through blood, blood products, and intravenous drug use. Hepatitis G infection is likely to be associated with progressive liver disease. Among children who have received multiple transfusions, there are marked variations in seroprevalence. The highest rates are reported in Egypt (24%) and Indonesia (32%), whereas the rate drops to 1 to 3% in developed nations. This infection has not been associated with travel.

Additional Readings

Hyams KC. Chronic liver disease among US military patients: the role of hepatitis C and G virus infection. Mil Med 2000;165:178–9.

HUMAN IMMUNODEFICIENCY VIRUS

Infectious Agent

Human immunodeficiency virus (HIV) is a lentivirus among the retrovirus family. Two types have been identified, HIV-1 and HIV-2, the latter being less pathogenic.

Transmission

HIV is transmitted in the same way as hepatitis B, through contact with semen and vaginal secretions during sexual activity and through exposure to contaminated blood on needles, syringes, etc. Transfusions also carry a risk. Tissue used in transplants may transmit HIV. Saliva, tears, urine, and bronchial secretions do not conclusively result in transmission, even with lower doses of HIV detected in these fluids. Transmission from mother to child is possible during or shortly after birth and by breastfeeding.

There is no risk of transmission from casual contact at home, at work, or socially. Insects do not transmit HIV.

Global Epidemiology

HIV infection occurs throughout the world. It is estimated that about 40 million men, women, and children are infected with HIV. In 2006, there were 3.4 million new infections with 65% of these in sub-Saharan Africa. The seroprevalence per 100,000 continues to be high in many countries of Africa (except for the Mediterranean countries), with rates of 500 to more than 15,000 in Botswana, Zambia, and Zimbabwe. In some of the Caribbean islands and several Central American countries (Guyana, Surinam), rates of 500 to 4,000 were found. Thailand, Cambodia, and Myanmar showed rates of 1,300 to 1,900. Extremely low rates (< 1) are observed in some of the New Independent States of the former Soviet Union, the Democratic Peoples Republic of Korea, and Afghanistan. The highest proportion of HIV infections worldwide is attributable to heterosexual intercourse rather than the commonly attributed risk factors—intercourse with homosexual or bisexual men, shared needles or syringes, or blood transfusions.

Risk for Travelers

Because travelers, not unlike the rest of the population, also engage in unprotected casual sex, HIV infection remains a primary concern for travel health professionals. Estimating the number of sexual exposures during a given length of stay and the proportion with condom use, as well as assuming a risk of infection of 1 per 500 through sexual intercourse with an infected person, it can be extrapolated that, of 100,000 male travelers having sex abroad, 19 will become infected if HIV prevalence among female partners is 1%. Further, 193 will become infected at a prevalence of 10%, and 576 will become infected at a prevalence of 30%. In various European countries, a previous trip abroad has been found to be the most important risk factor in new HIV infections among heterosexuals. Transmission rates from casual, unprotected sex far outweigh those from blood transfusions; transfusion abroad is rarely needed, and many centers now screen blood to be transfused.

Clinical Picture

HIV infection often manifests itself with a flu-like illness that resolves spontaneously. The infected person then remains without symptoms for up to 15 years or more. The proportion of persons not developing further symptoms is increasing with current antiviral therapy. Persons who gradually develop symptoms often experience fever, enlargement of lymph nodes, oropharyngeal or vulvovaginal candidiasis, oral hairy leukoplakia, herpes zoster, and peripheral neuropathy. In acquired immunodeficiency syndrome (AIDS), various serious opportunistic infections such as Kaposi's sarcoma and various lymphomas are possible symptoms. In addition, symptoms include loss of appetite, loss of weight, fatigue, and dementia. The CD4+ T-lymphocyte cell counts may gradually fall to < 200 per microliter. The disease is called "slim disease" in East Africa because of profound wasting. The ultimate fatal outcome is often due to an opportunistic infection.

Susceptibility and Resistance

Susceptibility is presumed to be general. Presence of other sexually transmitted diseases, particularly those with ulcerations, increases susceptibility. No post-infective immunity has been observed.

Minimized Exposure in Travelers

Provide all travelers with information about HIV risk and prevention, particularly those likely to engage in casual sex—persons traveling alone or in groups of the same sex, persons who are stressed or lonely, and those who will be away a long time. The following elements are essential:

- Knowledge of the facts
- Awareness of the implications of the risks and consequences
- Motivation to sustain a certain standard of behavior
- Skill to negotiate the conduct of sexual relations
- Support from family, colleagues, and community

Communicability

Presumed to start early after infection and persist for life.

Although a mutually monogamous sexual relationship with a noninfected partner is safe, condoms should be used for all other sexual intercourse. Note that condoms drastically reduce but do not eliminate the risk of infection. Intravenous drug use involving shared needles or syringes represents particularly high-risk behavior.

Transfusions of unscreened blood should be accepted only if medically essential.

Chemoprophylaxis

None before exposure. Postexposure prophylaxis is possible under specific circumstances.

Immunoprophylaxis

None available so far. Various candidate vaccines are being tested.

Self-Treatment Abroad

Postexposure prophylaxis ideally should be started within 4 hours; in travel medicine settings, even the longer margin of 48 hours is difficult to achieve in developing countries; in fact, medication may be unavailable and repatriation may not be immediately possible. Medical consultation required.

▌Principles of Therapy

Antiviral prophylaxis and, if necessary, therapy for complications.

▌Community Control Measures

Notification is mandatory in many countries. No isolation, but universal precautions should be taken.

Additional Readings

Apostolopoulos Y, et al. HIV-risk behaviors of American spring break vacationers: a case of situational disinhibition? Int J STD AIDS 2002;13:733–43.

Carey J, et al. Penicillium marneffei infection in an immunocompromised traveler: a case report and literature review. J Travel Med 2005;12:291–4.

Cavassini ML. Pharmacotherapy, vaccines and malaria advice for HIV-infected travellers. Expert Opin Pharmacother 2005; 6:891–913.

Furrer H, et al. Increased risk of wasting syndrome in HIV-infected travellers: prospective multicentre study. Trans R Soc Trop Med Hyg 2001;95:484–6.

Kaplan JE, et al. Guidelines for preventing opportunistic infections among HIV-infected persons—2002. Recommendations of the US Public Health Service and the Infectious Diseases Society of America. MMWR Recomm Rep 2002;51(RR-8):1–52.

Mahto M, et al. Knowledge, attitudes and health outcomes in HIV-infected travellers to the USA. HIV Med 2006;7:201–4.

Richens J. Sexually transmitted infections and HIV among travellers: a review. Travel Med Infect Dis 2006;4:184–95.

Schuhwerk MA, et al. HIV and travel. Travel Med Infect Dis 2006;4:174–83.

INFLUENZA, SEASONAL

Infectious Agent

Influenza A viruses are classified on the basis of two spike-like surface antigens: hemagglutinin (H, with usually three subtypes pathogenic in humans) and neuraminidase (N, with two subtypes). There is continuous and substantial antigenic variation, most frequently originating in China. Influenza B viruses are more stable. Influenza C so far has been virtually irrelevant in humans. So far, 16 hemagglutinins and nine neuraminidases have become known, most occurring only in the animal world. Since 1997, it is known that the avian H5N1 can be transmitted to humans and, very exceptionally, human-to-human transmission of this virus has been reported (see "Avian Influenza").

New variants because of minor antigenic drift result in small or intermediate epidemics. More substantial shifts may lead to major epidemics or pandemics when no immunity to distantly related, previously occurring subtypes exists. As of this writing, there are concerns about a pandemic threat basing on the spread of the H5N1; at the end of 2006, per the World Health Organization (WHO), the world was in phase 3 "Pandemic Alert" owing to the fact that there was a new virus that caused human cases but with no, or very limited, human-to-human transmission. Up until the end of 2006, no new pandemic influenza virus had been detected, so a pandemic might not necessarily originate from H5N1.

Transmission

Transmission of the human influenza virus is usually airborne and from person to person, occurring particularly in enclosed spaces. Viruses are spread in respiratory droplets caused by coughing or sneezing. Influenza can also be spread by contact with a contaminated surface when mucus membranes in the mouth or nose are touched thereafter. Influenza viruses may persist for hours to days in the environment, particularly in cold and low-humidity environments. So far, there is no proof that the virus replicates in the human intestine.

Global Epidemiology

Influenza occurs worldwide in the winter or early spring. In the northern hemisphere, transmission is highest from November to March. In the southern hemisphere, most activity occurs from April to September. Influenza can occur throughout the year in the tropics. Seasonal influenza affects 5 to 15% of the population, these annual epidemics are thought to result in between three and five million cases of severe illness and between 250,000 and 500,000 deaths every year around the world. Most deaths currently associated with influenza in industrialized countries occur among the elderly over 65 years of age.

Risk for Travelers

Influenza may be a travel-associated infection; the risk of exposure to influenza during foreign travel varies, depending on exposure (eg, close contacts on cruises), season, and destination. The incidence is 1% per month in developing countries, irrespective of season and destination. There are many reports on influenza outbreaks during or after cruises and group travel; the potential risk factors have not been formally evaluated.

Clinical Picture

Seasonal influenza is characterized by abrupt onset of fever, myalgia, sore throat, and nonproductive cough. It should not be confused with the common cold. Pneumonia is the most frequent serious complication. The case fatality rate is low, except in elderly patients and in those with preexisting illness.

Incubation

One to 3 days in seasonal influenza

Communicability

Viral shedding occurs 24 to 48 hours before onset of illness at low titers and extends 3 to 5 days from clinical onset in adults and usually 7 to up to 21 days in small children, even up to months in immunocompromised hosts.

Susceptibility and Resistance

There is universal susceptibility of nonimmune persons to new subtypes. Infection results in resistance to that specific virus.

Minimized Exposure in Travelers

To reduce the risk of seasonal influenza, avoidance of crowds is suggested, but this is difficult to practice during international travel (eg, at airports or in planes). Use of masks is not recommended against seasonal influenza.

WHO does not recommend travel restrictions to areas experiencing outbreaks of highly pathogenic H5N1 avian influenza in birds, including countries that have reported associated cases of human infection. Travelers to affected areas should avoid contact with live animal markets and poultry farms, and any free-ranging or caged poultry. Populations in affected countries are advised to avoid contact with dead migratory birds or wild birds showing signs of disease.

Chemoprophylaxis

Amantadine hydrochloride, 200 mg/d, is effective against influenza A with rapidly developing resistance. Neuraminidase inhibitors such as oseltamivir (Tamiflu) or zanamivir (Relenza), effective against influenza A and B, may help prevent infection. They are hardly ever indicated in travelers, except when a situation similar to a household contact with seasonal influenza occurs, or post-exposure prophylaxis for H5N1 is needed.

Immunoprophylaxis

The antigenic characteristics of new circulating strains are selected for planning for new vaccines each year. With 6-month intervals, WHO (and some national) expert groups determine which antigens should be included in the northern and southern hemisphere vaccines.

In the developed countries, there are a wide variety of trivalent influenza vaccines offering protection against type A and B infections, all based on current WHO recommendations. Although differing in their antigenic form, they all have a similar profile, and we describe these under one heading.

Immunology and Pharmacology

Viability: inactivated; in the U.S. also live attenuated intranasal vaccine.

Antigenic form: whole virus (now rare), split, virosomal, or subunit. Usually three antigens, 15 µg each in 0.5 mL

Strains: WHO revises yearly for the northern and southern hemispheres. Usually three strains named for the location, sequence number, and year of their isolation are selected in the spring for the northern hemisphere. That year's vaccine is then released in the autumn and vice versa for the southern hemisphere. Monovalent H5N1 vaccines are expected to be delivered in 2007, quadrivalent ones including H5N1 possibly in 2008.

Adjuvants: MF59 in Fluad (Novartis Vaccines) and in Inflexal V, the latter using liposomal technology, alum in some of the H5N1 vaccines.

Preservative: 0.01% thimerosal has been eliminated from most vaccines worldwide

Allergens/Excipiens: residual egg proteins / 0.05% gelatin, glycol p-iso-octylphenyl ether, polysorbate-80, tri(n)butylphosphate, not > 0.02% residual-free formaldehyde, in some vaccines polymyxin B, gentamicin, neomycin, propiolactone

Mechanism: induction of specific active immunity against influenza viruses

Application

Schedule and dosage: there are slight variations among national and product recommendations. Consult the package insert. The usual procedure is as follows:

Children age 6 to 12 months (depending on vaccine) to age 3 years (Europe) or age 9 years (United States)—2 doses of split or subunit vaccine only (0.25 mL) if unprimed; if primed, only a single dose. As dosages and regimens vary depending on the vaccine used and nationally approved registration, it is essential to consult the package insert.

Children age 6 to 12 years—one dose of split or subunit vaccine only (0.5 mL)

Children age > 12 years and adults—one dose of any vaccine (0.5 mL)

When two doses are given, they should be at least 1 month apart. Give the second dose before December 1 (northern hemisphere), if possible.

Booster: because of changing antigenicity of prevalent viral strains and waning immunity, give persons at risk of influenza a booster dose yearly. In travelers visiting the other hemisphere, a booster with the respective vaccine for this opposite hemisphere may be recommended after 6 months, where available.

Route: intramuscularly; some vaccines also subcutaneously (SC)

Site: use the deltoid muscle for adults and older children. For infants and young children, the anterolateral thigh is preferred.

Storage: store at 2 to 8 °C (35 to 46 °F). Discard frozen vaccine.

Availability: worldwide. There are a multitude of products marketed. In the United States, a live intranasal vaccine is available for persons aged 5 to 49 years (FluMist, MedImmune).

Protection

Onset: 2 to 3 weeks after application

Efficacy: vaccination will reduce influenza incidence by approximately 70% but it is less effective in elderly recipients. The vaccine is ineffective against common cold viruses. Influenza vaccine is more effective at preventing mortality and hospitalization than at preventing morbidity; it somewhat diminishes viral shedding in vacinees.

Duration: declines gradually from 4 months following the immunization

Protective level: hemagglutination inhibition (HI) antibody titers ≥ 1:40 correlates with clinical protection.

Adverse Reactions

Side effects of influenza vaccine are generally inconsequential in adults and occur at a low frequency but may be more common in pediatric recipients, in whom only subunit or split-virus vaccines should be used.

Up to two-thirds of recipients experience soreness around the vaccination site for 2 days.

Fever, malaise, myalgia, and other systemic symptoms occur infrequently and usually affect persons with no prior exposure to the antigens in the vaccine (such as young children). These effects usually begin 6 to 12 hours after vaccination and persist for 1 to

2 days. Immediate, probably allergic reactions such as hives, angioedema, allergic asthma, or systemic anaphylaxis occur extremely rarely following influenza vaccination.

Contraindications

Absolute: persons with an anaphylactoid or other immediate reactions (eg, hives, difficulty breathing, hypotension) to previous influenza vaccine doses. Do not vaccinate persons with a severe egg allergy or children below the age of 6 month.

Relative: any serious acute illness or unstable neurologic disorders. In multiple sclerosis (MS), uncertainty exists owing to an elevated risk of exacerbation 6 months following vaccination, but that risk is very small. In view of a much greater risk from influenza, there is consensus to vaccinate MS patients.

Children: not contraindicated. Vaccinate children and teenagers (age 6 months to 18 years) receiving long-term aspirin therapy; they are at risk of developing Reye's syndrome after influenza infection.

Pregnant women: category C. Vaccinating after the first trimester can minimize hypothetical risk of teratogenicity. Do not delay vaccination of pregnant women with high-risk conditions who will still be in the first trimester when the influenza season begins. It is unknown whether influenza vaccine or corresponding antibodies cross the placenta. Generally, most immunoglobulin G passage across the placenta occurs during the third trimester. Recommendations grossly vary in different countries; use if clearly needed.

Lactating women: it is unknown whether influenza vaccine or corresponding antibodies are excreted in breast milk. Problems in humans have not been documented. Use if clearly needed.

Immunodeficient persons: persons receiving immunosuppressive therapy or having other immunodeficiencies may experience a diminished antibody response to active immunization. Chemoprophylaxis of influenza A with amantadine or neuraminidase inhibitors may be indicated in such persons. Vaccination of persons infected with HIV is a prudent measure and will result in protective antibody levels in many recipients. However, antibody response to vaccine may be low in persons with advanced HIV-related illnesses. Booster doses have not improved the immune response in these individuals.

Interactions

Pneumococcal and influenza vaccines may safely and effectively be administrated simultaneously at separate injection sites. There is no indication that influenza vaccine should not be given simultaneously with any other travel vaccine.

Immunosuppressant drugs and radiation therapy may result in an insufficient response to immunization.

In patients receiving anticoagulants, give SC. Several patients treated with warfarin have shown prolonged prothrombin time after influenza vaccination.

Phenytoin plasma concentrations sometimes rise or fall after influenza vaccinations, and carbamazepine and phenobarbital levels sometimes rise.

Influenza vaccination may transiently lead to false-positive HIV serologic tests when particularly sensitive screening tests (ELISA, PERT for reverse transcriptase epitopes, etc.) are used. The latter is related to EAV-0, an avian retrovirus remaining in residual egg proteins.

Recommendations for Vaccine Use

Any traveler may elect immunization against influenza to avoid contracting it abroad. Influenza immunization is routinely recommended for persons aged > 65 years and for those with preexisting medical conditions that might increase complications. Several countries, including the United States, have expanded this recommendation to those over the age of 50 and to all children aged 6 to 23 months. This recommendation is particularly valid for those traveling in groups or passengers planning a cruise.

Self-Treatment Abroad

Supportive. Neuraminidase inhibitors (or amantadine) if prescribed before departure, to be used ideally within 36 (to 48) hours after onset of symptoms.

Principles Of Therapy

Supportive. Consider neuraminidase inhibitors (or amantadine) if patient consults within 48 hours after onset of symptoms.

▌Community Control Measures

None that relate to travel medicine.

Additional Readings

Center for Disease Control and Prevention. Influenza B virus outbreak on a cruise ship—Northern Europe, 2000. MMWR Morb Mortal Wkly Rep 2001;50:137–40.

Center for Disease Control and Prevention. Prevention and control of influenza. Recommendations of the Advisory Committee on Immunization Practices (ACIP). MMWR Recomm Rep. 2005;54(RR-8):1–40.

Miller JM, et al. Cruise ships: high-risk passengers and the global spread of new influenza viruses. Clin Infect Dis 2000;31:433–8.

Mutsch M, et al. Influenza virus infection in travelers to tropical and subtropical countries. Clin Infect Dis. 2005;40:1282–7.

JAPANESE ENCEPHALITIS

Infectious Agent

The Japanese encephalitis (JE) virus is a flavivirus.

Transmission

Japanese encephalitis is an arboviral infection transmitted by various Culex mosquitoes. In an endemic area, usually < 1 to 3% of the mosquitoes are infected. This vector feeds on various animal hosts (mainly pigs) and humans. The vector becomes infective by feeding on viremic swine and various wild birds. Agricultural regions, mainly rice fields, present the highest risk of transmission.

Global Epidemiology

Japanese encephalitis occurs only in Asia (Figure 29). In temperate regions, transmission is limited to summer and fall. Transmission occurs predominantly in rural areas, and children are at greatest risk of infection. About 50,000 cases are reported yearly, with an incidence rate reaching 10 per 10,000. The geographical distribution of JE is expanding, and now includes Northern Australia. An outbreak of JE occurred in Northern India in 2005 affecting thousands of people. Countries that have had major epidemics in the past, but that have controlled the disease primarily by vaccination include China, Korea, Japan, Taiwan, and Thailand. Other countries that still have periodic epidemics include Vietnam, Cambodia, Myanmar, India, Nepal, and Malaysia. JE is also decreasing as a result of replacing continuous irrigation by intermittent irrigation of rice fields. In addition, in all endemic countries, many small pig farms have disappeared, there are now fewer large pig farms, and these areas are rarely visited due to the very distinctive smell.

Risk for Travelers

The risk of JE for short-term travelers and long-term residents of urban centers is extremely low. Risk of JE for travelers depends

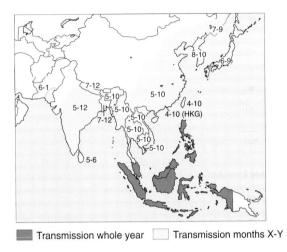

Transmission whole year ☐ Transmission months X-Y

Figure 29   Japanese encephalitis endemic areas

on destination, season, duration of travel, and activities. From 1978 to 1992, only 24 cases of JE had been diagnosed worldwide among travelers. Of these, six were American soldiers. Rates of JE infection of 1 to 21 per 100,000 weekly have been observed in military personnel. The rate of infection seems to be < 0.1 per 100,000 in tourists and business people.

Clinical Picture

Most infections (99.5%) are asymptomatic. Patients who develop clinical illness have a case fatality rate of 30%, and survivors experience neuropsychiatric sequelae in 50% of cases. The clinical course becomes more serious with age.

Incubation

The incubation period is usually 5 to 15 days.

Transmission

Whole year, predominantly during rainy season

Minimized Exposure in Travelers

Personal protective measures against mosquito bites in endemic areas.

Chemoprophylaxis

None available.

Immunoprophylaxis

Japanese Encephalitis Vaccine

Immunology and Pharmacology

Viability: inactive

Antigenic form: mouse-brain-derived inactivated, whole virus, Nakayama-NIH strain, or Beijing 1 strain

Adjuvants: none

Preservative: 0.007% thimerosal within the lyophilized powder

Allergens/Excipiens: < 50 µg mouse serum protein. No myelin basic protein can be detected at the lower threshold of the assay (< 2 ng/mL) per 500 microgram gelatin, < 100 µg formaldehyde

Mechanism: induction of protective antibodies

Application

Schedule: reconstitute the contents of single and multidose vials with 1.3 mL and 11 mL of diluent, respectively. Three doses of 1 mL for adults and children age > 3 years, normally on days 0, 7, and 30 for optimal immunogenicity. For children age < 3 years, give 0.5 mL each dose. Give the third dose on day 14 in urgent situations. Optimally, administer the third dose at least 10 days before arrival in endemic areas to allow protective antibody titers to develop. Residents of endemic areas may receive a schedule with only two doses separated by 7 days; preexisting exposure to flaviviruses may contribute to the immune response. Short-term travelers may receive a similar schedule.

Booster: a booster dose appropriate to the age group may be given 24 to 48 months after the first dose. In the absence of clear data, a definite recommendation on booster intervals cannot be made.

Route: subcutaneously

Site: over deltoid

Storage: store powder at 2 to 8 °C (35 to 46 °F). Do not freeze the reconstituted suspension. Protect from direct sunlight. Contact manufacturer regarding prolonged exposure to room temperature or elevated or freezing temperatures. Shipping data are not available. Refrigerate and use as soon as possible after reconstitution, preferably within 8 hours.

Availability: available in many countries as JE-Vax (Biken) distributed by Sanofi-Pasteur, but concerns about its safety resulted in withdrawal of this vaccine in various countries, at least for younger age groups. Also the World Health Organization no longer supports the use of vaccine made from neural tissues. In Japan, the Japanese Encephalitis Vaccine Seiken (Delta Seiken, Tokyo, Japan) is licensed and exported to a few European countries. Note that dosage differs from JE-Vax. Japanese Encephalitis Vaccine-GCVC from Rhein Biotech/Korean GreenCross Vaccine Corp. is also imported to several European countries. A live attenuated JE virus SA14-14-2 vaccine strain exists that was shown to be safe and immunogenic. It has been licensed in China since 1988, and millions of children have received the vaccine. This live vaccine is not registered outside Asia. A live attenuated flavivirus chimeric JE vaccine (Chimeri Vax JE, Acambis) and also an inactivated JE vaccine not requiring mouse brain (Intercell) are under development.

Biken JE Vaccine

Onset: 10 days after two doses, after the third dose in persons age ≥ 60 years

Efficacy: 78% after two doses, 99% after three doses

Duration: uncertain, but a substantial proportion of antibody is lost 6 months after two doses. Subsequent to a three-dose schedule, antibodies persist for at least 24 months and possibly up to 4 years

Protective level: based on challenge experiments in passively protected mice, neutralizing antibody levels ≥ 1:10 protected a 105 LD50 dose, which is the viral dose thought to be transmitted by infected mosquitoes

Adverse Reactions

Overall, 20% of vaccine recipients experience mild to moderate local side effects in the area of the injection, such as tenderness, redness, or swelling.

Systemic effects such as fever, headache, malaise, rash, chills, dizziness, muscle pain, nausea, vomiting, or abdominal pain may occur in 5 to 10% of cases. Hives and facial swelling were reported in 0.2% and 0.1% of vaccinees, respectively. Although JE vaccine is reactogenic, rates of serious allergic reactions (eg, generalized urticaria, angioedema) are rare (1 to 104 per 10,000). This may have been associated with a specific Biken vaccine lot. Two fatal cases of anaphylaxis have been recorded in the Republic of Korea. Persons with certain allergic histories are more likely to react adversely to vaccination. Observe vaccine recipients for 30 minutes and caution about delayed allergic reactions.

Several cases of encephalitis have been associated with JE vaccination, two of them fatal. Anecdotally, sudden death in a patient who also received plague vaccine and cases of Guillain-Barré syndrome have been reported, but association with JE vaccine is questionable.

Contraindications

Absolute: persons with hypersensitivity to any component of the vaccine or who experienced urticaria or angioedema after a previous dose of JE vaccine. There is no indication that prophylactic antihistamines or steroids prevent allergic reactions related to the vaccine.

Relative: any acute illness, history of urticaria, multiple allergies, chronic cardiac, hepatic, or renal disorders, generalized malignancies, diabetes

Children: safety and efficacy of JE vaccine in children age < 1 year have not been established.

Pregnant women: category C. It is unknown whether JE vaccine or corresponding antibodies cross the placenta. Generally, most immunoglobulin G passage across the placenta occurs during the third trimester. Japanese encephalitis infection acquired during the first or second trimester of pregnancy may cause intrauterine infection and fetal death. Infections during the third trimester have not been associated with adverse outcomes in newborns. Use only if the woman must travel and if the risk of infection clearly outweighs the risk of adverse reaction to vaccine.

Lactating women: it is unknown whether JE vaccine or corresponding antibodies are excreted in breast milk. Problems in humans have not been documented.

Immunodeficient persons: persons receiving immunosuppressive therapy or having other immunodeficiencies may experience diminished response to active immunization. They may remain susceptible to JE despite immunization.

Interactions

Immunosuppressant drugs and radiation therapy may cause an insufficient response to immunization.

Simultaneous application of JE vaccine with diphtheria-tetanus vaccines and with hepatitis A and B vaccines is apparently safe and immunogenic. No published data exist on concurrent use with other vaccines.

Risk to short-term tourists and business travelers is very low, even outside the urban areas. The vaccine has a considerable potential for adverse effects.

Recommendations for Vaccine Use

Japanese encephalitis vaccine is not recommended for all travelers to Asia. In general, vaccine should be offered to persons spending a month or longer in endemic areas during the transmission season, especially if travel will include rural areas. Under specific circumstances, vaccine should be considered for persons spending < 30 days in endemic areas (eg, travelers to rural areas experiencing epidemic transmission with extensive outdoor activities).

Community Control Measures

Notification is mandatory in many countries. No isolation or quarantine required.

Additional Readings

Bharati K, et al. Japanese encephalitis: development of new candidate vaccines. Expert Rev Anti Infect Ther 2006;4:313–24.

Monath TP. Japanese encephalitis vaccines: current vaccines and future prospects. Curr Top Microbiol Immunol 2002;267:105–38.

Padma TV. Encephalitis outbreak finds Indian officials unprepared. Nat Med 2005;11:1016.

Shlim DR, et al. Japanese encephalitis vaccine for travelers: exploring the limits of risk. Clin Infect Dis 2002;35:183–8.

WHO. Japanese encephalitis vaccines. Wkly epid Rec 2006;81:331-40.

Yang SE. The efficacy of mouse-brain inactivated Nakayama strain Japanese encephalitis vaccine-results from 30 years experience in Taiwan. Vaccine 2006;24:2669–73.

Lassa Fever

Infectious Agent

Arenavirus

Transmission

Rodents living in or near human dwellings excrete the virus; humans inhale it or ingest it with food. Laboratory infections have occurred.

Global Epidemiology

West Africa, probably from Senegal to Nigeria and Central African Republic

Risk for Travelers

There have been a few anecdotal cases imported to Europe, Japan, and the United States.

Clinical Picture

Gradual onset with fever, malaise, myalgia, conjunctival injection, sore throat, cough, chest and abdominal pain, vomiting, and diarrhea. The pharynx is often inflamed with patches or ulcers on the tonsils. This may resolve within 10 days or progress with facial and laryngeal edema, cyanosis, a mild bleeding diathesis, and shock. Neurologic complications carry a poor prognosis.

Incubation

5 to 21 days, with 7 to 14 days most common

Communicability

Lassa fever can be transmitted from person to person, and secondary cases have occurred with nosocomial spread, possibly by aerosol. Tertiary cases are rare. The virus is excreted in the urine for up to 9 weeks from onset of symptoms.

Susceptibility and Resistance

General susceptibility or immunity following infection is unknown.

Chemoprophylaxis

Not applicable.

Immunoprophylaxis

None available.

Self-Treatment Abroad

None. A physician should treat the patient.

Principles of Therapy

Supportive; case fatality rate reduced by ribavirin.

Community Control Measures

Reduce rodent reservoir.

Additional Readings

Isaacson M. Viral hemorrhagic fever hazards for travelers in Africa. Clin Infect Dis 2001;33:1707–12.

Macher AM, et al. Historical Lassa fever reports and 30-year clinical update. Emerg Infect Dis 2006;12:835–7.

Schmitz H, et al. Monitoring of clinical and laboratory data in two cases of imported Lassa fever. Microbes Infect 2002;4:43–50.

LEGIONELLOSIS

Infectious Agent

Bacteria of the *Legionella* genus, of which there are 35 species. The main infectious agent in legionellosis (also known as legionnaires' disease) is *Legionella pneumophila*, serogroup 1.

Transmission

Transmission is airborne, often attributed to showers. The organism may survive for months in warm water, air-conditioning cooling towers, humidifiers, jacuzzi-type baths, and decorative fountains. Immersion in a river has been associated with legionellosis.

Global Epidemiology

Worldwide distribution. Sporadic cases and outbreaks are more common in summer and autumn.

Risk for Travelers

There have been many anecdotal cases and documented outbreaks of the disease. An attack rate of < 0.1 per 100,000 has been found among Europeans visiting France, 0.1 to 1.0 in visits to Spain, Greece, and Italy, and 0.7 and 2.0 in two separate years in visits to Turkey.

Clinical Picture

Pneumonia develops after an initial phase of anorexia, malaise, myalgia, headache, and rapidly rising fever.

Incubation

Two to 10 days, with 5 to 6 days most common.
   Legionellosis is not directly transmitted from person to person.

Susceptibility and Resistance

Attack rates of 0.1 to 5% are seen in the population at risk, but unrecognized infections are common. Risk factors include age (most patients age > 50 years), gender (male to female incidence ratio is 2.5:1), smoking, history of diabetes, chronic illness.

Minimized Exposure in Travelers

Some experts recommend staying out of the bathroom for the first minute after turning on the warm water for showers.

Chemoprophylaxis

Not Applicable.

Immunoprophylaxis

None available.

Community Control Measures

Hot water temperatures above 60 °C inactivate the bacilli. This is rarely done in hotels, however, because of cost and risk of burns.

Additional Readings

Benin AL, et al. Trends in Legionnaires Disease, 1980–1998: declining mortality and new patterns of diagnosis. Clin Infect Dis 2002;35:1039–45.

Fields BS, et al. Legionella and Legionnaires' disease: 25 years of investigation. Clin Microbiol Rev 2002;15:506–26.

Huhn GD. Outbreak of travel-related pontiac fever among hotel guests illustrating the need for better diagnostic tests. J Travel Med 2005;12:173–9.

Ricketts KD. The impact of new guidelines in Europe For the control and prevention of travel-associated Legionnaires' disease. Int J Hyg Environ Health 2006;209:547-52.

LEISHMANIASIS

Infectious Agent

Leishmania parasites are protozoal pathogens that are found in many regions of the developing world. There are two morphologically different forms: intracellular amastigotes seen in humans and animals and extracellular promastigotes found in the intestine of the sandfly.

Transmission

Female sandflies are the vectors of the disease. Sandflies are found in poorly constructed housing and in forested regions. Insect saliva increases promastigote infectivity. The reservoir for cutaneous or mucosal leishmaniasis is often forest rodents. Humans become infected when visiting forested areas. Elsewhere, dogs, other animals, and humans serve as reservoirs.

Global Epidemiology

Visceral leishmaniasis (kala-azar) is endemic in the Middle East, Central and South America, India, Bangladesh, and Africa (Figure 30). Specific *Leishmania* are categorized depending on geographic occurrence (eg, *Leishmania aethiopica*, *L. mexicana*, *L. viannia peruviana*, *L. viannia braziliensis*). Cutaneous leishmaniasis is more widespread than is the visceral or mucosal form (Figures 31).

Risk for Travelers

Visceral leishmaniasis is occasionally contracted by visitors to endemic areas. In fact, US military personnel participating in Operation Desert Storm developed classic visceral disease. Cutaneous and mucosal involvement ("oriental sore") is the more common form.

The onset of visceral disease is insidious, leading to a chronic course with fever, malaise, anorexia, weight loss, and often abdominal swelling, resulting from hepatosplenomegaly. In the cutaneous form, a single or multiple lesion develops from the initial erythematous papule at the site of inoculation by the sandfly. The

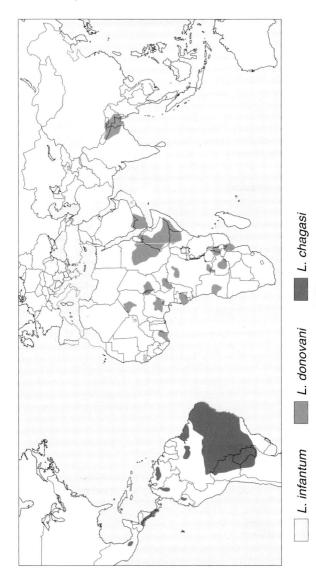

Figure 30   Geographic distribution of visceral leishmaniasis (WHO/CTD 1997, adapted)

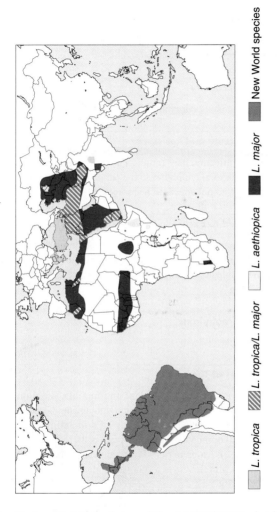

Figure 31 Geographic distribution of cutaneous leishmaniasis (WHO/CTD 1997, adapted)

nodule then ulcerates. Satellite lesions may then be seen. Cutaneous leishmaniasis may last months or years before healing. Regional adenopathy and systemic symptoms may develop.

Incubation

The incubation period for the visceral disease ranges from 3 to 8 months, and several weeks to months for the cutaneous form.

Communicability

The infection is not communicable from person to person.

Susceptibility and Resistance

Leishmania infection may stimulate a protective T cell immune response. Humoral antibodies to the parasite develop following infection but do not appear to be protective.

Minimized Exposure in Travelers

Travelers should use an insect repellent containing diethyltoluamide (deet) and wear permethrin treated clothing to minimize exposure to infected sandflies. Enclose sleeping areas with a fine mesh netting.

Chemoprophylaxis

Not applicable.

Principles of Therapy

Treat with one of the pentavalent antimonials—sodium stibogluconate (Pentostam) or meglumine antimoniate (Glucantime). Prescribe the following dose: 20 mg/kg/d of antimony for 28 days (visceral or mucocutaneous disease) or 10 to 20 days (cutaneous disease). Amphotericin B also appears to be effective in some cases. Miltefosine is a promising alternative, which can be given orally.

Community Control Measures

Not applicable.

Additional Readings

Antinori S. Cutaneous leishmaniasis: an increasing threat for travellers. Clin Microbiol Infect 2005;11:343–6.

Ahluwalia S. Mucocutaneous leishmaniasis: an imported infection among travellers to central and South America. BMJ 2004;329:842–4.

Lawn SD. New world mucosal and cutaneous leishmaniasis: an emerging health problem among British travellers. QJM 2004;97:781–8.

Magill AJ. Cutaneous leishmaniasis in the returning traveler. Infect Dis Clin North Am 2005;19:241–66.

Schwartz E, et al. New world cutaneous leishmaniasis in travellers. Lancet Infect Dis 2006;6:342–9.

Weitzel T, et al. Imported leishmaniasis in Germany 2001–2004: data of the SIMPID surveillance network. Eur J Clin Microbiol Infect Dis 2005;24:471–6.

LEPROSY

Leprosy is a chronic granulomatous infection of the skin and peripheral nerves with the intracellular bacterium *Mycobacterium leprae*. The damage to peripheral nerves results in sensory and motor impairment with characteristic deformities and disability. Host genetic factors have a partial effect on both the development of leprosy and the pattern of disease. The varying clinical forms of leprosy are determined by the underlying immunological response to *M. leprae*. At one pole, patients with tuberculoid leprosy have a vigorous cellular immune response to the mycobacterium, which limits the disease to a few well-defined skin patches or nerve trunks. At the other pole, lepromatous leprosy is characterized by the absence of specific cellular immunity. There is uncontrolled proliferation of leprosy bacilli with many lesions and extensive infiltration of the skin and nerves. The dynamic nature of the immune response to *M. leprae* leads to spontaneous fluctuations in the clinical state, which are termed leprosy reactions. Diagnostic signs of leprosy are hypopigmented or reddish patches with definite loss of sensation, thickened peripheral nerves, and acid-fast bacilli on skin smears or biopsy material. The first line drug against leprosy are rifampin, clofazimine, and dapsone. All patients should receive a multidrug combination with monthly supervision. Treatment for multibacillary leprosy is 12-24 months, for paucibacillary, 6 months.

Transmission is thought to be via respiratory droplets. Virulence is very low, and incubation very long (many years). Prolonged exposure is required for effective transmission. Therefore, the risk of leprosy is low amongst general travelers. Leprosy should be suspected in immigrants or refugees from leprosy endemic areas, if above signs and symptoms are present.

Additional Readings

Britton WJ, Lockwood DJ. Leprosy. Lancet 2004;363:1209–19.

Ooi WW, et al. Update on leprosy in immigrants in the United States: status in the year 2000. Clin Infect Dis 2001;32:930–7.

Schmiedel S, et al. A Thai patient with generalised inflammatory skin disease 18 years after migration to Europe. Lancet 2006;367:1458.

Van den Daele A. Leprosy in a backpacker. J Travel Med 2006;13:57.

LEPTOSPIROSIS

Leptospirosis, a spirochetal infection acquired on exposure to contaminated urine of wild and domestic mammals, may take an acute febrile form or a hemorrhagic form associated with jaundice, renal failure, and aseptic meningitis. Leptospirosis is endemic throughout the world. Tropical countries show the highest rates of endemicity, owing to humidity and heat. Infection can occur throughout the year in endemic areas. These include mainly Southeast and South Asia, Japan, Australia, and the Pacific Islands, specific areas in West and Central Africa, Central America, and Europe. The organism enters through breaks in mucous membranes or in the skin. Direct contact with infected animal urine places the individual at risk, as well as swimming or bathing in contaminated water.

The incubation period of the disease ranges from 2 days to 3 weeks, with an average of 7 to 12 days. Infections may be asymptomatic or range to Weil's syndrome, which is characterized by fever, jaundice, renal failure, neurologic disorders, and hemorrhage. Conjunctival suffusion is common in the acute form. Skin rash may be seen on the trunk and occasionally the extremities. Frank meningitis is common in the acute form of the disease. Leptospirosis in its classic form is a biphasic disease with a leptospiremic phase followed by a noninfectious immune phase. The infection is diagnosed by demonstration of a fourfold rise in anti-leptospira antibodies in paired serum samples. Antimicrobial therapy may benefit, if initiated within the first 4 days of clinical illness. Intravenous penicillin is generally considered the treatment of choice. Short-course corticosteroids may help control the bleeding and hemorrhaging caused by thrombocytopenia.

Minimize risk by immunizing domestic animals, controlling their access to human water supply, and eliminating rodent and other hosts. Travelers should avoid rivers, swamps, and ponds that may have been contaminated by animal urine. Likewise, they should wear clothing that prevents contact with surface water. In contaminated areas, weekly chemoprophylaxis with 200 mg of doxycycline may prevent the infection. Vaccines against some serotypes (eg, *Leptospira interrogans serovar icterohaemorrhagiae*) are available for human use in many countries. Spirolept, for instance, must be given subcutaneously at days 0, 14, 120, to

180, with boosters necessary every 2 years. Such vaccines are not indicated for the usual travelers, but play a role in occupational medicine (eg, sewage workers).

Additional Readings

Haake DA, et al. Leptospirosis, water sports, and chemoprophylaxis. Clin Infect Dis 2002;34:40–3.

Mortimer RB. Leptospirosis in a caver returned from Sarawak, Malaysia. Wilderness Environ Med 2005;16:129–31.

Sejvar J, et al. Leptospirosis in "Eco-Challenge" athletes, Malaysian Borneo, 2000. Emerg Infect Dis 2003;9:702–7.

LYME BORRELIOSIS

Lyme disease is a tick-borne disease caused by *Borrelia burgdorferi*. The disease occurs in the summer in endemic areas in the United States, Europe, and Asia (Figure 36). It is characterized in the early stages by an expanding skin lesion, often with central clearing (erythema migrans), followed weeks to months later by joint, cardiac, or neurologic manifestations. Early skin manifestations are often associated with nonspecific musculoskeletal complaints, such as fever, chills, malaise, myalgias, and headache. Some patients show clinical evidence of meningeal involvement. Central nervous system manifestations may occur within weeks to months after the onset of the illness, including meningitis and encephalitis. Bell's palsy may occur in the same period without other neurologic findings, as well as cardiac involvement including AV block and myopericarditis. Arthritis may develop up to 2 years after onset, involving one or two large joints at a time. This form of the illness may persist to resemble rheumatoid arthritis with pannus formation and erosion of bone and cartilage in 10% of patients. Lyme disease is diagnosed only when the characteristic clinical picture presents itself. The organism has rarely been isolated from the blood early in the disease. Serologic diagnosis is generally the most effective way to confirm the infection. Treat with antimicrobials, including amoxicillin, penicillin, doxycycline, or ceftriaxone for 14 to 28 days, depending on the clinical picture.

A vaccine consisting of recombinant *B. burgdorferi* outer surface lipoprotein A (LYMErix), introduced in the United States was removed from the market because of limited use and concern about side effect profiles.

Additional Readings

Jensenius M. Threats to international travellers posed by tick-borne diseases. Travel Med Infect Dis 2006;4:4–13.

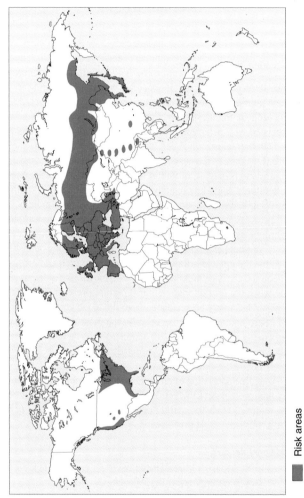

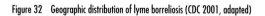

Risk areas

Figure 32 Geographic distribution of lyme borreliosis (CDC 2001, adapted)

MALARIA

Infectious Agent

Malaria, a protozoal infection, is caused by four species of the genus *Plasmodium*: *Plasmodium falciparum, P. vivax, P. ovale,* and *P. malariae.*

Transmission

These plasmodia are transmitted by the bite of an infected female Anopheles mosquito (Figure 33). Among 400 Anopheles species, some 80 will transmit malaria in different parts of the world, 45 of which are considered important vectors. Anopheles requires water for its early development, which can be found in rice fields, footprints, and lakes. The water may be fresh or salty, running or stagnant. The active flight range of an adult female is limited to about 1 mile, but passive dispersal by strong seasonal winds may transport Anopheles far from the place of origin. Biting times vary for these nocturnal mosquitoes, depending on the species, but bite protection should be used from dusk to dawn. Younger, uninfected mosquitoes may commence feeding at sunset. Anopheles will feed during the day only if unusually hungry. Following a latency period, the infected mosquito may inject plasmodial sporozoites from its salivary glands into the bloodstream of a human while feeding.

Malaria transmission occurs in most tropic and subtropic countries (Figure 34). About 40% of the world's population lives in

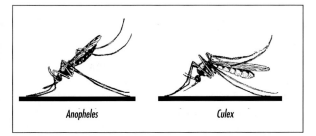

| Anopheles | Culex |

Figure 33   *Anopheles* and *Culex* mosquitoes

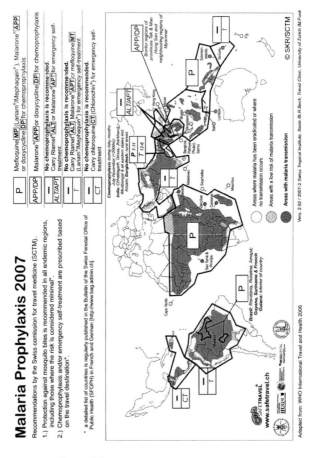

Figure 34 Malaria Prophylaxis 2007

areas afflicted with endemic malaria. There are more than 400 million new cases of malaria yearly, resulting in 1.5 to almost 3 million deaths, mainly in African infants and children but often in pregnant women. Mortality is related to the distribution of

P. falciparum, which is predominant in tropical Africa, eastern Asia, the South Pacific, and the Amazon Basin. The malaria situation is worsening in many areas of the world.

Although malaria is also transmitted in most urban centers in Africa and India, this is not the case for cities in Latin America and Southeast Asia, or for many tourist destinations in endemic regions (see Figure 38). Risk of malaria transmission decreases at altitudes over 1,500 meters but may occur at altitudes up to 3,000 meters in hotter areas. Transmission is highest at the end of the rainy season.

The United Arab Emirates succeeded in wiping out malaria; it was declared malaria-free at end of 2002.

Risk for Travelers

More than 15,000 cases of malaria are imported to non-endemic countries yearly. This is considered a low estimate, due to inadequate reporting. There are an additional unknown number of cases treated abroad. The risk of acquiring malaria depends on the area visited: the degree of endemicity, the predominant *Plasmodium* species, distribution of resistance, season, type of area visited (urban or rural), type of accommodation (air-conditioned or screened indoor versus outdoor) and, most importantly, duration of exposure, preventive measures taken, and individual behavior.

The risk for nonimmune travelers varies enormously among countries and even within a country (see country maps, Appendix B). Risk is highest in some Pacific islands, Papua New Guinea, and tropical Africa. For travelers with no chemoprophylaxis, the risk of symptomatic malaria infection is estimated to be 2.4% per month of stay in West Africa and 1.5% in East Africa. The incidence of malaria cases imported from West Africa varies: < 200 cases per 100,000 travelers in Senegal and Gabon; 200 to 399 in Burkina Faso, Ivory Coast, and Cameroon; and from 400 to more than 700 in Togo, Mali, Guinea, Benin, Congo-Zaire, and the Central African Republic.

Seroepidemiologic surveys using *P. falciparum* circumsporozoite antibodies indicate a high rate of infection in travelers returning from sub-Saharan Africa. Antibodies were detected in the sera of more than 20% of travelers who had visited Kenya for 2 to 16 weeks, with individual travelers at a 8.7 times greater risk (48.8%), compared with those on package tours (5.6%).

There is a low to intermediate risk on the Indian subcontinent. There is low risk of transmission in frequently visited tourist destinations in Latin America and Southeast Asia, but some areas of Brazil, India, and Thailand have a considerable risk. Differing meteorological conditions may cause annual and seasonal fluctuations.

There have been rare cases of malaria contracted by non-travelers living near international airports ("airport malaria"), by passengers aboard a plane touching down at an airport in an endemic area ("runway malaria"). Further, "harbor," "taxi," "minibus," and "luggage malaria" have been anecdotally described, and such unusual transmission cases are now collectively known as "Odyssean" malaria. Malaria may also be transmitted by infected blood, placing intravenous drug users, laboratory staff, and recipients of transfusions and transplants at risk.

Clinical Picture

Initial malaria symptoms may be mild, particularly in travelers who use chemoprophylaxis. There is usually fever and possibly headache, myalgias (muscular pain), vomiting, diarrhea, and cough. Malaria may be subjectively indistinguishable from influenza. Clinical symptoms such as fever are caused principally by the rupture of large numbers of erythrocytic schizonts in the erythrocytic cycle. Symptoms may or may not occur with classic periodicity. In the most serious forms, such as malaria tropica resulting from *P. falciparum* infection, complications may occur 24 hours after onset of symptoms or later. These include cerebral malaria with initial signs of confusion, drowsiness, and disorientation, followed by coma, or anemia, pulmonary edema, circulatory failure, renal failure, jaundice, acidosis, and hemorrhages. Infected red blood cells deform and rosette (become sticky) before rupturing, resulting in capillary clotting and some of the complications described. Immunologic responses, changes in regional blood flow, and biochemical systemic complications also occur. The case fatality rate for *P. falciparum* infections in developed countries ranges from 0.5 to 7%. It is close to zero for malaria caused by other *Plasmodium* species.

Incubation

Sporozoites infect hepatocytes in the human liver. There they develop and multiply. After a minimum incubation period of 6 days for *P. falciparum*, asexual parasites are released from the liver to invade red blood cells, where they grow and multiply cyclically (see Figure 14).

The incubation period usually ranges from 6 to 14 days for *P. falciparum*. For *P. vivax* the incubation period is longer; according to the experience of Soviet troops in Afghanistan, 60% became apparent within 20 weeks, and 97% within a year. There may be an incubation period exceeding 1 year for *P. ovale*.

Communicability

Untreated, or inadequately treated, patients can be a source of infection for 1 year or longer (eg, through blood transfusion).

Susceptibility and Resistance

Susceptibility is general, except for reduced susceptibility in those with certain genetic traits, such as sickle cell trait or the absence of Duffy factor in the erythrocytes. There is no complete immunity after infection but a semi-immunity as observed in the native population or in long-term residents with continuous exposure to parasites, may persist for approximately 1 year. Those leaving endemic areas soon lose their semi-immunity and become susceptible to malarial infection again. Some immunologic memory is, however, retained, which can reduce the severity of symptoms, if the individual becomes infected. Children born in non-endemic areas to settled immigrants have no semi-immunity and constitute a high-risk group for malaria acquisition.

Not only *P. falciparum* have become resistant to some of the antimalarials (eg, chloroquine-resistant *P. falciparum* [CRPF]) but also *P. vivax*.

Minimized Exposure in Travelers

Take personal protection measures against mosquito bites as described in Part 1 (see "Basics of Malaria Prophylaxis").

Chemoprophylaxis

Atovaquone and Proguanil

Pharmacology

Description: atovaquone is a hydroxynaphthoquinone used in a fixed-dose combination with the dihydrofolate antagonist proguanil (see "Proguanil" below). Available in tablet form as Malarone, containing 250 mg atovaquone and 100 mg proguanil hydrochloride. In the United States and in some European countries, pediatric tablets (62.5 mg atovaquone and 25 mg proguanil) are available for children weighing > 11 kg.

Mode of action: atovaquone affects mitochondrial electron transport leading to reduced pyrimidine nucleotide pools and decreased nucleic acid synthesis. Atovaquone is a schizonticide. Proguanil has a slow erythrocytic action but is highly effective against the pre-erythrocytic forms and has sporontocidal effects on *P. falciparum*. It is less active against *P. vivax*. Combining atovaquone and proguanil works synergistically against the erythrocytic stages of all Plasmodia parasites and the liver stage of *P. falciparum*. The combination is not active against the hypnozoites of *P. vivax* and *P. ovale*.

Pharmacokinetics: atovaquone is highly lipophilic with relatively poor oral bioavailability. The drug should be administered with food for increased absorption and bioavailability. In the plasma, atovaquone is highly protein bound (> 99%) and has a lengthy elimination half-life of 50 to 70 hours in adults and 24 to 48 hours in children. Persons with severe renal insufficiency (creatinine clearance < 30 mL/min) should not use atovaquone/proguanil, because of potentially elevated cycloguanil levels and decreased atovaquone levels. Excretion is almost exclusively through the feces (> 90%).

Administration

Dosage: one standard tablet daily for adults, starting 24 hours prior to arrival in the endemic area , during exposure in endemic areas, and for 7 days after leaving the malarious area only, due to the causal activity of the combination. Some countries have limits regarding the duration of intake. The individual should take the dose at the same time each day with food or a milky drink to ensure maximum absorption. In the event of vomiting within 1 hour of dosing, a repeat dose should be taken. Similarly, pediatric travelers should take 1 (if up to 20 kg of body weight), or 2 (if 21 to 30 kg body weight), or 3 (if 31 to 40 kg body weight) pediatric malarone junior tablets as a single dose daily.

Availability: the drug is currently approved in many countries for malaria treatment and prophylaxis.

Protection

Efficacy: the combination is effective against malaria isolates that are resistant to other drugs; three randomized, controlled chemoprophylaxis studies in semi-immune residents in Kenya, Zambia, and Gabon showed a 98% overall efficacy of atovaquone/proguanil in the prevention of *P. falciparum* (Pf) malaria. Atovaquone/proguanil was 100% effective in Pf malaria prevention in studies involving nonimmune travelers. Some isolated cases of therapeutic failures with treatment courses of atovaquone/proguanil have been reported, and resistance in such cases was viewed to be associated with the cytochrome b gene of *P. falciparum.*

Causal prophylaxis: yes. Volunteer challenge studies have confirmed the causal activity of the atovaquone/proguanil combination.

Adverse Reactions

Adverse reactions occurring can be attributed to the constituents or their combination. Proguanil has the reputation of being a very safe drug at standard chemoprophylactic doses. Mouth ulceration has been reported and mild epigastric discomfort may occur. To date, atovaquone has been well tolerated. The most common adverse reactions to atovaquone include headache, abdominal pain, anorexia, diarrhea, and coughing. In the chemoprophylactic studies performed to date, the drug combination was well tolerated, and in some comparative studies, was as well tolerated as placebo. Collectively, controlled trials in adults and children have shown that the tolerability of this combination is usually superior to other available regimens, and drug discontinuation rates are low, ranging from 2 to 5%. Serious adverse events include anaphylactic reaction, seizures in persons with a history of seizures, and hemolysis in a glucose-6-phosphate dehydrogenase (G-6P-D)-deficient individual.

Contraindications and Precautions

Absolute: the combination is contraindicated in persons with known hypersensitivity to atovaquone, proguanil, or any component of the formulation. The combination is also contraindicated in persons with severe renal impairment (creatinine clearance of < 30 mL/min). Safety in children weighing < 11 kg (in countries where no pediatric formulation is marketed, 40 kg) and in pregnant or lactating women has not been established.

Interactions

Avoid administering the combination concomitantly with tetracycline, rifabutin, metoclopramide or rifampin; this leads to significantly reduced plasma concentrations of atovaquone.

Pregnant women: category B. There is no evidence of teratogenicity in laboratory animals, but there have been no controlled clinical studies.

Lactating women: it is unknown whether atovaquone is excreted in breast milk; proguanil is excreted in small quantities. Do not recommend the combination for breastfeeding mothers.

Recommendations for Use

The atovaquone and proguanil combination is recommended increasingly for chemoprophylaxis in areas with chloroquine-resistant *P. falciparum* malaria. This option is particularly attractive for short exposure periods in view of superior tolerability and shorter duration of medication intake, compared with other chemoprophylactic regimens. For longer exposure periods, this option is expensive. This combination is one of two prophylactic drug regimens of choice in areas with multidrug resistance, such as the Thai-Myanmar and Thai-Cambodian borders, the other being doxycycline.

Azithromycin

Pharmacology

Description: semi-synthetic derivative of erythromycin with methyl-substituted nitrogen in the macrolide ring

Mode of action: inhibition of protein synthesis on 70S ribosomes. Azithromycin is a blood schizonticide and has been shown to have partial causal prophylactic activity in the human challenge model.

Pharmacokinetics: the drug is well absorbed, with 37% bioavailability after oral administration. Food may reduce the bioavailability of the suspension or sachet forms, but this is not clinically significant. Maximum plasma concentration is reached 2 to 3 hours after administration. Azithromycin has 10 to 100 times greater bioavailability in tissue than in serum. Protein binding is approximately 52%, and the drug is highly concentrated in the liver. Azithromycin has a half-life of 56 to 70 hours. Excretion is predominantly in the form of unchanged drug in the feces (88%) or urine (6 to 12%). Terminal plasma half-life ranges from 2 to 4 days.

Administration

Dosage: the dose for adults is 250 mg/d. Azithromycin can be administered with food. No data are available on pediatric doses for malaria chemoprophylaxis. Used as a malaria prophylactic, azithromycin requires daily dosing, starting the day before exposure, continued during exposure and for 4 weeks after departure from the malarial region.

Availability: available as Zithromax in capsule form (250 mg), suspension (5 mL containing 200 mg), and in powder sachets (100 mg, 200 mg, 300 mg, 400 mg, and 500 mg).

Protection

Efficacy: azithromycin had a causal prophylactic efficacy superior to doxycycline in rodents but only partial causal prophylactic efficacy in humans. One study has shown 100% efficacy for the regimen of 250 mg/d for 28 days after challenge, indicating that the combined causal and suppressive clinical efficacy of azithromycin is high. An efficacy trial in western Kenya showed 84% efficacy for azithromycin 250 mg/d versus 92% efficacy for doxycycline 100 mg/d. Studies conducted in Indonesia and Thailand have shown that the drug is particularly effective against *P. vivax* (98%).

Adverse Reactions

The overall incidence of adverse events with azithromycin is 12%, with < 1% of patients discontinuing treatment because of adverse reactions, including diarrhea (2 to 7%), abdominal pain (2 to 5%), nausea (1 to 5%), vomiting (up to 2%), allergic reactions (< 1%), and vaginitis (up to 2%). Photosensitivity, dizziness and headache have been reported.

Contraindications and Precautions

Absolute: azithromycin is contraindicated in persons with known hypersensitivity to the drug, with other macrolide antibiotics, or with adjuvants in the formulation, Likewise, it is contraindicated in patients receiving ergot alkaloids. Patients with liver or kidney insufficiency require dosage adjustments. Patients with severe hepatic disease should not receive the drug. Rare serious allergic reactions have been observed, as with erythromycin and other macrolides. Superinfection with resistant microorganisms is a possibility with all antibiotic treatments. Pseudomembranous colitis is possible in patients with diarrhea.

Interactions

Avoid administering azithromycin concomitantly with ergotamine or antacids. Monitor serum concentrations of cyclosporine and digoxin when administered with azithromycin. Like other macrolide antibiotics, azithromycin can potentially affect the cytochrome P450 system. No statistically significant interactions were observed, however, in pharmacokinetic studies with concomitant administration of theophylline, carbamazepine, methylprednisolone, terfenadine, or zidovudine.

Vaccination with live bacterial vaccines, such as oral live typhoid and cholera vaccines, should be completed at least 3 days before the first prophylactic dose of azithromycin.

Pregnant women: category B, with no evidence of teratogenicity in laboratory animals but no well-controlled clinical studies. It may be used during pregnancy if clearly required and if safer options are contraindicated.

Lactating women: no studies are available regarding excretion of azithromycin in breast milk.

Recommendations for Use

There is insufficient evidence to recommend azithromycin as an alternative stand-alone antimalarial prophylactic agent. Azithromycin presents an alternative option for children traveling to high-risk areas when chloroquine, mefloquine, or doxycycline are contraindicated. Pediatric dosage guidelines are required.

Future perspectives: it could be developed as a niche drug for target groups, such as pregnant women and young children, when other alternatives are contraindicated. The main disadvantage is the prohibitive cost of the extended prophylactic regimen.

Chloroquine

Pharmacology

Description: chloroquine is chemically classified as a 4-aminoquinoline. Preparations are available as phosphate, sulfate, and hydrochloride salts.

Mode of action: potent blood schizonticide. Highly active against the erythrocytic forms of sensitive strains of all four species of malaria. Gametocidal against *P. vivax*, *P. malariae*, and *P. ovale*. Activity is most likely due to the inhibition of the polymerization of toxic hemin into hemozoin.

Pharmacokinetics: oral bioavailability is approximately 90%. Peak plasma levels of chloroquine and the principal active metabolite desethylchloroquine are reached within 1 to 6 hours. Food increases the absorption and bioavailability of the drug. Chloroquine has a large volume of distribution and binds 50 to 65% to plasma proteins. The drug is eliminated in the urine. Elimination half-life is between 6 hours and 10 days. Terminal elimination half-lives of up to 2 months for chloroquine and desethylchloroquine have been reported.

Administration

Calculate dosage in terms of the base. Chloroquine base of 100 mg is approximately equivalent to 161 mg of chloroquine phosphate or 136 mg of chloroquine sulfate. Administer the recommended prophylactic regimen either weekly or daily. Pediatric solutions are available.

Weekly: the adult dose of 300 mg is administered once weekly. In infants and children, the weekly dosage is 5 mg/kg of body weight but, regardless of weight, it should not exceed the adult dose.

Daily: in some countries (mainly France), 100 mg base daily for adults or 1.5 mg/kg of body weight daily for children is prescribed.

Availability: worldwide. There are many well-known brand names such as Aralen, Avloclor, Bemaphate, Chinamine, Chlorquim, Cidanchin, Delagil, Gontochin, Imagon, Iroquine, Klorokin, Luprochin, Malarex, Matalets, Nivaquine, Nivaquine B, Resochin, Resochine, Resoquine, Sanoquin, Tanakan, Tresochin, and Trochin. — Also available as a combination tablet (chloroquine and proguanil) Savorine.

Protection

Efficacy: due to widespread chloroquine-resistant *P. falciparum*, chloroquine alone as a malaria prophylactic is limited to Central America, Haiti, the Dominican Republic, and the Near East. The effectiveness of the drug exceeds 95% in these areas. Chloroquine is active against other forms of plasmodia, with the exception of some resistant *P. vivax* strains in Oceania, India, Papua New Guinea, Southeast Asia (Indonesia and Myanmar), and parts of South America. In areas with considerable risk of CRPF, use an alternative chemoprophylaxis such as mefloquine.

Causal prophylaxis

None

Adverse Reactions

It is usually well tolerated at standard chemoprophylactic doses, although some studies have shown high rates of adverse events. Serious adverse events are rare.

Side effects include transient headache, gastrointestinal disturbances such as nausea, vomiting, diarrhea, abdominal cramps, pruritus, and macular, urticarial, and purpuric skin lesions. Itching of the palms, soles, and scalp is common in users with darker pigmentation.

Less frequent adverse events include loss of hair, bleaching of hair pigment, pigmentation of mucous membranes, tinnitus, hearing loss and deafness, photosensitivity, and neuromyopathy. Rare blood disorders, including aplastic anemia, agranulocytosis, thrombocytopenia, and neutropenia may occur. Hemolysis has been described in a few patients with G-6-PD deficiency.

Severe reactions include rare psychotic episodes, convulsions, hypotension, cardiovascular collapse, electrocardiographic changes, double vision, and difficulty in focusing. Corneal and retinal damage may occur, usually with prolonged usage or high dosages as used in rheumatology. Pigmented deposits and opacities in the cornea are often reversible if the drug is withdrawn early enough, but retinal damage with macular lesions, defects of color vision, pigmentation, optic nerve atrophy, scotomas, field defects, and blindness are usually irreversible.

Those using chloroquine long term should have ophthalmologic checks every 6 months, particularly when the total cumulative dose exceeds 100 g. Changes may occur after the drug is withdrawn.

Contraindications and Precautions

Absolute: use of chloroquine is contraindicated in persons with known hypersensitivity to 4-aminoquinoline compounds. Similarly, it is also contraindicated in persons with preexisting retinopathy, diseases of the central nervous system, myasthenia gravis, or disorders of the blood-producing organs. Persons with a history of epilepsy, psychosis, or retinopathy should not take chloroquine.

Caution is necessary when administering the drug to patients with hepatic disease, alcoholism, impaired renal function (dosage reduction may be required in patients with kidney impairments), porphyria, or psoriasis.

Chloroquine is toxic if the recommended dose is exceeded. Immediately induce vomiting if an overdose occurs. Admission to an intensive care unit may be indicated.

Pregnant women: category C, chloroquine is considered safe for pregnant women, either alone or in combination with proguanil.

Lactating women: the drug is excreted in breast milk but not in sufficient quantities to harm the infant or to protect against malaria.

Interactions

Concomitant use with proguanil increases the incidence of mouth ulcers.

Cimetidine inhibits the metabolism of chloroquine and may cause elevated levels of the drug in the plasma.

Administering live bacterial vaccines, such as oral live typhoid vaccines, should be completed at least 3 days before the first pro-phylactic dose of chloroquine. Chloroquine can suppress the antibody response to intradermal primary pre-exposure rabies vaccine, which should therefore be administered intramuscularly.

Avoid concurrent administration of chloroquine with drugs capable of inducing blood disorders, such as gold salts. Other possible interactions can occur with monoamine oxidase inhibitors, digoxin, and corticosteroids. The activity of methotrexate and other folic acid antagonists is increased by chloroquine use.

Recommendations for Use

Chloroquine, the drug of choice in areas without CRPF, is cheap and relatively well tolerated. See "Proguanil" below for the rec-ommendation of combination with proguanil.

Doxycycline

Pharmacology

Description: base doxycycline monohydrate. A 100 mg base is approximately equivalent to 115 mg doxycycline hydrochlo-ride. It is administered in tablets or capsules as the hydrochloride, or in syrup and suspension as calcium chelate or monohydrate. The gastrointestinal tolerance to doxycycline hyclate is clearly inferior, and thus this agent is not recommended.

Mode of action: slow but effective blood schizonticide of *P. vivax* and multidrug-resistant strains of *P. falciparum*. Weak activity against the pre-erythrocytic stages of *P. falciparum*.

Pharmacokinetics: doxycycline is highly lipophilic. After oral administration, the drug is almost fully absorbed and peak plasma levels are achieved within 2 hours. Thereafter, the drug is strongly bound to plasma proteins (90%). The half-life of doxycycline ranges from 15 hours after a single dose to 22 hours after repeated doses. Doxycycline is not significantly metabolized and is eliminated from the body in feces and urine. There is no significant accumulation of the drug in patients with reduced kidney function. Unlike other tetracyclines, concomitant administration of food or milk does not significantly decrease absorption of doxycycline.

Administration

Dosage: the dosage for malaria chemoprophylaxis in adults and children over age 12 years is 100 mg base daily. Daily doses of 50 mg doxycycline as used for acne treatment are probably inadequate against *P. falciparum*. Children aged 8 to 12 years, however, may receive 1.5 mg/kg daily.

Individuals should take doxycycline with plenty of liquid to avoid esophagitis.

Availability: worldwide under many brand names, including Vibramycin, Doxyclin, Biociclina, Doxacin, and Nordox

Protection

Efficacy: limited data are available regarding the efficacy of doxycycline for malaria chemoprophylaxis. Two trials have evaluated the efficacy of doxycycline in semi-immune persons in Kenya, and three trials examined nonimmune populations in Oceania. The overall protective efficacy in these trials ranged from 92 to 100%. In areas of multidrug resistance, such as the Thai-Cambodian border provinces of Tak and Trat, doxycycline is considered to be one of the most effective chemoprophylactic agents available. In the US Military Operation in Somalia, most malaria cases occurred in persons who missed at least one dose of medication, and parasite resistance to doxycycline does not appear to be a problem in malaria endemic areas.

Causal prophylaxis: insufficient causal activity. A human challenge study has shown that the agent's causal prophylaxis is inadequate against *P. falciparum* malaria.

Other: although the protective efficacy of doxycycline against travelers' diarrhea is small at most destinations, it may offer protection against less frequent infections, such as leptospirosis.

Adverse Reactions

Overall, in randomized controlled trials (RCTs), doxycycline is well tolerated, and serious adverse events are rare. Most commonly reported adverse events are gastrointestinal symptoms such as nausea, vomiting, and diarrhea, as well as rare, esophageal ulceration associated with older hyclate formulations. Other events include dizziness, headache, and skin rash. Overgrowth of resistant coliform organisms such as Proteus species, Pseudomonas species, and Campylobacter enteritis may occur and should be considered a possibility in persons with diarrhea who have been taking doxycycline. Reported diarrhea should also be distinguished from pseudomembranous colitis because of superinfection with *Clostridium difficile.*

Using doxycycline may result in overgrowth of nonsusceptible organisms such as fungi. Candidiasis, vulvovaginitis, and pruritus in the anogenital region may result due to proliferation of *Candida albicans.* Photosensitivity of the skin has frequently been reported, but the risk may be reduced by using appropriate sunscreens.

Permanent brown discoloration of teeth in children under age 8 years has been observed. Blood disorders have been reported occasionally. Hepatotoxicity, nephrotoxicity, erythema multiforme, intracranial hypertension, and lupus erythematosus have been associated with the use of tetracyclines.

Contraindications and Precautions

Absolute: the drug is contraindicated in persons who have shown previous hypersensitivity to any of the tetracyclines. The use of tetracyclines during periods of tooth development may cause permanent staining of the teeth and should be avoided in pregnant women during breastfeeding and in children under age 8.

Caution: advise doxycycline users to use an effective sunscreen (SPF > 15 and protective against both ultraviolet A and ultraviolet B rays) because of increased photosensitivity. The drug should be discontinued at the first sign of skin erythema. Individuals should avoid taking doxycycline before lying down; there is a theoretical danger of esophagitis associated with the drug.

Interactions

Concomitant administration of preparations containing aluminum, iron, calcium, or magnesium reduces absorption of doxycycline.

Complete vaccination with live bacterial vaccines such as oral live typhoid and cholera vaccines at least 3 days before the first prophylactic dose of doxycycline.

The mean half-life of doxycycline is reduced by concomitant use of alcohol, phenobarbital, phenytoin, or carbamazepine. Reduced dosages of anticoagulants may be necessary due to reduced plasma prothrombin activity. There are unconfirmed reports suggesting reduced activity of oral contraceptives during doxycycline intake. Fatal nephrotoxicity has been reported with concomitant use of methoxyflurane.

Pregnant women: contraindicated in pregnancy, due to interference with fetal bone and teeth formation. Evidence of embryotoxicity has been noted in animals treated early in pregnancy.

Lactating women: the drug is readily excreted in breast milk.

Recommendations for Use

Recommended as an alternative priority chemoprophylactic regimen in areas with considerable risk of CRPF, particularly when mefloquine or atovaquone/proguanil are contraindicated. The safety of long-term use of doxycycline (> 1 year) at the dosage of 100 mg daily is unknown; smaller doses have been used in acne therapy for years. Anecdotal experience from Spain in patients with Q fever endocarditis shows that doxycycline 100 mg daily is well tolerated for 5 years or more. Doxycycline is a prophylactic drug of choice in areas of multidrug resistance such as the Thai-Myanmar and Thai-Cambodian borders (see Figure 15). The use of doxycycline is currently increasing, and this will provide more tolerability and efficacy data required for civilian travelers, particularly women.

Mefloquine

Pharmacology

Description: mefloquine is a 4-quinolone methanol derivative structurally related to quinine. It is used clinically as a 50:50 racemic mixture of the erythroisomers. The commercial form is available as mefloquine hydrochloride in oral preparations only.

Mode of action: mefloquine is a potent, long-acting blood schizonticide that targets trophozoites and schizonts in particular and is effective against all malarial species. It is ineffective against mature gametocytes and intrahepatic stages. There is some evidence for sporontocidal activity. The exact mechanism is unclear, but the most plausible hypothesis points to hemoglobin degradation. Mefloquine is thought to compete with the complexing protein for heme binding. The resulting drug-heme complex is toxic to malarial parasites.

Pharmacokinetics: there is significant variation among individuals. Bioavailability of the tablet formulation is approximately 89%. Food increases the rate and extent of absorption, causing a 40% increase in bioavailability. The mean peak concentration in whole blood or plasma is reached in a mean time of 17.6 hours after a single dose. Mefloquine is distributed in the tissues, with extensive binding to plasma proteins (98.2%) and high lipid solubility. The mean volume of distribution is 20 L/kg, and the drug is cleared slowly from the body, resulting in a long terminal half-life of about 18 days. Studies in animals have shown that the drug is excreted primarily in the bile and feces. Carboxylic acid is the main metabolite, the concentrations of which exceed those of the parent compound by a factor of three to four. This metabolite is devoid of antimalarial activity. The pharmacokinetics of mefloquine are highly stereospecific, but its potential to cause adverse events does not appear to depend on the stereochemistry of the enantiomers or the concentration of the carboxylic acid metabolite.

Administration

Mefloquine has a bitter, slightly burned taste and should be taken after food to maximize bioavailability and thus optimize prophylactic efficacy. The food-enhanced drug absorption has been attributed to stimulated gastric acid secretion and delayed gastric emptying, enhanced intestinal motility, and increased bile flow. Individuals should swallow the tablets whole, but tablets can be divided, crushed, and mixed with milk or jam for small children or for those with difficulties swallowing.

Dosage: the US mefloquine tablet formulation contains 250 mg hydrochloride, which is equivalent to 228 mg base, whereas elsewhere the tablets contain 250 mg base.

The recommended adult dose for chemoprophylaxis in adults > 45 kg is 250 mg base weekly as a single dose, translating to 228 mg base in the United States. Some concern exists that heavy

Table 11 Mefloquine and Survival

Risk in 21 Million Users in Africa, according to ROCHE files

No fatality associated with convincing evidence
20 probably / possibly associated cases

Benefit per 1,000,000 Users in Africa (assuming average 2 week duration)

Risk of Malaria (conservative estimate)	Infection (P.f.)		Death (CFR 1%)	
• without chemoprophylaxis	5000	⟍	50	⟍
• with mefloquine (efficacy 90%)	500	⟋ △ 4500	5	⟋ △ 45
• with CQ + PG (efficacy 75%)	1250	⟋ △ 750	12	⟋ △ 7

CQ = chloroquine, PG = proguanil

individuals may require more than one 250 mg tablet weekly to attain the required protective plasma concentration within the required time frame. This issue needs clarification.

Adults weighing < 45 kg and children weighing > 5 kg should take a single weekly dose of 5 mg/kg.

Travelers with last-minute bookings who are unable to take a first dose 5 days or more prior to departure may require a loading dose to attain levels of prophylactic efficacy. This consists of one 250 mg tablet daily for 3 days, followed thereafter by the usual weekly dosage.

Mefloquine can be used for long-term travelers, and good tolerability has been shown during use over 3 years and more. There is no limit to the duration of intake.

Mefloquine intake may begin at 2 to 4 weeks before travel, if the prescriber feels tolerability is questionable in a patient or if the compatibility of coadministered medications requires monitoring.

Availability: available worldwide as Lariam, Mephaquine

Protection

Efficacy: mefloquine is recognized as a highly effective antimalarial against *P. falciparum* strains resistant to other antimalarials. The minimal inhibitory chemosuppressive plasma concentration of mefloquine is estimated at 600 μg/L. Resistance to mefloquine has been reported and are lates of only 30% has been reported in the Thai provinces of Trat and Tak. Mefloquine resistance is also slowly developing in other areas of Southeast Asia, the Amazon Basin, and, to a lesser extent, in central and

West Africa. There are sporadic pockets of resistance in endemic regions of East Africa, although the effectiveness probably still exceeds 90% at tourist destinations. Failure of mefloquine prophylaxis despite proven adequate drug concentrations has been documented in some African countries.

Mefloquine is fairly effective against other *Plasmodium* species, primarily *P. vivax*, although it does not prevent relapse infections.

Causal prophylaxis
None

Adverse Reactions
Similar to other malaria chemoprophylactics, high rates of perceived adverse reactions (24 to 90%) have been reported. There is some controversy with respect to the tolerability of this drug. A meta-analysis of 10 RCTs found that rates of withdrawal and overall incidence of adverse events with mefloquine were not significantly higher than those observed with comparator regimens, but media claims have highlighted certain adverse events. The most frequent reactions to mefloquine are dizziness, nausea, and vomiting. So-called neuropsychiatric adverse events, such as vivid dreams, mood changes, and depression, have often been reported, particularly in women. Other reported reactions include muscle weakness and cramps, myalgia, arthralgia, fatigue, asthenia, malaise, fever, chills, and loss of appetite. Laboratory abnormalities, including transient elevation of transaminases, leukopenia or leukocytosis, and thrombocytopenia, have also been reported.

Several studies, including RCTs, suggest mefloquine causes fewer dermatologic reactions than do other antimalarials. Skin photosensitivity among American troops in Somalia was significantly lower for mefloquine users than for doxycycline users.

Neurologic reactions include vertigo, disturbed balance, headache, sleep disturbances, nightmares, and, less frequently, auditory and visual disturbances. Psychiatric events such as neurosis, affective disorders, hallucinations, delusions, paranoia, anxiety, agitation, and suicidal ideation have also been observed. Isolated cases of encephalopathy have been known to result from taking mefloquine.

The frequency of serious adverse central nervous system (CNS) reactions to mefloquine was 1 in 607 in a British study, 1 in 10,000 to 13,000 among European travelers, and 1 in 20,000 in Canadians surveyed. Reactions included seizures, disorientation, and toxic encephalopathy; the risk of attributable suicide is debated but is extremely rare. Rare severe cutaneous adverse reactions have been reported, including erythema multiforme and Stevens-Johnson syndrome.

Persons with a personal or family history of neurologic or psychiatric disorders appear to be at higher risk for such events. Women appear to have significantly more CNS events, compared with men, which may reflect higher mg/kg dosing for women. Persons receiving the standard weekly mefloquine regimen, with or without adverse events, show similar levels of mefloquine and its carboxylic acid metabolite. Other reports suggest that concurrent alcohol and/or drug abuse may play a role in those events. Reported cardiovascular events include circulatory disturbances, tachycardia, bradycardia, irregular pulse, extrasystoles, and other transient alterations in cardiac conduction.

Due to the long half-life of the drug, events attributable to mefloquine may occur up to several weeks after the last dose, but most adverse events occur early on in prophylaxis, and approximately 75% of these are apparent by the third dose.

Contraindications and Precautions

Mefloquine is contraindicated in persons with a history of hypersensitivity to mefloquine or related substances such as quinine, and is also contraindicated for those with epilepsy, psychiatric disorders, or active depression.

The World Health Organization (WHO) and various national expert groups advise persons involved in tasks requiring fine coordination and spatial discrimination (eg, pilots) to avoid using mefloquine prophylaxis. Studies, however, have shown no impact on fine coordination in healthy subjects who tolerated the drug.

Users experiencing anxiety, depression, confusion, or uneasiness during mefloquine prophylaxis should discontinue the regimen and seek medical advice and use another chemoprophylaxis. If mild AE occur, a biweekly dosage of 125 mg may be considered.

Interactions

Mefloquine and related substances (eg, quinine, halofantrine) should not be used concomitantly or consecutively due to an increased risk of cardiotoxicity—a life-threatening prolongation of the corrected QT interval—and convulsions.

Concomitant use of mefloquine with antiarrhythmic agents, β-adrenergic blocking agents, calcium channel blockers, antihistamines including H1-blocking agents, and phenothiazines could theoretically contribute to the prolongation of the QTc interval, but this does not constitute a contraindication.

Complete vaccination with oral live typhoid or cholera vaccines at least 3 days before the first dose of mefloquine.

Both a slight increase and decrease of the effects of anticoagulants have been noted but not to the extent that concomitant use would be contraindicated.

Pregnant women: category C. Studies of mefloquine prophylaxis during the second and third trimesters have shown no evidence of elevated maternal or fetal toxicity. The potential for teratogenicity in the first trimester requires further clarification, and mefloquine should only be used during this period if benefits outweigh potential risks. Women of childbearing age should avoid conception during mefloquine prophylaxis and for 3 months thereafter. However, a termination is not indicated if pregnancy occurs in this time frame.

Lactating women: mefloquine is excreted in breast milk. No adverse effects have been observed in breast-fed infants, but the amount is insufficient to protect the breast-fed infant.

Recommendations for Use

Mefloquine prophylaxis is recommended by the WHO, the Center for Disease Control and Prevention, and several European and other North American expert groups for travelers visiting high-risk areas with CRPF. It is particularly useful for long-term travelers.

Proguanil

Pharmacology

Description: available as proguanil hydrochloride. Tablets contain 100 mg hydrochloride, which equals 87 mg base. Dosage is expressed in terms of the hydrochloride. Chlorproguanil, a long-acting analogue of proguanil, has also been extensively used.

Mode of action: both proguanil and chlorproguanil are pro-drugs. Their activity results from the action of the metabolites cycloguanil and chlorcycloguanil, respectively. The drug is a dihydrofolate reductase inhibitor that acts by interfering with the folic-folinic acid systems. The main effect occurs at the time of nuclear division. The drug is a slow-acting blood schizonticide that acts on the erythrocytic forms of all malaria parasites. It is highly effective against the primary exoerythrocytic (hepatic) forms and thus makes an effective causal prophylactic. It also interferes with malaria transmission through sporontocidal effects against *P. falciparum*. It is less active against *P. vivax*.

Pharmacokinetics: proguanil is only available in oral formulations. It is rapidly absorbed, and peak plasma concentrations are reached in approximately 4 hours. Peak plasma levels of about 140 ng/mL are attained after a single oral dose of 200 mg proguanil hydrochloride. Proguanil is metabolized to cycloguanil and 4-chlorophenylbiguanide. The active triazine metabolite cycloguanil reaches a maximum serum concentration of 75 ng/mL after 5 hours. Plasma protein binding of proguanil is approximately 75%, and high concentrations occur in the erythrocytes. Blood concentrations decline rapidly, and proguanil is excreted largely unchanged (60%) in the urine, with about 30% as the metabolite cycloguanil and 10% as chlorophenylbiguanide. The elimination half-life of proguanil is 11 to 20 hours, and concentrations fall to an undetectable level one week after administration. Proguanil is metabolized in the liver to cycloguanil by the cytochrome P-450 system. There is considerable variation in individual ability to convert the prodrug to the active metabolite. About 3% of Caucasians are considered to be poor metabolizers of proguanil, and in some subpopulations in Kenya, the proportion is estimated to be as high as 35%. The prophylactic efficacy of the drug is therefore limited for certain groups due to inadequate circulating concentrations of the active metabolite.

Administration

Dosage: the adult dosage is usually 200 mg daily when combined with chloroquine (or 100 mg if in combination with atovaquone) and should be taken with water after meals. Several different dosage regimens are used for children, but the WHO recommends 3 mg/kg daily in combination with chloroquine. Tablets can be crushed and mixed with milk, honey, or jam.

Use of proguanil alone is not recommended. The current British guidelines indicate the only exception to that rule: proguanil (200 mg/d) can be used alone in areas without chloroquine resistance when that drug is contraindicated, as in epilepsy.

In some countries, Savarine, a combination tablet containing 100 mg chloroquine base and 200 mg proguanil hydrochloride combined in a single tablet taken daily is available. This should increase acceptability of, and compliance with, the combined chloroquine and proguanil regimen.

Malarone, a fixed combination containing 250 mg atovaquone and 100 mg proguanil is used for chemoprophylaxis and treatment of malaria (see "Pharmacology" under "Atovaquone and Proguanil" above).

Availability: proguanil is available in many countries (except the United States), usually as Paludrine. Combinations are available as above.

Protection

Efficacy: proguanil-resistant *P. falciparum* is widespread, which limits the drug's usefulness as monoprophylaxis at most destinations. Cross-resistance occurs with other antimalarials. There is improved protection with combination proguanil sulfonamide regimens, although a proguanil and dapsone combination on the Thai-Cambodian border resulted in unacceptably high infection rates. There is a high degree of proguanil resistance in Papua New Guinea and Southeast Asia. In East Africa, poor protective efficacy with 100 mg proguanil daily was experienced in 1984, but an increase to 200 mg daily resulted in a protective efficacy of 91%, which led the manufacturer to increase the recommended dosage to that amount. Publications estimate a protective efficacy in West Africa of only 50% for chloroquine alone (300 mg weekly or 100 mg daily), compared with 66 to 78% for the chloroquine/proguanil combination regimen. Studies in Kenyan school children showed varying protective efficacy, ranging from 36 to 77%. Dutch travelers to East, Central, and southern Africa in a randomized study showed no significant difference in the number of prophylaxis failures with three different proguanil regimens: 200 mg/d proguanil monoprophylaxis, 300 mg/week chloroquine with 100 mg/d proguanil, and 300 mg/week chloroquine with 200 mg/d proguanil.

Causal prophylaxis: yes. Proguanil is effective against preerythrocytic forms of *P. falciparum*.

Adverse Reactions

Proguanil is considered a safe antimalarial drug. Mouth ulcers in up to 25% of cases may occur, and some experts believe the addition of chloroquine exacerbates this tendency. Abdominal discomfort and nausea are also frequently reported. Other reactions include hair loss and scaling and a significant drop in neutrophils. Users of the chloroquine plus proguanil regimen experienced a 30% incidence rate of adverse events in a retrospective study of returning travelers, compared with an incidence of approximately 17% in users of monochloroquine regimens. Most RCTs have shown that the chloroquine plus proguanil combination is significantly less well tolerated than atovaquone plus proguanil, doxycycline, or mefloquine. Most of these events were minor.

Serious adverse events with the combination regimen are estimated to occur in 1 of 10,000 users.

Contraindications and Precautions

There is no known absolute contraindication for proguanil. Dosage adjustments are necessary in patients with acute kidney failure.

Pregnant women: category B. Proguanil has been used safely for over 40 years without any association with teratogenicity. Most experience has been with the older 100 mg daily regimen.

Lactating women: Both proguanil and its metabolite are excreted in breast milk.

Interactions

Use with chloroquine may increase the incidence of mouth ulcers. Complete vaccination with live oral typhoid or cholera vaccines at least 3 days before commencing chemoprophylaxis with proguanil combinations.

Recommendations for Use

Use in combination with chloroquine in areas where CRPF is a risk (other than Southeast Asia) only where more effective regimens are contraindicated. In the future, proguanil will most likely be used with atovaquone. Use of proguanil monoprophylaxis is rarely indicated.

Obsolete or Withdrawn Agents

Maloprim (a combination of dapsone and pyrimethamine) is sometimes used as a chemoprophylactic drug, especially among British and Australian travelers. Potentially fatal agranulocytosis has been associated with this regimen.

Other regimens previously used in malaria chemoprophylaxis include amodiaquine, frequently associated with agranulocytosis, quinacrine hydrochloride, and sulfonamide-pyrimethamine combinations (Metakelfin and Fansidar), which frequently caused serious adverse cutaneous reactions.

Immunoprophylaxis

Various candidate malaria vaccines are being investigated, but none are expected to be ready for travel health protection in the near future.

Self-Treatment Abroad

Most travelers are able to obtain prompt medical attention when malaria is suspected. Standby emergency treatment (SBET) is an option when malaria symptoms (fever, chills, headache, malaise) occur and medical attention cannot be obtained within 24 hours. Travel health professionals prescribing antimalarials for self-administration must instruct the traveler on the following:

- Recognition of malaria symptoms
- The importance of first seeking medical attention if symptoms occur no earlier than 7 days after reaching the endemic area
- That SBET is a temporary measure and that medical evaluation is imperative as soon as possible

Provide standby emergency treatment to travelers using agents of limited prophylactic efficacy, such as chloroquine with or without proguanil, for travel to areas where plasmodia are resistant to chloroquine. Travelers with no chemoprophylaxis visiting low-risk areas can also be provided with SBET, as well as those making very short, often repeated visits into malarious areas (eg, airline crews). Although the travel medicine expert should strongly recommend chemoprophylaxis for travelers visiting high-risk areas, the traveler sometimes refuses this option. They may have had a previous adverse reaction, the cost of the drug may be prohibitive, or their planned stay may be long-term. These individuals should be provided with SBET. Choice and dosages of SBET are given below.

Antifolate and Sulfa Drug Combinations

Fansidar, Fansimef, Metakelfin. These are no longer recommended as SBET.

Artemisinin (Qinghaosu) and Derivatives

Artemether, artesunate, arteether (see "Co-artemether" below)

Pharmacology

Description: these compounds are derived from the leaves of the Chinese traditional herb *Artemisia annua*, which has been used as a treatment for fever in China for over 2,000 years. The antimalarial properties of the qinghaosu compounds were rediscovered in 1971. Artemisinin is available as capsules or in suppository form. Artesunate is formulated in tablets or used parenterally for severe malaria. Artemether and arteether are oil soluble ethers that are suitable for intramuscular injection. Artemether is also formulated for oral administration.

Mode of action: chemically, these compounds are sesquiterpene lactones which contain an endoperoxide linkage, which is essential for their antimalarial activity. Artemisinin has been shown to be a schizonticide, but the exact mechanism of action of this drug and its more potent derivatives is poorly understood. Studies have shown that this group of drug compounds give faster parasite and fever clearance than any other antimalarial drugs. One property of the artemisinins that is important is their gametocidal effect, which could result in reduced transmission.

Pharmacokinetics: the compounds bind strongly to plasma proteins and red blood cells. In vivo, the derivatives of artemisinin are converted to the biologically active metabolite dihydroartemisinin, which reaches peak plasma levels in about 3 hours. Current data suggest a short half-life for artesunate (minutes) and

Table 13 Dosage for the Treatment of Uncomplicated Malaria in Adults and in Children Older Than 6 Montths

Artesunate (oral)	
Day 1	5 mg/kg as a single dose
Day 2	2.5 mg/kg as a single dose + mefloquine 15 to 25 mg base/kg
Day 3	2.5 mg/kg as a single dose
Artemisinin (oral)	
Day 1	25 mg/kg as a single dose
Day2	12.5 mg/kg as a single dose + mefloquine 15 to 25 mg base /kg
Day3	12.5 mg/kg as a single dose

longer half-lives (hours) for the oil soluble derivatives. Metabolites of dihydroartemisinin are excreted in the urine.

Administration

Oral preparations of artemisinin and derivatives are widely available in Asia and Africa, but their optimal use needs clarification. A possible combination with a long-acting schizonticide, such as mefloquine, would provide the initial fast artemisinin response, coupled with the prolonged action of mefloquine, to clear residual parasites. The national authorities in Thailand recommend a first-line treatment of mefloquine plus artesunate or artemether in areas with highly mefloquine-resistant malaria, and a new combination, Artequin, contains artesunate and mefloquine in a prepacked single blister for simultaneous coadministration once daily for 3 days (Table 11).

Availability: oral preparations for uncomplicated malaria are available in Asia and Africa, but there is concern regarding counterfeit drugs. Riamet is registered in Switzerland and in the UK.

Efficacy

Several studies have confirmed the accelerated parasite clearance and rapid defervescent action of this group of agents against *P. falciparum* and have shown a more rapid therapeutic response with the artemisinin group than with the combination drugs, which included quinine and mefloquine. A recurring and major problem with artemisinin and derivatives is the high recrudescence rate (45 to 100%) which occurs within 1 month after treatment. This problem can be reduced by combining a short course of artemisinin with a longer-acting antimalarial such as mefloquine. Resistance to these drugs can be induced in animal models, and treatment failures have been reported. Recent in vitro sensitivity tests indicated that isolates of *P. falciparum* from the Chinese Hainan and Yunnan provinces were resistant to this group of drugs. Use of these agents should be tightly controlled to minimize the potential for the development of resistance.

Adverse Reactions

This is considered to be a very safe group of drugs. Treatment of several thousand patients has failed to reveal any significant toxicity. Mild transient gastrointestinal symptoms, headache, and dizziness have been reported. Several studies have reported a drug-induced fever. Cardiotoxicity and dose-related decreases in reticulocyte counts have been observed, as have transient reductions in neutrophil counts. High doses produce neurotoxicity in large animals, and this is the main reason why regulatory authorities in some developed countries hesitate to approve these compounds.

Contraindications and Precautions

There are no known contraindications.

Pregnancy: qinghaosu compounds can cause rodent fetal resorption, even at relatively low doses. Experience in humans is limited.

Lactation: no data available regarding secretion in breast milk.

Interactions

There are no known interactions.

Recommendations for Use

Use of these valuable compounds must be controlled. They usually cannot be recommended in the developed countries because they are not licensed. When used as advised by medical professionals in the developing countries, however, they appear promising for safe and rapid treatment of malaria, particularly in sequential combination with a slower-onset, longer-acting antimalarials, such as mefloquine. In view of the short half-life, artemisinin compounds are never recommended for prophylaxis.

Atovaquone and Proguanil

(See "Pharmacology," "Contraindications and Precautions," "Adverse Reactions," and "Interactions," under "Chemoprophylaxis" above.)

Administration

The combination therapy with 250 mg atovaquone and 100 mg proguanil (Malarone) or with pediatric formulation (Malarone junior, 62.5/25 mg) has been approved in several countries for the treatment of acute, uncomplicated *P. falciparum* infection in adults and children who weigh more than 10 kg. The therapy dose of Malarone is divided over 3 days (Table 14). Persons should take the daily dose at the same time each day with a meal or a glass of milk. Pediatric tablets are available in some countries.

Efficacy

Several studies have confirmed the efficacy.

Recommendations for Use

This is an option for SEBT for all regions with endemicity of malaria, but in the few areas without CRPF, chloroquine is cheaper.

Table 14 Therapeutic Dosage of the Atovaquone Plus Proguanil Combination

Weight (kg)	Day 1	Day 2	Day 3
5 to 8*	2 tablets	2 tablets	2 tablets
9 to 10*	3 tablets	3 tablets	3 tablets
11 to 20**	1 tablet	1 tablet	1 tablet
21 to 30**	2 tablets	2 tablets	2 tablets
31 to 40**	3 tablets	3 tablets	3 tablets
> 40**	4 tablets	4 tablets	4 tablets
Adult**	4 tablets	4 tablets	4 tablets

*all tablets are pediatric strength
**all tablets are adult strength

Chloroquine

(See "Pharmacology," "Contraindications and Precautions," and "Interactions," under "Chemoprophylaxis" above.)

Administration

The total dose for the treatment of uncomplicated, chloroquine-sensitive malaria is 25 mg base/kg over 3 days (Table 15).

Efficacy

Chloroquine remains the drug of choice for the treatment of susceptible malaria; however, only *P. malariae* and *P. ovale* remain fully sensitive to it. The use of this drug as an agent for emergency self-treatment is currently limited due to widespread CRPF and *P. vivax*.

Table 15 WHO Treatment Schedule for Chloroquine

Weight (kg)	Age	Number of Tablets (100 mg base)			Number of Tablets (150 mg base)		
		Day 1	Day 2	Day 3	Day 1	Day 2	Day 3
5 to 6	< 4 mo	0.5	0.5	0.5	0.5	0.25	0.25
7 to 10	4 to 11mo	1	1	0.5	0.5	0.5	0.5
11 to 14	1 to 2 yr	1.5	1.5	0.5	1	1	0.5
15 to 18	3 to 4 yr	2	2	0.5	1	1	1
19 to 24	5 to 7 yr	2.5	2.5	1	1.5	1.5	1
25 to 35	8 to 10 yr	3.5	3.5	2	2.5	2.5	1
36 to 50	11 to 13 yr	5	5	2.5	3	3	2
50+	14+ yr	6	6	3	4	4	2

Adverse Reactions

The standard treatment dosage is comparatively well tolerated. Minor events include gastrointestinal symptoms, dizziness, and visual disturbances. Itching, rash, and psoriasis may occur. Rare neuropsychiatric reactions have been reported, including epileptic seizures.

Recommendations for Use

Indicated for the treatment of malaria caused by chloroquine-susceptible plasmodia. Chloroquine can be provided for standby treatment to travelers with destinations in Hispaniola, Central America, and the Near East.

Co-artemether

Pharmacology

Description: co-artemether (formerly CGP56697) is an orally administered fixed combination of 20 mg artemether, the methyl ether of dihydroartemisinin and 120 mg lumefantrine (formerly benflumetol), a novel aryl amino alcohol. This combination was developed in the 1970s in China by the Academy of Military Medical Sciences, Beijing, and is now produced by Novartis Pharma, Switzerland. For travelers' self-treatment, the combination artemether/lumefantrine Riamet is available and registered for emergency self-treatment indication. This combination is also on the WHO list of antimalarial drugs recommended for the treatment of uncomplicated malaria in travelers.

Mode of action: this new treatment agent has effective schizonticidal and gametocytocidal activity against *P. falciparum.* Potentiation between artemether and lumefantrine was detected in combination experiments, and it is proposed that use of the combination should reduce the speed of development of resistance.

Pharmacokinetics: artemether is rapidly absorbed, and there is improved bioavailability after postprandial administration. A broad inter- and intra-individual variability of the plasma concentrations of both components has been observed. Artemether is rapidly metabolized into the active dihydroartemisinin. Whereas artemether has a brief half-life of 2 hours, that of lumefantrin is 2 to 3 days in healthy volunteers and 4 to 6 days in patients.

Administration

Dosage: in nonimmune adults, 4 tablets each at 0, 8, 24, 36, 48, and 60 hours, for 24 tablets in total. In semi-immune adults, a course of 16 tablets at 0, 8, 24, and 48 hours is sufficient in areas without multiresistant *P. falciparum*. In children, the recommended dosage is as follows:

- 10 to 15 kg: 1 tablet each at 0, 8, 24, 36, 48, and 60 hours; 6 tablets total
- 15 to 25 kg: 2 tablets each at 0, 8, 24, 36, 48, and 60 hours; 12 tablets total
- 25 to 35 kg: 3 tablets each at 0, 8, 24, 36, 48, and 60 hours; 18 tablets total

Availability: Riamet is available in a few European countries. The same drug is available in many developing countries under the name of Co-Artem, but there are only 16 tablets per package, which is sufficient for semi-immunes, whereas nonimmunes need the full 24-tablet course. Note that shelf life is limited to a maximum of 2 years.

Efficacy

Dose-finding studies usually indicate good efficacy with a four-dose regimen, except in an area of multidrug resistance in Thailand, but six dose regimens were highly effective there. An RCT of co-artemether versus pyrimethamine and sulfadoxine showed that co-artemether is safe in African children with acute, uncomplicated falciparum malaria, that it clears parasites more rapidly than the comparator, and that it results in fewer gametocyte carriers. In mixed infections with *P. vivax*, additional therapy with 8-aminoquinoline is indicated to eliminate exoerythrocytic forms of the parasites.

Adverse Reactions

Frequent adverse events ($\geq 10\%$) include headache, dizziness, insomnia, abdominal pain, and anorexia. Less frequent (1 to 10%) were palpitations, prolongation of QTc without any clinical symptoms (7%), diarrhea, nausea and vomiting, pruritus, exanthema, arthralgia and myalgia, and, rarely ($< 1\%$), cough. Ototoxicity has been reported from Mozambique, but another study in Thailand did not confirm this effect. A slight elevation of alamine transaminase has been observed. Because of tiredness and asthenia, the ability to drive a car or to handle machines may be impaired.

Contraindications and Precautions

Relative contraindications in serious renal or hepatic insufficiency, known congenital QT prolongation, or conditions that may result in QT prolongation, such as specific cardiac conditions, hypokalemia, hypomagnesemia; for medication see "Interactions" below. Contraindicated also in severe malaria, as bioavailability, mainly of lumefantrine, may be insufficient.

Pregnancy: category C, no data available.

Lactation: contraindicated

Interactions

There are no known interactions, but avoid using Riamet concomitantly with halofantrine, quinine, antiarrhythmic agents (classes IA, III), H1-blockers such as terfenadine or astemizole. In contrast, no interaction with mefloquine has been noted.

Recommendations for Use

This is a novel option for treatment of uncomplicated malaria caused by *P. falciparum*. This combination treatment will be useful for the emergency self-treatment indication in travelers and is likely to offer fastest relief of all SBTs because of the artemisinin component.

Mefloquine

(See "Pharmacology," "Contraindications and Precautions," and "Interactions," under "Chemoprophylaxis" above.)

Administration

The split dose is administered as a first dose of 15 mg base/kg on day 1, followed by a second dose of 10 mg base/kg, 6 to 24 hours later. The table that follows shows the recommended WHO dosages (Table 16). Tablets for children can be crushed and added to jam or yogurt to disguise the bitter taste.

Adverse Reactions

The rate of adverse events in higher doses used for treatment are markedly elevated, compared with the ones in prophylaxis. There is an incidence of 30 to 50% of severe nausea and dizziness, but use of the split dosage reduces the incidence of dose-related adverse events, especially vomiting. Serious adverse events, particularly neuropsychiatric events, show a higher incidence after treatment (1 of 216) than after prophylactic use of the drug. The mechanism for serious neurotoxicity is unknown but may be dose-related, although serious adverse events have also occurred at relatively low plasma mefloquine concentrations. Because mefloquine has a long and variable half-life of up to 33 days, treatment with mefloquine or quinine in persons who are using mefloquine prophylaxis should only be performed under close medical supervision.

Table 16 Recommended Treatment Dosages for Mefloquine

Weight (kg)	Age	Single dose (15 mg base/kg)	Split dose (25 mg base/kg) First dose (15 mg base/kg)	Second dose (10 mg base/kg)
< 5	< 3 mo	NR	NR	NR
5 to 6	3 mo	0.25	0.25	0.25
7 to 8	4 to 7 mo	0.5	0.5	0.25
9 to 12	8 to 23 mo	0.75	0.75	0.5
13 to 16	2 to 3 mo	1	1	0.5
17 to 24	4 to 7 mo	1.5	1.5	1
25 to 35	8 to 10 yr	2	2	1.5
36 to 50	11 to 13 yr	3	3	2
51 to 59	14 to 15 yr	3.5	3.5	2
60 +	15+ yr	4	4	2

NR = not recommended

Recommendations for Use

Indicated for the treatment of uncomplicated malaria caused by CRPF, mefloquine can be provided for standby treatment to travelers with destinations in South Asia or in South America. When the destination is in tropical Africa, mefloquine is indicated as prophylaxis rather than an SBET drug. Exceptions would include the possibility of travelers using the less effective chloroquine plus proguanil chemoprophylaxis or in travelers using no chemoprophylaxis (eg, short trips as in airline crews, long-term residents, or refusal of chemoprophylaxis).

Quinine

Pharmacology

Description: quinine is the main cinchona alkaloid and has been used for more than 300 years in malaria therapy. Quinidine is a stereoisomer of quinine. It is available as the quinine salts, most commonly quinine hydrochloride, quinine dihydrochloride, and quinine sulfate. Each 10 mg salt contains approximately 8 mg quinine base. Quinine is most valuable in the treatment of severe falciparum malaria, when it must be administered parenterally. This section is concerned with the treatment of uncomplicated malaria only.

Mode of action: quinine is a highly active blood schizonticide and is also gametocyticidal against *P. vivax, P. ovale,* and *P. malariae.*

Pharmacokinetics: good oral bioavailability and peak plasma levels are achieved within 1 to 3 hours. Quinine is metabolized in the liver and excreted as the parent drug (20%) or its metabolites in the urine. The mean elimination half-life varies from approximately 11 hours (healthy volunteers) to 16 hours (uncomplicated malaria patients).

Administration

Quinine is no longer recommended as an SBET.

Availability: worldwide. Numerous preparations containing quinine salts are marketed.

Efficacy

Resistance to quinine is developing in some parts of the world, especially in Southeast Asia (mainly Vietnam and Thailand), where quinine is administered in a 7-day course with tetracycline. Despite the two-pronged approach, increasing recrudescence rates and decreased in vitro sensitivity have been noted. In a standby treatment setting, the probable success of a complex combination regimen therapy over a prolonged period of 7 days is questionable due to projected poor compliance. Rather, this treatment option is for malaria treatment under a physician's supervision.

Adverse Reactions

The adverse events associated with this agent are collectively known as "cinchonism," which consists of high-tone deafness, tinnitus, nausea, vomiting, dizziness, malaise, and vision disturbances. Other potential adverse reactions include hypoglycemia in persons with a high level of *P. falciparum* parasitemia. CNS and cardiovascular reactions have been reported, especially in cases of overdose. Other less frequent adverse events include skin reactions (eg, erythema multiforme), asthma, agranulocytosis, thrombocytopenia, hemolysis, and liver damage.

Contraindications and Precautions

Absolute: hypersensitivity to the drug and in the presence of hemoglobinuria during malaria or in persons with optic neuritis or myasthenia gravis.

Relative: caution is required in patients with atrial fibrillation or other heart disease. Avoid combining quinine with digoxin, and give with caution to persons who have been taking mefloquine prophylaxis or to persons who have received mefloquine therapy in the preceding 2 weeks because of possible cardiovascular toxicity. Quinine has been associated with hemolysis in persons with a G-6-PD deficiency. Caution is advised with diabetics and in persons with impaired liver function.

Pregnancy and lactation: quinine can stimulate uterine contractions and may cause abortion at high doses. Quinine is, however, considered a safe agent for the treatment of malaria in pregnant women who should, if at all possible, seek prompt medical attention for all febrile episodes. Quinine is secreted in breast milk.

Interactions

Interactions have been reported for digoxin, cimetidine, and mefloquine (see above).

Recommendations for Use

Quinine is no longer recommended for SBET; compliance and tolerability are delimiting factors.

Primaquine

Primaquine phosphate may be considered for radical cure of established infection with *P. vivax* or *P. ovale* malaria, also for presumptive anti-relapse therapy (PART), possibly also for primary prophylaxis where the drug is available. Persons using primaquine must demonstrate that they are not G-6-PD deficient. The adult dose is 30 mg per day for 14 days in PART, in prophylaxis starting 1 day before, during and 7 days after leaving the endemic area.

Obsolete Therapeutic Agents

Halofantrine (Halfan), a phenanthrene methanol antimalarial, is available in tablet form (250 mg) and as an oral suspension (20 mg/mL). Clinical trials have repeatedly established the efficacy of this agent against chloroquine-sensitive and chloroquine-resistant *P. falciparum*. Originally considered to be a very safe drug, one disadvantage was the agent's poor and erratic absorption. Mainly, however, the cardiotoxic potential of halofantrine has been established; sudden deaths have been associated with the therapeutic use of this drug, which led to the issue of the WHO statement "halofantrine is no longer recommended for standby treatment following reports that it can result in prolongation of the QTc intervals and ventricular dysrhythmias in susceptible individuals. These changes can be accentuated if halofantrine is taken with other antimalarial drugs that can decrease myocardial conduction." An electrocardiogram with normal QTc interval prior to departure apparently does not preclude the risk of a fatal adverse event with this drug.

Future Prospects

Pyronaridine, a blood schizonticide, is highly effective against multiresistant strains. Pharmacokinetic data indicate poor bioavailability. This drug has yet to be registered outside China.

Chlorproguanil/dapsone, a synergistic, low-cost combination, has been shown to be effective against pyrimethamine/sulfadoxine-resistant *P. falciparum* in healthy human volunteers.

Agents in early clinical development include tafenoquine (formerly etaquine, WR 238605), also deferoxamine (an iron chelating agent) and calcium antagonists including verapamil and promazine.

Agents in preclinical development include inhibitors of phospholipid metabolism and protease inhibitors that have blocked in vitro parasite development and cured malaria-infected mice. Malaria vaccines are many years away and are unlikely to offer sufficient efficacy for travelers. Studies in Mozambique evaluated a promising candidate malaria vaccine for children. However, they will be important—even with protective efficacy of just 50%. Approximately one million lives could be saved, mainly among African infants and children.

Principles of Therapy

The mainstay of malaria therapy is speed. Make the patient aware of symptoms to minimize "patient delay," and the consulted medical professional should promptly conduct diagnostic tests (not confusing malaria with influenza) to minimize "doctor delay." Provide therapy according to the circumstances, availability of drugs, and instructions in the specific country. Details of management are not discussed here, which a specialist in tropical medicine or infectious diseases should conduct after a definite species diagnosis has been established.

Community Control Measures

Notification to authorities (is required in most countries).

▊ Isolation or Quarantine

None.

▊ Contacts

Examine travel partners; they are often infected.

Additional Readings

Baird JK et al. Primaquine for prevention of malaria in travelers. Clin Infect Dis 2003;37:1659-67.

Chen LH, et al. Prevention of malaria in long-term travelers. JAMA 2006;296:2234–44.

Chiodini P et al. Guidelines for malaria prevention in travelers from the United Kingdom. HPA 2007. http://www.hpa.org.uk/publications/PublicationDisplay.asp?PublicationID=87

Hill DR, et al. Primaquine: report from CDC expert meeting on malaria chemoprophylaxis. Am J Trop Med Hyg 2006; 75:402–5.

Kain KC, et al. Malaria chemoprophylaxis in the age of drug resistance. I. Currently recommended drug regimens. Clin Infect Dis 2001;33:226–34.

Keystone JS. Reemergence of malaria: increasing risks for travelers. J Travel Med 2001;8 (Suppl 3):42–7.

Schlagenhauf P, et al. Tolerability of malaria chemoprophylaxis in non-immune travelers to sub-Saharan Africa: a randomised, double-blind, four-arm study. Brit Med J 2003;327:1078.

Schlagenhauf P. Travelers' malaria, 2nd ed. Hamilton (ON): BC Decker Inc; 2007.

Shanks GD, et al. Malaria chemoprophylaxis in the age of drug resistance. II. Drugs that may be available in the future. Clin Infect Dis 2001;33:381–5.

MEASLES

Infectious Agent

Measles is caused by the measles virus, a member of the genus Morbillivirus of the family Paramyxoviridae. It is the most infectious virus known to humans.

Transmission

Measles is transmitted by droplet spread and occasionally by freshly soiled articles.

Global Epidemiology

Measles occurs throughout the world but has become rare in the Americas due to vaccination campaigns. It has been possible to eradicate the American serotype, but imported serotypes still may result in outbreaks. During 2005, local and state health departments in the United States reported 66 confirmed cases of measles to the Center for Disease Control and Prevention (CDC), an incidence of less than one case per 1 million population. Thirty-four of those cases were from a single outbreak in Indiana associated with infection in a traveler returning to the United States. Only 2,106 cases were confirmed in Europe in 1996, but there was a resurgence in 1997, with 88,485 cases reported, 27,635 of them confirmed. Overall, 44 million cases were estimated by the World Health Organization to have occurred in 1995 (only 580,287 reported in 2005 due to incomplete reporting); 454,000 died in 2004, mostly children. Insufficient vaccination coverage was responsible for epidemic outbreaks in several European countries from 2002 to 2007, including deaths in the Netherlands, Germany, and the United Kingdom.

Risk for Travelers

In the United States from 1980 to 1985, approximately 100 measles cases were imported annually, accounting for 0.7 to 6.9% of the annual number of reported measles cases. Of these, secondary spread of infection occurred in approximately 20%. About 43% of reported cases were epidemiologically linked to exposure to an imported case. The importation rate varied from one to three cases in 1 million travelers when the destination had been Europe or Mexico to > 30 in 1 million when travelers had been to India or the Philippines. Cases in non-US citizens were considered non-preventable. Of the remainder, 44% had not been vaccinated, and 28% had occurred in children younger than the recommended age for vaccination or in people with a history of adequate vaccination. There have been reports of suspected transmission of measles during international and domestic flights.

Clinical Picture

Measles initially causes fever, conjunctivitis, coryza, and Koplik's spots. These initial symptoms are followed in 3 to 5 days by a red blotchy rash, beginning in the face. Complications include otitis media, pneumonia, croup, diarrhea, and encephalitis, more often observed in infants and adults than in children and more often in malnourished individuals. The case fatality rate is 0.3% in developed nations and usually 3% in the developing countries, but may reach 30% in some localities.

Incubation

There is an incubation period of 7 to 18 days before the onset of fever. The rash develops a few days later.

Communicability

The communicable period extends from slightly before the beginning of prodromal symptoms until 4 days after the appearance of the rash.

Susceptibility and Resistance

General susceptibility; permanent immunity occurs after illness.

Immunology and Pharmacology

Viability: live, attenuated
Antigenic form: whole virus strains—Edmonston-Enders, Edmonston-Zagreb EZ19. Schwarz strains usually used, minimum 1000 TCID50
Adjuvants: none

Preservative: none

Allergens/Excipients: variable, some with residual egg or human proteins, 25 µg neomycin per dose. Sorbitol and hydrolyzed gelatin added as stabilizer.

Mechanism: induction of a modified measles infection in susceptible persons. Antibodies induced by this infection protect against subsequent wild virus infection.

Application

Schedule: 0.5 mL subcutaneously (SC), preferably at age 12 to 15 months. Usually, a combined measles, mumps, rubella (MMR) vaccine is used.

Booster: a second dose is recommended in most countries not earlier than 4 weeks after the first dose or at age 4 to 7 years or 11 to 15 years. Routine revaccination with MMR is recommended.

Route: SC

Site: preferably over deltoid

Storage: store at 2 to 8 °C (35 to 46 °F). Freezing does not harm the vaccine but may crack the diluent vials. Store the diluent at room temperature or in the refrigerator. The vaccine should be transported at 10 °C (50 °F) or cooler and protected from light. The vaccine powder can tolerate 7 days at room temperature. Reconstituted vaccine can tolerate 8 hours in the refrigerator.

Availability: many products are available worldwide.

Protection

Onset: 2 to 6 weeks

Efficacy: induces neutralizing antibodies in at least 97% of susceptible children. Seroconversion is somewhat less in adults. Disease incidence is typically reduced by 95% in family and classroom cohorts.

Possibly, attenuated rubella vaccine given within 72 hours after exposure to natural measles virus will prevent illness but, if available, specific hyperimmune immunoglobulins are more effective in such situations. There is no contraindication to vaccinating children already exposed to natural measles.

Duration: antibody levels persist 10 years or longer in most recipients, with possible lifelong protection granted.

Protective level: specific measles neutralizing antibody titer of > 1:8 is considered immune, ≥ 300 mIU/mL (EIA) is now more commonly used.

Adverse Reactions

Burning or stinging of short duration at the injection site is frequently reported. Local pain, induration, and erythema may also occur at the injection site.

Symptoms similar to those following natural measles infection may occur, such as mild regional lymphadenopathy, urticaria, rash, malaise, sore throat, fever, headache, dizziness, nausea, vomiting, diarrhea, polyneuritis, and arthralgia or arthritis (usually transient and rarely chronic). Reactions are usually mild and transient. Moderate fever occurs occasionally, high fever (> 39.4 °C [103 °F]) less commonly.

Erythema multiforme has been reported rarely, as well as optic neuritis. Isolated cases of polyneuropathy, including Guillain-Barré syndrome, have been reported after immunization with vaccines containing measles. Encephalitis and other nervous system reactions have occurred rarely in subjects given this vaccine, but no causal relationship has been established.

Contraindications

Absolute: persons with known hypersensitivity to the vaccine or any of its components.

Relative: any acute illness. Persons with a history of anaphylactoid or other immediate reactions following egg ingestion for the vaccines with traces of egg protein (see below).

Children: safe and effective for children age ≥ 12 months. Vaccination is not recommended for children age < 12 months because remaining maternal measles-neutralizing antibodies may interfere with the immune response.

Pregnant women: contraindicated. Advise postpubertal women to avoid pregnancy for 3 months on theoretical grounds.

Lactating women: the vaccine-strain virus is secreted in milk and may be transmitted to infants who are breast-fed. In infants with serologic evidence of measles infection, none exhibited severe symptoms.

Immunodeficient persons: do not use in immunodeficient persons, including persons with immune deficiencies, whether due to genetic disease, malignant neoplasm, or drug or radiation therapy. Routine immunization of asymptomatic HIV-infected persons with MMR is recommended.

Interactions

To avoid hypothetical concerns over antigenic competition, administer measles vaccine simultaneously with other live vaccines or 1 month apart. Routine immunizations may be given concurrently.

Measles vaccination may lead to false positive HIV serologic tests when particularly sensitive assays (eg, product-enhanced reverse transcriptase assay) are used. This is related to the presence of EAV-0, an avian retrovirus remaining in residual egg proteins of most measles vaccines.

Recommendations for Vaccine Use

Children are routinely immunized against measles throughout the world, usually with the preferred combined MMR vaccine administered at age 12 to 15 months. In most countries, a second dose is recommended, the interval varying in the national programs.

In view of the increased risk of infection in developing countries resulting from complications in malnourished local populations, the age limit for children traveling to these areas should be lowered to 6 months for preferably a single measles antigen vaccine dose. Children vaccinated before their first birthday must be revaccinated (standard recommendations), ideally at age 12 to 15 months and upon starting school. Infants under age 6 months are usually protected by maternal antibodies.

For admission to schools in the United States, it is usually compulsory to provide proof of immunization against measles or of natural immunity. Recently, the Center for Disease Control and Prevention also recommended administration of MMR to all crew members of cruise ships lacking documented immunity to rubella. All adults should be immune to measles as well, but respective recommendations vary from country to country. In most countries, those born prior to 1956 or 1964 are considered immune. Almost all expert groups agree that adults with professional risk (eg, those working with children; health professionals) should be immune.

Self-Treatment Abroad

Supportive

Principles of Therapy

There is no specific treatment.

Community Control Measures

Notification is mandatory in some countries. Isolation is not practical in the community at large, but if possible, persons should avoid contact with nonimmunes for 4 days after the appearance of rash. Quarantine is not practical. Immunization of contacts may provide protection, if given within 72 hours of exposure. In addition, specific IG may be used within 3 to 6 days of exposure (plus vaccine 6 months later) in contacts who have a high risk of complications, such as infants age < 1 year, pregnant women, or immunocompromised persons.

Additional Readings

Center for Disease Control and Prevention. Measles United States 2005. MMWR 2006;55:1348–51.

Coughlan S, et al. Suboptimal measles-mumps-rubella vaccination coverage facilitates an imported measles outbreak in Ireland. Clin Infect Dis 2002;35:84–6.

De Barros FR, et al. Measles transmission during commercial air travel in Brazil. J Clin Virol 2006;36:235–6.

Rota PA, et al. Molecular epidemiology of measles viruses in the United States, 1997–2001. Emerg Infect Dis 2002;8:902–8.

MENINGOCOCCAL MENINGITIS
(MENINGOCOCCAL DISEASE)

Neisseria meningitidis, gram-negative, aerobic diplococci, are classified into serogroups according to the immunologic reactivity of their capsular polysaccharides, which are the basis for currently licensed meningococcal vaccines. Thirteen serogroups are recognized, but only five—A, B, C, Y and W135—are clinically important.

Transmission

Humans are the only natural reservoir of *N. meningitidis*. The nasopharynx is the site from which meningococci are transmitted by aerosol or secretions to others, from either cases or asymptomatic carriers. Rates of transmission and carriage are much higher among populations living in confined areas (military recruits, dormitories). The ability of rapid acquisition of meningococcal carriage due to close social mixing has been demonstrated among British students within as short a period as the first week at university.

Global Epidemiology

Globally, there are about 500,000 cases yearly, and, by far, more cases occur during epidemics. Serogroups A, B, and C are the predominant cause of meningococcal disease throughout the world, with serogroup W135 playing an increasing role, mainly in Africa.

Meningococci group A has caused two pandemic waves: the first affected China, northern Europe, and Brazil between the 1960s and the 1970s; a second wave began in China and Nepal in the early 1980s, hit New Delhi in 1985, and extended to Mecca, Saudi Arabia, during the annual hajj of 1987 when almost 2000 pilgrims developed meningococcal disease serogroup A. In the mid-1990s, an outbreak occurred in Mongolia. The most explosive epidemics have occurred in sub-Saharan Africa, with the highest number ever reported in 1996 with about 200,000 cases and 20,000 deaths. More recent epidemics occurred in the year 2000—2,549 cases in Sudan and 1,000 cases in Ethiopia. In 2002, a large outbreak was reported in Burkina Faso, with more than

13,000 cases and 1,500 deaths. The sub-Saharan meningitis belt appears to be extending further south. In 2002, the Great Lakes region was affected by outbreaks in villages and refugees camps, which caused more than 2,200 cases, including 200 deaths.

Serogroups B and C are the main causes of endemic disease in Europe, Northern America, and New Zealand. Rates of disease in the United States are about 1 per 100,000; in the United Kingdom, about 4 to 5 per 100,000; and in New Zealand, it has reached over 20 per 100,000. Before a nationwide vaccination campaign targeted on the dominating serogroup B strain was launched in 2003. Serogroup Y is increasingly reported in the United States, accounting now for about one-third of cases. Group Y disease causes pneumonia more frequently than strains of other groups.

Serogroup W135 was responsible for an outbreak in hajj pilgrims in 2000 and 2001. This outbreak generated particular interest, as W135 was not known to cause major outbreaks. Later, W135 was the origin of major outbreaks in the meningitis belt regions. The current distribution of the various serogroups is shown in Figure 36.

Risk for Travelers

Data on the risk of meningococcal infection for travelers are limited. In a questionnaire survey directed to health authorities in industrialized nations, the estimated risk among travelers to countries with hyperendemic disease was 0.4 per million travelers monthly. This reflects an overall small risk for travelers. From 1982 to 1984, an epidemic affecting over 4,500 local people occurred in Nepal. During that period, six cases of meningococcal disease occurred in tourists, with two deaths. All these individuals had trekked with, and been in close contact with, the local population. The best documented risk of meningococcal disease among travelers has been in pilgrims for Mecca and Medina in Saudi Arabia. In 1987, an outbreak affecting more than 1,400 pilgrims was reported (serogroup A). Upon return to their countries of origin, W135 disease occurred, in both 2000 and 2001, in contacts of returning pilgrims and also within the wider community. As a result of strict vaccination requirements in the Kingdom of Saudi Arabia, no more cases associated with the hajj have been reported in the past few years.

Clinical Picture

N. meningitidis causes a broad spectrum of diseases that range from transient fever and bacteremia to fulminant septicemia and meningitis. Despite treatment with appropriate antimicrobial agents, the overall case fatality rates have remained relatively stable over the past 20 years (at about 10%), with a rate of up to 40% among patients with meningococcal sepsis. Of survivors, 11 to 19% have sequelae such as hearing loss, neurologic disability, or loss of a limb. Symptoms of meningitis include sudden onset of fever, intense headache, vomiting, and frequently the appearance of a rash. Subsequently, delirium and coma may occur. Prompt initiation of antibiotic treatment is paramount.

Incubation

The incubation periods are 3 to 4 days, and, rarely, 2 to 10 days.

Communicability

Communicability persists until no meningococci are present in the discharge from the nose and mouth, which is the case within 24 hours following initiation of adequate antimicrobial treatment.

Susceptibility and Resistance

Susceptibility to the clinical disease is low and decreases with age. Underlying immune defects that may predispose to invasive meningococcal infection include functional or anatomic asplenia, a deficiency of properdin, and a deficiency of terminal complement components. Although persons with these conditions have a substantially elevated risk of meningococcal infection, infections in such persons account for only a small proportion of cases. In household contacts of cases with invasive disease, the risk of invasive disease is increased by the factor of 400 to 800. Smoking, as well as concurrent viral infection of the upper respiratory tract, increases the risk of transmission. Group-specific immunity follows even subclinical infections for an unknown duration.

Minimized Exposure in Travelers

Immunization and avoidance of crowded situations

Chemoprophylaxis

Possible with various agents (eg, rifampin, ceftriaxone, ciprofloxacin).

Immunoprophylaxis by Meningococcal Vaccines

Two different types of vaccines are available, polysaccharide and conjugate vaccines. A third type—based on outer membrane vesicles (OMV) against the epidemic strain-specific Group B—began testing in New Zealand.

Polysaccharide Vaccines

The traditional meningococcal vaccines are polysaccharide vaccines. They are either bivalent (A and C) or tetravalent (A, C, Y and W135). Both group A and group C vaccines have documented short-term efficacy levels of 85 to 100% in older children and adults. Group C vaccines, however, do not prevent disease in children under 2 years of age, and the efficacy of group A vaccine in children under 1 year of age is unclear. Group Y and W135 polysaccharides have been shown to be immunogenic only in children over 2 years of age.

Polysaccharide meningococcal vaccines such as the currently available bivalent and quadrivalent vaccines have several shortcomings. First, they induce only a relatively short-life, T cell independent antibody response with short-life protection. Second, they are not effective in children under age 2 years. Third, they can induce hyporesponsiveness to serogroup C after repeated vaccination, but the clinical significance of this is unclear. Fourth, they do not prevent meningococcal carriage and, thus, do not increase herd immunity.

Immunology and Pharmacology

Viability: inactivated

Antigenic form: capsular polysaccharide fragments from *N. meningitidis*, groups A, C, in some vaccines also Y, and W135 containing 50 µg each.

Adjuvants: none

Preservative: 0.01% thimerosal in some vaccines

Allergens/Excipiens: none / 2.5 to 5 mg lactose per 0.5 mL

Mechanism: induction of protective bactericidal antibodies

Application

Schedule: 0.5 mL as a single dose. Some manufacturers recommend a second dose in small children age < 18 months where no conjugate vaccines are available.

Booster: revaccination may be indicated, particularly in children at high risk who were first immunized at an age < 4 years. Revaccinate such children after 2 or 3 years if they remain at high risk. Subsequent doses will reinstate the primary immune response but not evoke an accelerated booster.

Route: subcutaneously, some intramuscularly; see package insert.

Site: over deltoid

Storage: store at 2 to 8 °C (35 to 46 °F); discard if frozen. Lyophilisate can tolerate 12 weeks at 37 °C (98.6 °F) and 6 to 8 weeks at 45 °C (113 °F). Shipping data are not provided. Some vaccines must be reconstituted. Use the single-dose vial within 24 hours after reconstitution. Refrigerate the multidose vial after reconstitution, and discard within 5 days.

Availability: various vaccines are marketed worldwide, either against groups C, A and C, or A, C, Y, and W135. No group B vaccine is yet commercially available, except in Cuba.

Protection

Onset: 7 to 14 days

Efficacy: group A vaccine reduces disease incidence by 85 to 95% and group C vaccine by 75 to 90%. Clinical protection from the Y and W135 strains has not been directly determined. Immunogenicity has been demonstrated in adults and children age > 2 years. Meningococcal vaccine is unlikely to be effective in infants and very young children because of insufficient immunogenicity at this age. The vaccine is not effective against serogroup B, the most common form of meningococcal infection in many developed countries, specifically in New Zealand, but also frequently occurring in parts of Asia and South America.

Vaccination does not substitute for chemoprophylaxis in individuals exposed to meningococcal disease because of the delay in developing protective antibody titers. However, the meningococcal polysaccharide vaccine has been effective against serogroup C meningococcal disease in a community outbreak.

Duration: antibodies against group A and C polysaccharides decline markedly over the first 3 years following vaccination. The decline is more rapid in infants and young children than in adults, particularly with respect to group C. In a group of children age > 4 years, 3 years after vaccination, the seroprotective rate declined to 67% from > 90%. Duration is 3 to 5 years, but most likely, only 2 years in young children.

Protective level: estimated to be 1 µg/mL anti-polysaccharide antibodies; not well established.

Adverse Reactions

Reactions to vaccination are generally mild and infrequent, consisting of localized erythema lasting 1 to 2 days. Up to 2% of young children develop fever transiently after vaccination.

Contraindications

Absolute: none

Relative: any acute illness

Children: not recommended for children under age 2 years, because they are unlikely to develop an adequate antibody response (see above for schedule). Serogroup A polysaccharide vaccine induces antibodies in some children as young as age 3 months, although a response comparable to that seen in adults is not achieved until age 4 or 5 years.

Pregnant women: category C. The manufacturer recommends that this vaccine not be used in pregnant women, especially in the first trimester, on theoretical grounds. It is unknown whether the meningococcal vaccine or corresponding antibodies cross the placenta. Generally, most immunoglobulin G passage across the placenta occurs during the third trimester. Use only if clearly needed.

Lactating women: it is unknown whether the meningococcal vaccine or corresponding antibodies are excreted in breast milk.

Immunodeficient persons: persons receiving immunosuppressive therapy or those with other immunodeficiencies may have diminished response to active immunization. Nevertheless, this vaccine is indicated for asplenic patients.

Interactions

Meningococcal vaccine efficacy was slightly suppressed following measles vaccination in one study. If possible, separate these vaccines by 1 month for optimal response.

Immunosuppressant drugs and radiation therapy may result in an insufficient response to immunization.

Conjugate Vaccines

The newer conjugate vaccines, in contrast to polysaccharide vaccines, induce a T cell dependent immunological memory. Therefore, the duration of protection is longer, and they can be administered to infants. In addition, they can overcome hyporesponsiveness, reduce carriage, and increase herd immunity. Monovalent serogroup C conjugate vaccines were first licensed for use in 1999 and are now incorporated in national vaccination programs in an increasing number of countries, but they are of little relevance in travel medicine and thus not discussed in detail in this manual. In contrast to group C polysaccharide vaccines, the group C conjugate vaccine elicits adequate antibody responses and immunological memory even in infants who are vaccinated at 2, 3, and 4 months of age. However, they do not protect against other serogroups.

More recently, a tetravalent conjugate vaccine (A, C, Y, W135) was licensed for the age group of 11 to 55 years in a limited number of countries. The advantage is coverage against a broader range of serogroups.

Immunology and Pharmacology

Viability: inactivated

Antigenic form: polysaccharide diphtheria toxoid conjugate vaccine that contains *N. meningitidis* serogroup A, C, Y and W135 capsular polysaccharide antigens individually conjugated to diphtheria toxoid protein.

Adjuvants: none

Preservative: none

Mechanism: induction of protective bactericidal antibodies

Application

Schedule: single 0.5 mL injection by the intramuscular (IM) route, preferably in the deltoid region. At the time of publication, the vaccine is only licensed for the age group of 11 to 55 years.

Booster: the need for, or timing of, a booster dose has not yet been determined.

Route: IM, in contrast to polysaccharide vaccines—not subcutaneously

Site: over deltoid

Storage: store at 2 to 8 °C (35 to 46 °F); discard if frozen.

Availability: at the time of publication, ACW135Y available only in North America

Protection

Onset: 7 to 14 days

Efficacy: vaccine efficacy was inferred from the demonstration of immunologic equivalence to polysaccharide meningococcal vaccine. Results from comparative clinical trials showed that the immune response to all four serogroups to the conjugate meningococcal vaccine was similar to that of the polysaccharide vaccine, for the age group of 11 to 55 years.

Vaccination does not substitute for chemoprophylaxis in individuals exposed to meningococcal disease because of the delay in developing protective antibody titers.

Duration: not well established yet.

Adverse Reactions

Reactions to vaccination are generally mild and infrequent, consisting of localized erythema lasting 1 to 2 days. The most commonly reported solicited adverse reactions were local pain, headache, and fatigue. In the United States, eight confirmed cases of Guillain-Barré Syndrome (GBS) after receipt of meningococcal conjugate vaccine (Menactra, MCV4) were reported to the Vaccine Adverse Events Reporting System (VAERS). Because available evidence neither proves nor disproves a causal relation between MCV4 and GBS, further monitoring and studies are ongoing within VAERS and the Vaccine Safety Datalink (VSD). The Center for Disease Control and Prevention continues to recommend use of MCV4 for persons for whom vaccination is indicated; the additional reported cases have not resulted in any change to that recommendation.

Contraindications

Absolute: none

Relative: any acute illness

Children: safety and effectiveness in children under 11 years (and adults older than 55 years) are in the process of getting established for the ACW135Y vaccine.

Pregnant women: category C. The manufacturer recommends that this vaccine not be used in pregnant women, especially in the first trimester, on theoretical grounds. Use only if clearly needed. Health care providers are encouraged to register pregnant women who receive the meningococcal conjugate vaccine.

Lactating women: it is unknown whether the meningococcal vaccine or corresponding antibodies are excreted in breast milk.

Immunodeficient persons: persons receiving immunosuppressive therapy or those with other immunodeficiencies may have diminished response to active immunization. Nevertheless, this vaccine is indicated for asplenic patients.

Interactions

Concomitant administration of Menactra vaccine with tetanus-diphtheria (Td) or with Typhim Vi vaccine did not result in reduced antibody responses to any of the vaccine antigens. The safety and immunogenicity of concomitant administration of Menactra vaccine with other vaccines have not been determined.

Immunosuppressant drugs and radiation therapy may result in an insufficient response to immunization.

Group B Vaccines

The polysaccharide capsule of the group B meningococcus is poorly immunogenic and, due to antigenic similarities with human tissue glycoproteins, concerns have been raised regarding possible autoimmune reactions following vaccination. Consequently, there has been considerable research into alternative vaccines to prevent group B meningococcal disease. Antibodies to outer membrane proteins (OMPs) that have bactericidal activity are present in convalescent sera, supporting the logic of vaccine development utilizing OMPs. Studies on the efficacy of group B OMV vaccines have so far mainly been produced by the Norwegian Institute of Public Health against the Norwegian epidemic strain (B:15:P1.7,16), by the Finlay Institute against the Cuban epidemic strain (B:4:P1.19,15), and by the Walter Reed Army Institute of Research against the Chilean epidemic strain (B:15:P1.3). The tailor-made New Zealand vaccine (based on the national specific serotype) is produced using similar technology to that used for the Norwegian vaccine. New Zealand has had more than a decade of widespread epidemic of group B meningococcal disease dominated by a single PorA subtype (P1.7b,4). Currently, a public health intervention is going on in order to control this epidemic in New Zealand, but this vaccine is not licensed internationally.

Recommendations for Vaccine Use

Vaccination with the ACWY quadrivalent vaccine is required for pilgrims visiting Mecca in Saudi Arabia for the hajj. Vaccination is indicated for travelers to the African meningitis belt (extending from Senegal to Somalia), especially during the dry season (December through June). Although bivalent meningococcal vaccine (against A and C) was recommended to general travelers in the past, in view of the recent W135 outbreaks, most advise giving

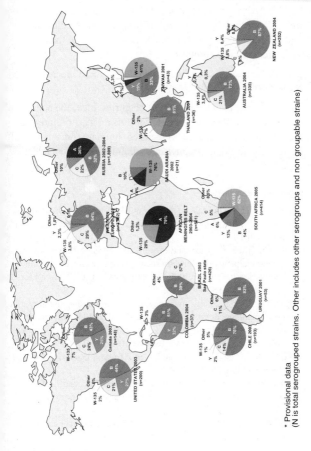

Figure 35   Global meningococcal serogroup distribution in the early 2000's.

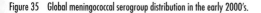

preference to quadrivalent meningococcal vaccine against A, C, W135, and Y in all travelers. Likewise, meningococcal vaccine is indicated in countries with recent or current meningococcal disease epidemics caused by a vaccine preventable subgroup. Offer immunization to all travelers with special risks (ie, asplenia, properdin deficiency; also to aid workers in refugee camps).

The American Committee of Immunization Practices recommends conjugate quadrivalent meningococcal vaccination for college students, especially first-year students and those living in catered-hall accommodation.

▌ Community Control Measures

Notification is mandatory in most countries. Place the patient in respiratory isolation for 24 hours following start of antimicrobial therapy. No quarantine is required. Intimate contacts should be actively traced for prophylactic administration of an effective antimicrobial agent.

Additional Readings

Aguilera JF, et al. Outbreak of serogroup W135 meningococcal disease after the Hajj pilgrimage, Europe, 2000. Emerg Infect Dis 2002;8:761–7.

Center for Disease Control and Prevenetion. Guillain-Barré syndrome among recipients of Menactra meningococcal conjugate vaccine—United States, October 2005-February 2006. MMWR Morb Mortal Wkly Rep 200;55:364–6.

Keyserling H, et al. Safety, immunogenicity, and immune memory of a novel meningococcal (groups A, C, Y, and W-135) polysaccharide diphtheria toxoid conjugate vaccine (MCV-4) in healthy adolescents. Arch Pediatr Adolesc Med 2005;159:907–13.

WHO. Risk of epidemic meningitis in Africa: a cause for concern. Wkly epid Rec 2007;82:79-87.

Wilder-Smith A, et al. Acquisition of W135 meningococcal carriage in Hajj pilgrims and transmission to household contacts. BMJ 2002;325:365–6.

Wilder-Smith A. Meningococcal disease in international travel: vaccine strategies. J Travel Med 2005;12:S22–9.

MONKEYPOX

Human monkeypox is a viral zoonotic disease that occurs mostly in the rain forests of central and western Africa. Monkeypox virus is similar to smallpox. The discontinuation of general smallpox vaccination in the 1980s has given rise to increasing susceptibility to monkeypox virus infection in the human population. With decreasing immunity to smallpox resulting, the incidence of monkeypox infection seems to increase as illustrated by an epidemic in remote parts of Congo-Zaire in 1997. The disease recently emerged in the United States in imported wild rodents from Africa. Monkeypox has a clinical presentation very similar to that of ordinary forms of smallpox, including flu-like symptoms, fever, malaise, back pain, headache, and characteristic rash. Given this clinical spectrum, differential diagnosis to rule out smallpox is very important. There are no licensed therapies for human monkeypox, although the smallpox vaccine can protect against the disease. Effective prevention relies on limiting the contact with infected patients or animals and limiting the respiratory exposure to infected patients.

Additional Readings

Meyer H, et al. Outbreaks of disease suspected of being due to human monkeypox virus infection in the Democratic Republic of Congo in 2001. J Clin Microbiol 2002;40:2919–21.

Nalca A, et al. Reemergence of monkeypox: prevalence, diagnostics, and countermeasures. Clin Infect Dis 2005;41:1765–71.

Norovirus/Norwalk Agent Disease

Infectious Agent

Norovirus (formerly Norwalk), a calicivirus; various genotypes have been identified. Another genus of the calicivirus family that can also cause gastroenteritis in humans is Sapovirus, formerly described as "sapporo-like virus" (SLV).

Transmission

Noroviruses are highly contagious, and as few as 10 viral particles may be sufficient to infect an individual. The viruses are transmitted essentially through the fecal oral route, but also environmental and airborne transmission from fomites has been suggested (eg, on cruise ships). No evidence suggests that infection occurs through the respiratory system.

Global Epidemiology

Worldwide, probably increasing, in industrialized countries reported mainly from hospitals, nursing homes, and cruise ships.

Risk for Travelers

The risk for travelers has not been systematically assessed, but it seems substantial, mainly during cruises. It also may be associated with the consumption of raw shellfish or other contaminated food or beverages.

Clinical Picture

Norovirus infection usually presents as acute-onset vomiting (mainly in children), watery non-bloody diarrhea with abdominal cramps, and nausea. Low-grade fever occasionally occurs. Dehydration is the most common complication, especially among the young and elderly, and may require medical attention. Symptoms usually last 24 to 60 hours. Recovery is usually complete, and there is no evidence of any serious long-term sequelae. Asymptomatic infection may occur in as many as 30% of infections.

Incubation

Commonly 24 to 48 hours; exceptionally, 10 to 50 hours

Communicability

During acute illness and up to 48 hours after diarrhea stops

Susceptibility and Resistance

Susceptibility is general, people of blood group O being at greatest risk for severe infection. There is variable, possibly strain-specific, resistance after infection limited to some months; serum antibody to norovirus does not correlate with resistance

Minimized Exposure in Travelers

Avoid contact with patients (see "Essentials of Maritime Medicine" in "General Strategies in Environment-Related Special Risks").

Chemoprophylaxis

None

Immunoprophylaxis

None

Self-Treatment Abroad

Supportive

Principles of Therapy

Antiemetics, fluids and electrolytes in severe cases

Communicability Control Measures

Provision of safe food and water is paramount. Noroviruses are able to survive freezing, temperatures as high as 60 °C, and have been associated with illness after being steamed in shellfish. Moreover, noroviruses can survive in up to 10 parts per million of chlorine, well in excess of levels routinely present in public water systems.

Despite these features, it is likely that hygienic measures, such as correct handling of cold foods, strict hand washing after using the bathroom and before handling food items, and paid sick leave, may substantially reduce food-borne transmission of noroviruses.

Prevention of norovirus disease spread via droplets from vomitus (person-to-person transmission) should focus on methods to limit transmission, including isolation precautions (eg, on cruise ships) and environmental disinfection.

Additional Readings

Isakbaeva ET, et al. Norovirus transmission on a cruise ship. Emerg Infect Dis 2005;11:154–8.

Ko G, et al. Noroviruses as a cause of traveler's diarrhea among students from the United States visiting Mexico. J Clin Microbiol 2005;43:6126–9.

Kroneman A, et al. Increase in norovirus activity reported in Europe. Eurosurveillance 2006;11:E061214.1.

PERTUSSIS

Infectious Agent

Bordetella pertussis

Transmission

Highly communicable respiratory illness—transmission by respiratory droplets

Global Epidemiology

Pertussis occurs worldwide, with disease rates being highest among young children in countries where vaccination coverage is low. Vaccination has reduced the rate of reported pertussis in the United States from 157 per 100,000, in the pre-vaccine era to less than 3 in 100,000. In the pre-vaccine era, virtually all reported cases occurred in unvaccinated children. Recently, the age of infected persons has increased, with about half of reported cases occurring in adolescents and adults. Recent studies have estimated the incidence of pertussis in adolescents and adults to be around 400 cases per 100,000 person-years in industrialized countries. In several series, pertussis was found as causative agent in 25% of cases presenting with prolonged cough. Pertussis is often underdiagnosed in adolescents and adults because it is not considered by general practitioners and it is often difficult to diagnose.

Risk for Travelers

The risk for travelers has not been studied, except in hajj pilgrims. There are anecdotal reports on pertussis in adopted children. The risk in adolescent or adult travelers is likely to be similar to that of the non-traveling population, but may be higher due to travel in crowded conditions or travel to developing areas where vaccine coverage against pertussis is suboptimal.

Clinical Picture

In classic disease, mild upper respiratory tract symptoms are followed by the development of a prolonged cough that becomes paroxysmal. Coughing paroxysms in children are often associated with vomiting; in younger infants, with apnea, hypoxia, and feeding difficulties. Fever is absent or minimal. In adolescents and adults, the signs and symptoms are less classical. The most common presentation is a persistent cough with a mean duration of 36 to 48 days. Complications in adults can arise from mechanical problems due to persistent coughing, which include rib fracture, hernia, incontinence, or back pain. Other complications are sinusitis, otitis media and pneumonia, or, rarely, encephalopathy.

Incubation

Commonly 5 to 10 days with an upper limit of 21 days

Communicability

Approximately 3 weeks

Susceptibility and Resistance

Susceptibility is general; usually, there is resistance after infection, but reinfection may rarely occur.

Minimized Exposure in Travelers

Avoid contact with patients.

Chemoprophylaxis

Prophylaxis with antibiotics for close contacts and high-risk contacts of such cases is generally recommended within 3 weeks of exposure, regardless of the age and vaccination status of the contacts.

Immunoprophylaxis with Pertussis Vaccines

Many combination vaccines against pertussis (either whole cell or acellular) exist; mainly the travel related issues will be discussed hereunder.

Immunology and Pharmacology

Viability: inactivated

Antigenic form: most acellular vaccines contain equal or similar parts of pertussis toxin (PT, inactivated to toxoid) and filamentous hemagglutinin (FHA).

Application

Immunization for infants and children up to the seventh birthday consists of five doses of DTaP (or tetra-, penta- hexavalent) vaccine. The first three doses are usually given at ages 2, 4, and 6 months; the fourth dose at age 15 to 18 months, and the fifth dose at age 4 to 6 years. If an accelerated schedule is required, the schedule may be started at 6 weeks of age, with the second and third doses given 4 weeks after each preceding dose. The fourth dose should not be given before the child is age 12 months and should be separated from the third dose by at least 6 months. The fifth dose should not be given before the child is age 4 years.

Adolescents and adults: the whole cell pertussis vaccine is contraindicated in this age group due to its reactogenicity. Acellular pertussis vaccine has been shown to be highly immunogenic, safe, and well tolerated in adolescents and adults. During spring 2005, two tetanus toxoid, reduced diphtheria toxoid, and acellular pertussis (DTaP) vaccine products formulated for use in adolescents (and, for one product, use in adults) were licensed in the United States (BOOSTRIX, GlaxoSmithKline Biologicals, Rixensart, Belgium [licensed May 3, 2005, for use in persons aged 10 to 18 years], and ADACEL, Sanofi Pasteur, Toronto, Ontario, Canada [licensed June 10, 2005, for use in persons aged 11 to 64 years]). Pre-licensure studies demonstrated safety and efficacy against tetanus, diphtheria, and pertussis when DTaP was administered as a single booster dose to adolescents. To reduce pertussis morbidity in adolescents and maintain the standard of care for tetanus and diphtheria protection, the Advisory Committee on Immunization Practices recommends that: 1) adolescents aged 11 to 18 years should receive a single dose of DTaP instead of tetanus and diphtheria toxoids (Td) vaccine for booster immunization against tetanus, diphtheria, and pertussis if they have completed the recommended childhood diphtheria and tetanus toxoids and whole-cell pertussis vaccine (DTP)/diphtheria and tetanus toxoids and acellular pertussis vaccine (DTaP) vaccination series (five doses of pediatric DTP/DTaP before the seventh birthday; if the fourth dose was administered on or after the fourth birthday, the fifth dose is not needed) and have not received Td or DTaP. The preferred age for DTaP vaccination is 11 to 12 years; 2) adolescents aged 11 to 18 years who received Td, but not DTaP, are encouraged to receive a single dose of DTaP to provide protection against pertussis if they have completed the recommended childhood DTP/DTaP vaccination series. An interval of at least 5 years between Td and DTaP is encouraged to reduce the risk of local and systemic reactions after DTaP vaccination.

Schedule: a primary series consists of three 0.5 mL doses.

Route: see package insert

Site: in the deltoid region. In infants and children the preferred site is the anterolateral thigh.

Storage: store at 2 to 8 °C (35 to 46 °F); do not freeze.

Availability: available in most countries, often included in five- or six-valent childhood vaccines; trivalent DTaP for adults.

Contraindications

Absolute: persons with a history of hypersensitivity to any component of the vaccine. Whole-cell pertussis is contraindicated for persons 7 or more years of age. Also see package inserts for the various products.

Relative: any acute illness

Pregnant women: category C. Use only if clearly needed.

Lactating women: problems in humans have not been documented.

Recommendations for Vaccine Use

The travel clinic may provide the opportunity to update the immunization status against pertussis for adolescents and adults.

Self-Treatment Abroad

None; medical diagnosis is needed for specific measures.

Principles of Therapy

Antibiotic therapy with a macrolide may ameliorate the cough illness if given during the catarrhal stage. Once paroxysmal cough has developed, however, antibiotics usually have no effect on the course of the illness but are recommended to limit transmission to others.

Additional Readings

Broder KR, et al. Preventing tetanus, diphtheria, and pertussis among adolescents: use of tetanus toxoid, reduced diphtheria toxoid and acellular pertussis vaccines recommendations of the Advisory Committee on Immunization Practices (ACIP). MMWR Recomm Rep 2006;55(RR-3):1–34.

Ward JI, et al. Efficacy of an acellular pertussis vaccine among adolescents and adults. N Engl J Med 2005;353:1555–63.

Wilder-Smith A, et al. Adult pertussis vaccine booster in travelers: knowledge, attitude and practices. J Travel Med 2007;14:145–50.

Wilder-Smith A, et al. High incidence of pertussis among Hajj pilgrims. Clin Infect Dis 2003;37:1270–2.

PLAGUE

Infectious Agent

Yersinia pestis

Transmission

Plague is an acute bacterial illness transmitted to humans by the bites of infected fleas, direct contact with infected animals (rodents, cats), or transmission of infected droplets between persons.

Global Epidemiology

Plague occurs infrequently on all continents, except Europe, Australia, and the Antarctic (Figure 36). Worldwide, 2,118 cases (including 118 deaths) were reported from nine countries to the World Health Organization (WHO) in 2003; however, there is considerable underreporting. The WHO Weekly Epidemiological Record regularly reports infected areas. The main foci currently are in:

Africa: Algeria, Democratic Republic of Congo, Madagascar, Malawi, Mozambique, Tanzania, Uganda;

the Americas: Peru; a few cases also occur in the United States each year; and

Asia: China, Kazakhstan, Mongolia, Vietnam.

An alleged plague epidemic in India in 1994 was extensively covered by the media and resulted in considerable hysteria in the developed countries. The epidemic, however, was due to a large extent not to plague but to various other infections. Such inadequacies in diagnosis mostly result from limited laboratory facilities.

Risk for Travelers

Plague is extremely rare among international travelers. Between 1970 and this writing, only a single internationally imported case had been reported, and that was in an American researcher who was investigating rats in Bolivia. Plague has occasionally been associated with recreational activities in California and, within the United States, a couple imported plague from Santa Fe, NM, to New York in 2002.

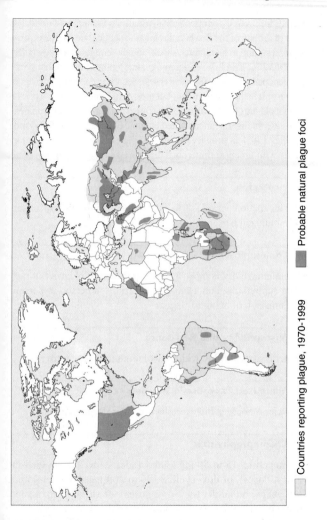

Figure 36 Geographical distribution of plaque

Clinical Picture

More than 80% of *Y. pestis* infections result in bubonic plague. Initial signs include unspecific fever, headache, myalgia, nausea, and sore throat, followed by lymphadenitis, usually in the inguinal drainage area of the site of the flea bite. Progress to septicemic plague is possible, resulting in meningitis, shock, and disseminated intravascular coagulation. Primary septicemic plague without detectable lymphadenopathy is rare (10% of all cases). Secondary pneumonic plague may result in the uncommon—but most dangerous—primary pneumonic plague (10% of all cases) by direct person-to-person transfer. The case fatality rate in untreated bubonic plague exceeds 50%, and reaches 100% in primary pneumonic plague. The prognosis is far better with timely antimicrobial therapy.

Incubation

The incubation period is 1 to 7 days and possibly slightly longer in immunized persons.

Communicability

Communicability is most feared in pneumonic plague, but pus from suppurating buboes may rarely result in person-to-person transmission of bubonic plague.

Susceptibility and Resistance

General susceptibility with limited immunity after recovery.

Minimized Exposure in Travelers

Travelers should avoid overcrowded areas during outbreaks.

Chemoprophylaxis

Tetracycline, 15 to 50 mg/kg/day (adults 1 to 2 g, divided in 2 or 4 doses), or doxycycline 100 to 200 mg/day in children > 9 years and adults (in 1 or 2 doses), or sulfamethoxazole/ trimethoprim 1.6 g/ day in 2 doses for adults, and 40 mg/kg/day for children above 2 months during and for 1 week once exposure ceases.

▌ Immunoprophylaxis by Plague Vaccine

The inactivated, whole bacterium *Y. pestis* vaccine is no longer commercially available. It is still routinely used in Kazakhstan and in some military settings.

Antibodies against capsular fraction 1 (F1) antigen were thought to be key in protection, but other factors may play a role. The schedule consisted of three doses in a primary series, with doses of 1 mL on day 0, 0.2 mL, days 30 to 90, 0.2 mL 3 to 6 months after the second dose being injected intramuscularly. Booster were given at 1- to 2-year intervals if risk persisted. The vaccine was not recommended for children because insufficient data were available.

Protective titers were recorded 2 weeks following the second dose in 90% of recipients and a 90% reduction in the incidence of bubonic plague occurred after the second dose. Efficacy against pneumonic plague was unknown. Vaccination often limited the severity of infection but did not completely prevent it.

Mild local reactions frequently followed primary immunization, with increasing incidence and severity following repeated doses. Sterile abscess occasionally occurred. Systemic effects were noted in 10% of cases.

Immunization is not required by any country as a condition for entry.

▌ Community Control Measures

Notification is mandatory according to International Health Regulations. Isolate patients, and give contacts chemoprophylaxis and place under surveillance.

Additional Readings

Fritz CL, et al. Surveillance for pneumonic plague in the United States during an international emergency: a model for control of imported emerging diseases. Emerg Infect Dis 1996;2:30–6.

Hardiman M. The revised International Health Regulations: a framework for global health security. Int J Antimicrob Agents 2003;21:207–11.

Williamson ED. Plague vaccine research and development. J Appl Microbiol 2001;91:606–8.

WHO. Standard case definition of plague. Wkly epid Rec 2006;81:279.

POLIOMYELITIS ("POLIO")

Infectious Agent

The infection is caused by types 1, 2, or 3 of the poliovirus, all of which can cause paralysis. Type 1 has most often been associated with epidemics or paralysis.

Transmission

The virus is usually transmitted through oral contact with feces, but where sanitation is good, pharyngeal spread becomes more important. Food and beverages contaminated by feces have occasionally been implicated.

Global Epidemiology

After the 1988 World Health Assembly resolution to eradicate poliomyelitis globally, the number of polio-endemic countries decreased from 125 in 1988 to six (Afghanistan, Egypt, India, Niger, Nigeria, and Pakistan) in 2003. However, during 2002 to 2005, a total of 21 previously polio-free countries were affected by importations of wild poliovirus (WPV) type 1 from the six remaining countries (primarily Nigeria) where WPV was endemic; four countries (Indonesia, Somalia, Sudan, and Yemen) had outbreaks of > 100 polio cases. By the end of 2005, WPV transmission in all 21 countries except Somalia had been interrupted or substantially curtailed. The current distribution of polio is shown in Figure 37; note that only Afghanistan, India, Nigeria, and Pakistan at no time had stopped polio transmission.

Risk for Travelers

Although it was estimated that, from 1975 to 1984, 1 in 100,000 travelers would be infected by poliovirus and that 1 in 3,000,000 would be paralyzed, the risk currently now is minimal. In the developed nations, poliomyelitis was occasionally diagnosed in immigrants. Two travelers imported polio to Germany in 1991, one returning from Egypt and one from India. The recent resurgence in the year 2005 of polio in Indonesia, Yemen, etc. is thought to have been due to importation and international travel, most

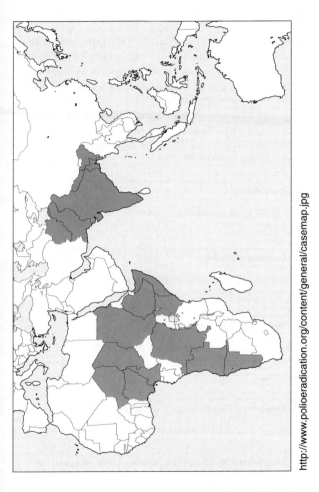

http://www.polioeradication.org/content/general/casemap.jpg

Figure 37   Countries reporting indigenous wild virus poliomyelitis (February 2006 to February 2007) Note: no poliomyelitis in the Americas and Europe

likely from countries that are still endemic, such as Nigeria, or through hajj.

Clinical Picture

Poliovirus infection occurs primarily in the gastrointestinal tract, spreads to regional lymph nodes and, in a minority of cases, to the nervous system to cause flaccid paralysis in < 1% of all infections. Infections may be accompanied by fever and, occasionally, by headache, vomiting, and muscle pain. Poliomyelitis, in many languages known as "infantile paralysis," is not limited to children. It may cause an even higher rate of paralysis and death in adults; the oldest patient diagnosed with a travel-acquired polio infection was over age 80.

Incubation

The incubation period for polio is 3 to 35 days (usually 7 to 14 days).

Communicability

Communicability extends from 36 hours to 6 weeks after exposure but rarely beyond that.

Susceptibility and Resistance

Susceptibility is common, but paralysis rarely occurs. Lifelong type-specific immunity results from clinical and subclinical infection.

Minimized Exposure in Travelers

Travelers should be immunized.

Inactivated Poliomyelitis Vaccine (Salk Vaccine)

Immunology and Pharmacology

Viability: inactivated

Antigenic form: whole viruses: serotypes 1 (Mahoney strain), 2 (MEF-1 strain), 3 (Saukett strain). Enhanced inactivated poliomyelitis vaccine (e-IPV) is a more potent formulation.

Adjuvants: none

Preservative: 0.5% 2-phenoxyethanol, < 0.02% formaldehyde

Allergens/Excipiens: < 5 μg neomycin, 200 μg streptomycin, or polymyxin B, each per 0.5 mL / none

Mechanism: induces protective virus neutralizing antipoliovirus antibodies, reducing pharyngeal and possibly fecal excretion of poliovirus after exposure to the wild virus.

Application

Schedule: a primary series consists of three 0.5 mL doses.

Children: most countries have national recommendations to follow (eg, in EPI schedules 6, 10, and 14 weeks). Essentially, separate the first two doses by at least 4 weeks, but preferably 8 weeks; they are in developed countries commonly given at age 2 and 4 months. Give the third dose at least 6 months (but preferably 12 months) after the second dose, commonly at age 15 months. Give all children who received a primary series of e-IPV or a combination of e-IPV and oral poliomyelitis vaccine (OPV) a booster dose of OPV or e-IPV before they enter school, unless the third dose of the primary series was administered on or after the fourth birthday. Most industrialized countries have changed to IPV-only schedules.

Adults: for non-vaccinated adults at increased risk of exposure to poliovirus, give a primary series of e-IPV—two doses given at a 1- to 2-month interval with a third dose given 6 to 12 months later. If < 3 months but > 2 months remain before protection is needed, give three doses of e-IPV at least 1 month apart. Likewise, if only 1 or 2 months remain, give two doses of e-IPV 1 month apart.

Give at least one dose of e-IPV to adults at increased risk of exposure who have had at least one dose of OPV that is equal to three doses of conventional IPV (available before 1988; in some countries, still the only available Salk vaccine). Or give a combination of conventional e-IPV and OPV, totaling an equivalent of three doses. Give any additional doses needed to complete a primary series, if time permits. Adults who have completed a primary series with any poliovirus vaccine and who are at increased risk of exposure to poliovirus should be given a single dose of e-IPV.

To complete a series of primary and booster doses, a total of four doses is required. Give incompletely immunized children and adolescents sufficient additional doses to reach this number.

Booster: the need to routinely administer additional doses is not apparent, except for exposed persons, such as travelers to endemic areas, who should receive booster doses every 10 years.

Route: subcutaneously or intramuscularly; see package insert

Site: in the deltoid region. In infants and children, the preferred site is the anterolateral thigh.

Storage: store at 2 to 8 °C (35 to 46 °F); do not freeze. Contact manufacturer regarding prolonged exposure to room temperature or elevated or freezing temperatures.

Availability: available in most countries, often included in fiv- or six-valent childhood vaccines.

Protection

Onset: antibodies develop within 1 to 2 weeks following several doses.

Efficacy: 97.5 to 100% seroconversion to each type after two doses. This e-IPV formulation is more potent and more consistently immunogenic than previous IPV formulations. Cases of existing or incubating poliomyelitis cannot be modified or prevented by e-IPV.

Duration: many years, precise duration still uncertain

Protective level: ≥1:8 serum virus neutralizing antibody titer

Adverse Reactions

IPV/e-IPV administration may result in erythema, induration, and pain at the injection site. Body temperatures at 39 °C (102 °F) or higher were reported in up to 38% of e-IPV vaccinees. No paralytic reactions to e-IPV are known to have occurred.

Contraindications

Absolute: persons with a history of hypersensitivity to any component of the vaccine

Relative: any acute illness

Children: e-IPV is safe and effective in children as young as age 6 weeks

Pregnant women: category C. It is unknown whether e-IPV or corresponding antibodies cross the placenta. Generally, most immunoglobulin (Ig) G passage across the placenta occurs during the third trimester. Use only if clearly needed.

Lactating women: it is unknown whether e-IPV or corresponding antibodies are excreted in breast milk. Problems in humans have not been documented.

Immunodeficient persons: e-IPV is the preferred product for polio immunization of persons who reside with an immunodeficient person. Use of e-IPV in children infected with the HIV virus outweighs the theoretical risk of adverse immunologic effects. Persons receiving immunosuppressive therapy or with other immunodeficiencies may experience diminished antibody response to active immunization with e-IPV.

Interactions

Use of routine pediatric vaccines and travel vaccines does not interfere with e-IPV. All immunosuppressant drugs and radiation therapy may cause an insufficient response to immunization.

Oral Poliomyelitis Vaccine (Sabin Vaccine)

Immunology and Pharmacology

Viability: live, attenuated
Antigenic form: whole viruses, Sabin strains 1, 2, 3
Adjuvants: none
Preservative: none
Allergens/Excipiens: < 25 µg neomycin per dose, 25 µg streptomycin per dose, calf serum / Sorbitol, phenol red, polygeline
Mechanism: the oral poliomyelitis vaccine (OPV) administration simulates natural infection, inducing active mucosal and systemic immunity.

Application

Children: this vaccine is used in most World Health Organization eradication campaigns but has become obsolete in most industrialized countries; even a minimal risk of vaccine that associates with paralytic poliomyelitis is unacceptable in countries that are polio-free. A primary series consists of three doses, starting optimally at age 6 to 12 weeks. Separate the first two doses by at least 6 weeks, but preferably 8 weeks; they are commonly given at age 2 and 4 months. Give the third dose at least 8 months, but preferably 12 months after the second dose, commonly at age 18 months. An optional additional dose of OPV may be given at age 6 months in areas where poliomyelitis disease is endemic. Give older children (up to age 18 years) two OPV doses, not < 6 weeks (and preferably 8 weeks) apart, followed by a third dose 6 to 12 months after the second dose. Give children entering elementary school who have completed the primary series a single follow-up dose of OPV. All others should complete the primary series. This fourth dose is not required in those who received the third primary dose on or after their fourth birthday. The multiple doses of OPV in the primary series are not administered as boosters but as catch-up doses to ensure that immunity to all three types of virus has been achieved in all who have not previously responded to any constituent of the vaccine.

Adults: the e-IPV (or where unavailable, IPV) is preferred for the primary series because adults are even more likely to develop OPV-induced poliomyelitis than children.

Booster: the need for routine additional doses of poliovirus vaccine has not been determined, except in exposed persons, such as travelers to endemic areas, in whom booster doses should be administered every 10 years.

In some countries, e-IPV is preferred if persons older than age 18 years need additional vaccination.

Route: oral

Storage: store in a freezer. After thawing, use vaccine within 30 days. Vaccine is not stable at room temperature. Do not expose to more than 10 freeze-thaw cycles, with none exceeding 8 °C (46 °F). If the cumulative period of thaw is > 24 hours, use the vaccine within 30 days. During this time, it must be stored at between 2 °C to 8 °C (35 ° to 46 °F). The vaccine is shipped at −18 °C (0 °F) or colder in insulated containers with dry ice.

Availability: worldwide

Protection

Onset: antibodies develop within 1 to 2 weeks following several doses.

Efficacy: > 95% of children who were studied 5 years after immunization had protective antibodies against all three types of poliovirus. Type-specific neutralizing antibodies will be induced in at least 90% of susceptible persons. The OPV is not effective in modifying or preventing cases of existing or incubating poliomyelitis.

Duration: the vaccine is effective for many years, although symptomatic poliomyelitis has occurred in travelers who had completed their primary OPV series and had the last dose at least 17 years prior to infection.

Protective level: ≥1:8 virus neutralizing serum antibody titer

Adverse Reactions

Poliovirus is shed for 6 to 8 weeks in vaccinees' stools and by the pharyngeal route.

Some report tiredness or fever.

According to US data, paralysis associated with polio vaccine occurs with a frequency of 1 case in 2.6 million OPV doses distributed. Of 105 cases of paralytic poliomyelitis recorded from 1973 to 1984 (in this period, 274.1 million OPV doses were distributed), 35 cases occurred in vaccine recipients, 50 in household and non-household contacts of vaccinees, 14 in immunodeficient recipients or contacts, and 6 in persons with no history of vaccine exposure.

Contraindications

Absolute: immunosuppressed patients or their household contacts. Use e-IPV in these cases, except in endemic countries where OPV may be preferred.

Relative: any acute illness, diarrhea, or vomiting

Pregnant women: category C. Use OPV in pregnancy if exposure is imminent and immediate protection is required.

Lactating women: breast-feeding does not generally interfere with successful immunization of infants, despite IgA antibody secretion in breast milk. In certain tropical endemic areas where the infant may be vaccinated at birth, the manufacturer suggests the OPV series be completed when the infant reaches age 6 months.

Immunodeficient persons: do not use in immunodeficient persons, including persons with congenital or acquired immune deficiencies, whether due to genetic disease, medication, or radiation therapy. Avoid use in HIV-positive persons, whether symptomatic or asymptomatic. Use IPV or e-IPV if available.

Interactions

There is no evidence of interaction between routine or travel-related vaccines (including oral Ty21a) and OPV, except that after co-administration with the first dose of an oral rotavirus vaccine, the seroconversion rate was reduced.

Recommendations for Vaccine Use

Polio immunization is routine worldwide. Until complete eradication is achieved, vaccination remains important for travelers visiting endemic countries. After completion of a primary series, administer a booster dose every 10 years to travelers going to countries where transmission of wild polio virus is still a risk (see Figure 38). Infected travelers may shed the virus while visiting areas where polio had previously been eradicated, which may lead to a resurgence of endemicity.

The Global Polio Eradication Initiative focuses now on 1) interrupting wild poliovirus transmission worldwide, 2) limiting the international spread of circulating polioviruses, and 3) refining the program of work for eventual cessation of immunization with oral poliovirus vaccine. There is no international unanimity about whether OPV or IPV is preferable. Travel health professionals should follow the recommendations that are valid in their country. In general, there is a trend toward IPV (or e-IPV where available) for several reasons: 1) to reduce the small, yet unacceptable, risk of vaccine-associated paralytic poliomyelitis from OPV; 2) to reduce environmental contamination with vaccine or wild virus; and 3) to reduce the risk of mutation of vaccine virus to wild virus.

Table 17 Advantages and Disadvantages of IPV and OPV

	IPV	OPV
Administration	Injection possibly combined with other pediatric vaccines	Oral, easy, cheaper
Cold chain	Less temperature sensitive	Cold chain needed
Effectiveness	Better in young infants in tropical areas	Serological response less in very young infants
Immunity, onset	≥ 2 doses needed	Rapid
Intestinal resistance	Low	High
Herd immunity	Limited	Yes
Vaccine related paralysis	None	Yes, rare — in recipients and contacts
Immunocompromised	Can be used	Contraindicated

Advantages and disadvantages of both vaccines are shown in Table 17.

Community Control Measures

Notification is mandatory by the revised International Health Regulations, thus, also in each country. Enteric precautions should be taken in hospitals. No quarantine. Immunization of contacts, and tracing the source of infection are required.

Additional Readings

Aylward RB. Eradicating polio: today's challenges and tomorrow's legacy. Ann Trop Med Parasitol 2006;100:401–13.

Center for Disease Control and Prevention. Imported vaccine-associated paralytic poliomyelitis—United States, 2005. MMWR Morb Mortal Wkly Rep 2006;55:97–9.

Center for Disease Control and Prevention. Resurgence of wild poliovirus type 1 transmission and consequences of importation—21 countries, 2002-2005. MMWR Morb Mort Wkly Rep 2006;55:145–50.

World Health Organization. Conclusions and recommendations of the Advisory Committee on Poliomyelitis Eradication, Geneva, 11–12 October 2006, Part II. Wkly epid Rec 2006;81:465–8.

World Health Organization. Progress towards interruption of wild poliovirus transmission. Weekly epid Rec 2006;81:165–72.

Rabies

Infectious Agent

The rabies virus belongs to the genus Lyssavirus and occurs primarily in the animals as listed below.

Transmission

Humans contract rabies by being bitten or, occasionally, by being scratched by an infected animal. The rabies virus is introduced into wounds or through mucous membranes. Airborne infection is rare but has been contracted in caves from infected bats and also has occurred in laboratory settings. Person-to-person transmission is very rare, and saliva may contain the virus. Rabies has occurred after corneal transplant from a donor with an undiagnosed fatal central nervous system (CNS) disease.

Global Epidemiology

Rabies occurs throughout the world with several exceptions (Figure 38). There are an estimated 40,000 to 60,000 human deaths yearly from rabies (15,000 to 35,000 in India), mostly in the developing countries where transmission by dog bites in urban areas is common. Fox rabies predominates in Europe and is usually transmitted in rural areas. Bat rabies cases have been reported in Europe (Denmark, Holland, Germany, Spain, Switzerland, and the United Kingdom), Africa, Asia, and the Americas. Rabies in North America primarily involves bats, raccoons, skunks, foxes, coyotes, wolves, and, occasionally, dogs and cats. It is likely that several million persons receive postexposure prophylaxis annually around the world.

The risk of rabies and subsequent death for travelers is unknown, but many anecdotal cases have been reported, particularly after exposure in India and Southeast Asia. The annual incidence of animal bites in expatriates is approximately 2%, according to two studies, with most of the animals potentially infected. The number of these individuals receiving postexposure rabies vaccination is unknown.

Initial rabies symptoms include a sense of apprehension, headache, fever, malaise, and indefinite sensory changes in the

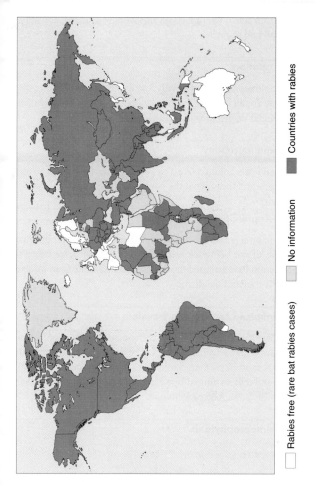

Figure 38   Geographic distribution of rabies (WHO 2002, adapted)

area of the wound. These are followed by excitability, aeropho-
bia, and later hydrophobia, due to spasms of the swallowing
muscles, delirium, and convulsions. Death occurs after several
days because of respiratory paralysis. Case fatality rate is close
to 100% in patients who develop symptoms; there are less than

one dozen anecdotal reports on survivors worldwide, and apparently all had sequelae.

Incubation

The incubation period is usually 3 to 8 weeks but may be as short as 4 days or as long as 7 years, depending on the severity of the wound and its distance from the brain.

Communicability

Dogs and cats are infective 3 to 14 days before the onset of clinical signs and throughout the course of the clinical disease.

Susceptibility and Resistance

Some natural resistance has wrongly been claimed in Iran, where in spite of not being treated, only 40% among those bitten by rabid animals developed the disease. Not all bites from infected animals transmit the disease.

Minimized Exposure in Travelers

Travelers should avoid contact with animals that are not known to be immunized against rabies. Make travelers aware which animals are most likely to transmit rabies in the host country (usually dogs) and that no animal bite can be ignored with respect to the possibility of rabies transmission.

Chemoprophylaxis

None

Pre-Exposure Immunoprophylaxis by Rabies Vaccine

Various rabies vaccines exist in the developed countries. These include:

- Human diploid cell vaccines (HDCV; Chiron Vaccines, Sanofi Pasteur, Lyon, France), strain Pitman-Moore, cultivated on human cells WI38 or MRC5
- purified chick embryo cell vaccine (PCECV; Chiron Vaccine)

- purified duck embryo vaccine (PDEV; Zydus Cadila, India; formerly by Berna Biotech Ltd.)
- vero cell rabies vaccine (PVRV; Sanofi Pasteur)
- chromatography purified rabies vaccine (CPRV, purified vero-cell—Sanofi Pasteur) not yet licensed, marketing pending in many countries

These vaccines have a similar profile and are described under a single heading below. Additional vaccines that are more reactogenic and less immunogenic are available, particularly in developing countries.

Immunology and Pharmacology

Viability: inactivated

Antigenic form: whole virus

Adjuvants: none

Preservative: none

Allergens/Excipiens: Rabies Pasteur Merieux Connaught—Neomycin <150 µg, human serum albumin < 100 mg/mL dose / Rabies Pasteur Merieux Connaught 3 µg phenol red

Mechanism: induction of neutralizing antibody, cellular immunity, and perhaps interferon

Application

Pre-exposure prophylaxis: three doses (each 1 mL, except PVRV 0.5 mL) IM on days 0, 7, and 21 or 28 — or at 0, 1, 2 months.

Postexposure prophylaxis: see below.

Booster: for persons at continuous high risk (such as rabies research workers, rabies biologics production workers), serologic testing every 6 months is required after completion of the primary course. If antibody titer is below the acceptable level (≥ 0.5 IU/mL required for protection), a booster vaccination is required. For persons with frequent exposure (cavers, veterinarians, wildlife workers, etc.), serologic testing every 2 years is required, and booster vaccination given if the titer is below acceptable level. For those with infrequent exposure (such as travelers), the Center for Disease Control and Prevention (CDC) in Atlanta (GA) does not specify serologic testing or booster vaccination. In Europe, a booster is given at one year after primary series.

Route: intramuscularly (IM). The intradermal (ID) route that was previously 0.1 mL ID (not subcutaneously) for HDCV only is no longer available or approved.

Site: the deltoid area is the only acceptable site for rabies vaccination of adults and older children (IM and ID). In younger children, use the anterolateral thigh. Never administer the rabies vaccine in the gluteal area.

Storage: store at 2 to 8 °C (35 to 46 °F). Do not freeze.

Availability: high quality, modern tissue culture rabies vaccines are now available almost worldwide. In the developing countries, some embassies (eg, Sweden, Canada) have the vaccine. Travelers should contact their embassy first if they require rabies vaccine while abroad. In some developing countries, particularly in rural areas, often only suboptimal vaccines are available.

Protection

Onset: antibodies appear 7 days after IM injection and peak within 30 to 60 days. Adequate titers usually develop within 2 weeks after the third pre-exposure dose.

Efficacy: essentially 100%. Note that pre-exposure immunization does not eliminate the need for prompt postexposure prophylaxis if bitten by a potentially rabid animal. Pre-exposure immunization only eliminates the need for rabies immune globulin (RIG) and reduces the number of vaccine injections required after an incident.

Duration: antibodies persist for at least 1 and usually 5 years.

Protective level: two alternate definitions are used for minimally acceptable antibody titers in vaccinees. The CDC considers a 1:5 titer by rapid fluorescent focus inhibition test to indicate an adequate response to pre-exposure vaccination. The World Health Organization (WHO) specifies an antibody titer of 0.5 IU/mL (comparable to a dilution titer of 1:25) as adequate for postexposure vaccination.

Adverse Reactions

Rabies vaccination can cause transient pain, erythema, swelling, or itching at the injection site in 25% of cases (up to 70% occasionally). These reactions can be treated with simple analgesics. Mild systemic reactions, including headache, nausea, abdominal pain, muscle aches, and dizziness, are seen in 8 to 20% of cases.

Serum–sickness-like reactions occur 2 to 21 days after injection in < 1 to 6% of those receiving HDCV booster doses. These reactions may result from albumin in the vaccine formula rendered allergenic during manufacturing by β-propiolactone.

Contraindications

Absolute: previous hypersensitivity reactions to components of pre-exposure prophylaxis vaccine. None in postexposure prophylaxis.

Relative: any acute illness (pre-exposure prophylaxis)

Children: not contraindicated; pediatric dosage is the same as for adults. Safety and efficacy for children are established.

Pregnant women: category C. It is unknown whether rabies vaccine or corresponding antibodies cross the placenta. Generally, most immunoglobulin G passage across the placenta occurs during the third trimester. Use only if clearly needed.

Lactating women: it is unknown whether rabies vaccine or corresponding antibodies are excreted in breast milk. Problems in humans have not been documented.

Immunodeficient persons: immunosuppression and immunodeficiency may interfere with development of active rabies immunity and may predispose the patient to develop the disease following exposure. Avoid administering the immunosuppressive agents during postexposure therapy unless essential for treatment of other conditions.

Interactions

In postexposure prophylaxis, simultaneous administration of RIG may slightly delay the antibody response to rabies vaccine. Recommendations for postexposure prophylaxis must be followed closely.

Chloroquine may suppress the immune response to rabies vaccines. Complete pre-exposure vaccination should be done 1 to 2 months before chloroquine administration. Other travel-related vaccines may be administered simultaneously.

Immunosuppressant drugs and radiation therapy may cause an insufficient response to immunization.

In all IM administration, caution is indicated in patients receiving anticoagulants.

Recommendations for Vaccine Use

Pre-exposure prophylaxis should be considered for prolonged stays (> 1 [WHO] to 3 months depending on the available recommendations) in countries where rabies is endemic—remember that the risk is highest in India. Veterinarians, animal handlers, field biologists, spelunkers, and certain laboratory workers are known to be at high risk. Anecdotal reports suggest that children, teenagers, and young adults riding a bicycle, hikers, walkers, and joggers are at greater risk because they more often come in contact with animals.

Pre-exposure prophylaxis does not eliminate the need for additional therapy after a rabies exposure. It simplifies postexposure treatment, however, as RIG is not required and the number of doses of vaccine required is reduced. Vaccines produced in the developing countries may have an elevated risk of adverse reactions and of lower efficacy.

Self-Treatment Abroad and Postexposure Prophylaxis

Bites and wounds received from animals must be cleaned and flushed immediately with soap and water. Apply either ethanol (70%) or tincture or aqueous solution of iodine or povidone iodine. A physician must decide the need for postexposure immunization, taking into account the following:

- The animal species involved
- Circumstances of the bite (unprovoked?) or other exposure (touching, licking)
- Immunization status of the animal
- Whether the animal can be kept under observation for 10 days (start postexposure prophylaxis, and stop if animal does not develop symptoms) or sacrificed for appropriate laboratory evaluation (usually within 24 hours)
- Presence of rabies in the region
- That persons not previously (or incompletely) immunized with high-risk exposure should be given:
  - RIG, (preferably human 20 IU/kg, otherwise equine RIG, 40 IU/kg body weight). As much as possible should be infiltrated into and around the bite sites (the rest deep IM at a site distant from the vaccine injection site). If a finger or toe needs to be infiltrated, care must be taken not to cause a compartment syndrome.

- rabies vaccine IM (eg, deltoid area) starting as soon as possible: either on days 0, 3, 7, 14, and 28, or two doses on day 0, plus one each on days 7 and 21. Also intradermal regimens are recommended by WHO, such as the 2.2.2.0.1.1 (or 2.2.2.0.2) 0.1 mL ID dose regimens (when two doses at different locations) of PVRV or PCECV on days 0, 3, 7, 30, and 90.
- That persons previously immunized with a complete pre- or postexposure course (or who had a documented titer of > 0.5 IU/mL rabies neutralizing antibody previously) should receive two doses of vaccine, one each on days 0 and 3. No RIG is required.

Rabies is a notifiable disease in most countries. Danger of transmission from saliva and respiratory secretions requires the patient to be isolated from contacts. Immunization of contacts is necessary only if they have open wounds or mucous membrane exposure. Check whether other persons may have been exposed.

Additional Readings

Blanton JD. Rabies postexposure prophylaxis, New York, 1995-2000. Emerg Infect Dis 2005;11:1921–7.

Meslin FX. Rabies as a traveler's risk, especially in high-endemicity areas. J Travel Med 2005;12:S30–S40.

Pandey P, et al. Risk of possible exposure to rabies among tourists and foreign residents in Nepal. J Travel Med 2002;9:127–31.

Sudarshan MK, et al. Assessing the burden of human rabies in India. Internat J Infect Dis 2007;11:29–35.

Wilde H, et al. Rabies update for travel medicine advisors. Clin Infect Dis 2003;37:96–100.

World Health Organization. Rabies vaccines. Wkly Epidem Rec 2002;77:109–19.

RELAPSING FEVER

Relapsing fever, also known as recurrent fever or tick-bite fever, is caused by *Borrelia recurrentis* or *B. duttonii*. It is transmitted by lice or ticks and occurs mainly in tropical Africa but also in foci in Asia and South America. The incubation period is 5 to 15 days. Characteristically, it includes periods of fever of 2 to 9 days in duration, alternating with free intervals. There may be more than 10 relapses. Petechial rashes are common. Untreated by antibiotics, the case fatality rate may be up to 10%. In a study in Israel, doxycycline was shown to be effective as postexposure treatment in tick-borne relapsing fever due to *B. persica*. Anecdotal cases in travelers have been reported.

Additional Readings

Colebunders R, et al. Imported relapsing fever in European tourists. Scand J Infect Dis 1993;25:533–6.

Hasin T, et al. Postexposure treatment with doxycycline for the prevention of tick-borne relapsing fever. N Engl J Med 2006;355:148–55.

Vial L, et al. Incidence of tick-borne relapsing fever in west Africa: longitudinal study. Lancet 2006;368:37–43.

RESPIRATORY TRACT INFECTIONS

Most upper respiratory tract infections are caused by viruses and are uncomplicated. Recognition of group A streptococcal infection is important to prevent post-streptococcal complications, particularly acute rheumatic fever. The presence of enlarged anterior cervical lymph nodes, inflamed tonsils with exudates, fever, and pain on swallowing are suggestive of streptococcal pharyngitis.

Infectious Agents

Although there are regional differences in endemic pathogens, the similarity of pathogens found in all regions of the world is more impressive than are the differences in distribution. There are many causes of acute respiratory tract infection. Most of these are not identified in patients with acute illness. The common pathogens in acute upper respiratory tract infection include:

- viruses: rhinoviruses, adenoviruses, coronaviruses, enteroviruses, Epstein-Barr virus, influenza (see "Influenza" and "Avian Influenza" above), parainfluenza, respiratory syncytial virus
- bacteria: group A, C, and G streptococci; *Mycoplasma* and *Chlamydia* cause lower, rather than upper, respiratory tract infections.

The important causes of lower respiratory tract infection include adenoviruses, enteroviruses, influenza viruses, parainfluenza viruses, respiratory syncytial virus, Chlamydia, *Haemophilus influenzae*, *Legionella pneumophila*, *Mycobacterium tuberculosis*, *Mycoplasma pneumoniae*, and *Streptococcus pneumoniae*.

Transmission

Virtually all the infectious agents are spread by the airborne route in large droplets, droplet nuclei, aerosols (ø ≤ 5μm, small enough to remain airborne for prolonged periods) or by direct contact. Spread as aerosol has been discussed. Respiratory tract infections occur worldwide. Occurrence rates are higher during dry winter seasons and in China, northern Europe, and North America.

Risk for Travelers

Acquisition of an upper respiratory tract infection during international travel is a common problem. This is especially true for travel in China and other regions during dry, cool periods. Respiratory tract infection is the most common illness among travelers to the developed regions and is second in importance to diarrhea among travelers to the developing tropical areas.

Group travelers acquire acute respiratory tract infection in a range between 1 and 88%, depending on the group. The average incidence for all travelers ranges from 6 to 12%.

Clinical Picture

Patients with acute respiratory tract infection present with runny nose, nonproductive cough, sore throat, headache, malaise, and muscle aches and pains. In acute streptococcal pharyngitis, patients experience abrupt onset of sore throat with pain on swallowing, tender swollen anterior cervical lymph nodes, and pharyngeal and tonsillar inflammation, occasionally with patchy exudates. Laryngitis is common in those with viral respiratory tract infection. Uncomplicated illness lasts between 3 and 7 days. Lower respiratory tract infection typically presents with sudden onset of fever, chills, productive cough, and systemic symptoms, including myalgias. Lower respiratory tract infection may progress and have a more serious outcome. These cases, therefore, require emergency evaluation and therapy.

The incubation period for most respiratory tract infections is short—between 12 and 72 hours.

Communicability

Many of the viral agents causing upper respiratory tract infection are highly communicable to susceptible (previously unexposed) persons in close proximity to infected individuals. Recirculated air in aircrafts may facilitate the spread of respiratory pathogens, including viruses and *M. tuberculosis*. Bacterial pathogens, including *Legionella*, are not normally highly communicable.

Susceptibility and Resistance

Previous exposure to viral respiratory pathogens with resulting infection induces protective immunity in most persons. The many agents present in the environment explain repeated bouts of infection. Cigarette smokers, particularly those older than age 50 years, are at increased risk for certain pathogens such as *Legionella* and *S. pneumoniae*.

Minimizing Exposure in Travelers

Patients at high risk for health problems, such as those with diabetes mellitus and cardiopulmonary disease, should avoid large groups of people during viral seasons (eg, winter, when the disease is prevalent). The only other practical way to prevent exposure to respiratory tract infections is to practice frequent hand washing when in contact with other persons.

Chemoprophylaxis

For the most part, this is not applicable. Antimicrobials (eg, rifampin) may be used in the short term for prevention of meningococcal infection when exposed to an active case.

Immunoprophylaxis

Immunization with diphtheria toxoid is important to prevent diphtheria in international travelers. Before travel, give pneumococcal and influenza vaccines to those at high risk (see those respective chapters).

Self-Treatment Abroad

Travelers with upper respiratory tract infection can usually treat symptoms themselves. Take acetaminophen, paracetamol, or acetylsalicylic acid for relief of headache and sore throat; nose drops can be used in the short term (< 48 hours) to relieve severe nasal congestion, (particularly if flying). Antitussives may relieve dry cough with no fever, and interrupting sleep to consume adequate fluids will ensure adequate hydration. Watch for complications of respiratory tract infection, including group A streptococcal pharyngitis, adenitis, epiglottitis, pneumonia, mastoiditis, otitis media, periorbital cellulitis, retropharyngeal or peritonsillar abscess, sinusitis, and bronchitis. If complications occur, the patient should seek local medical attention for evaluation and consideration for antibacterial or other therapy. Fluoroquinolones, which a traveler may have for possible diarrheal disease, may not be appropriate for therapy of bacterial infection of the respiratory tract because they may not be active against some of the *Streptococcus* strains.

Principles of Therapy

Symptomatic treatment and consumption of fluids should be undertaken for acute upper respiratory tract infection, and antimicrobial therapy should be reserved for group A *Streptococcus* infection and lower respiratory tract infection.

Community Control Measures

For the most part, community control measures are not practical to control the broad array of respiratory pathogens. Decontamination of industrial cooling water and proper disinfection of spas and hot tubs in recreational areas will minimize *Legionella* infection.

Notification of authorities, isolation, quarantine, and contact study are not applicable, except for *Legionella* in some countries.

Additional Readings

Freedman DO, et al. Spectrum of disease and relation to place of exposure among ill returned travelers. N Engl J Med 2006;354:119–30.

Leder K, et al. Respiratory infections during air travel. Intern Med J 2005;35:50–5.

Leder K, et al. Respiratory tract infections in travelers: a review of the GeoSentinel Surveillance Network. Clin Infect Dis 2003;36:399–406.

RICKETTSIAL INFECTIONS

Rickettsial infections are transmitted to humans by various insect vectors, including ticks, mites, lice, and fleas, or by aerosol from animals and animal products. Rickettsiaceae are bacteria, and the species of the genus Rickettsia is divided into:

- Typhus group
  - *Rickettsia prowazekii*: classical epidemic typhus—transmitted by the human body louse
  - *R. typhi* (*R. mooseri*): endemic murine typhus—transmitted by the rat flea
- Spotted fever group, with *R. rickettsii*, *R. conorii*—transmitted from rodents and other animals by ticks
- Scrub typhus, caused by *Orientia tsutsugamushi*—transmitted by larval trombiculid mites

The reclassified genus Bartonella (formerly Rochalimaea) is divided into:

- *Bartonella quintana*, the cause of trench fever
- *B. henselae*, the cause of cat-scratch fever
- South American, classical bartonellosis, also named Oroya fever

Coxiella burnetii, the only species of its genus, causes Q-fever. Ehrlichia can cause various febrile infections in humans.

The relevance of rickettsial infections for travelers is undetermined because many imported cases remain undiagnosed. Serologic surveys among travelers show that this group of diseases is underdiagnosed. Rickettsia africae is the most common rickettsiosis in Southern Africa, often affecting travelers.

Skin rash is common in rickettsial infection, although it may be faint or not present in ehrlichiosis and is not present in Q fever. Epidemic typhus, Brill-Zinsser disease, flying squirrel-associated typhus, and scrub typhus are more prevalent worldwide than are other rickettsial infections. In Rickettsia and Ehrlichia rickettsial infections, the illnesses are clinically similar; skin rash, however, is prominent only in the former. Diagnosis is made by serology and is treated with antirickettsial drugs. Adults are treated primarily with doxycycline, but chloramphenicol is also used. Typhus vaccine was available in the United States from 1941 to 1981. Rocky Mountain spotted fever vaccine is also no longer available.

Additional Readings

Isaksson HJ, et al. Acute Q fever: a cause of fatal hepatitis in an Icelandic traveller. Scand J Infect Dis 2001;33:314–5.

Jelinek T, et al. Clinical features and epidemiology of tick typhus in travelers. J Travel Med 2001;8:57–9.

Jensenius M, et al. Seroepidemiology of Rickettsia africae infection in Norwegian travellers to rural Africa. Scand J Infect Dis 2002;34: 93–6.

Owen CE et al. African tick-bite fever: a not-so-uncommon illness in international travelers. Arch Dermatol 2006;142:1312–4.

Rift Valley Fever

This arboviral infection is caused by the Rift Valley fever virus, a Phlebovirus belonging to the Bunyaviridae family. It is transmitted by various mosquitoes or through blood or body fluids during slaughter of animals, most often sheep and goats, and less frequently horses and camels. Consumption of sick animals or drinking unpasteurized milk can also lead to the disease. Incubation time is 2 to 4 days, and infectivity persists for 4 to 6 days. Epidemics occur mainly after heavy rainfall and flooding, such as that which occurred in Kenya and Somalia in 1997 and 2007. The endemicity areas now include regions in East and West Africa, Egypt, and on the Arabian peninsula. Infected mosquito eggs can survive many years in the soil and, with flooding, new infected mosquitoes can start a new epizootic cycle. The risk for travelers is minimal; apparently the infection has only been described in a few United Nations soldiers. Symptoms resemble those of flu or dengue, and nausea and vomiting may occur. Late manifestations of a hemorrhagic fever may occur, mainly in malnourished populations, with a 1- to 3-week delay. Prevention includes protection against mosquito bites, avoidance of unpasteurized milk, and avoidance of sick animals and their products. Animals may be immunized. Inactivated and live human vaccine candidates are under study.

Additional Readings

Durand JP, et al. Rift Valley fever virus infection among French troops in Chad. Emerg Infect Dis 2003;9:751–2.

Gubler DJ. The global emergence/resurgence of arboviral diseases as public health problems. Arch Med Res 2002;33:330–42.

Isaacson M. Viral hemorrhagic fever hazards for travelers in Africa. Clin Infect Dis 2001;33:1707–12.

SANDFLY FEVER

Infectious Agent

Several members of the Bunyaviridae family.

Transmission

Sandfly, mainly phlebotomus papatasii. Thus also labeled Phlebotomus fever, Papatasi fever, Toscana fever, Chandipura fever (here Rhabdovirus), etc..

Global epidemiology

Subtropical and tropical areas with long periods of hot, dry weather, also rainforests in Southern Europe, northern Africa, Asia (central, western, also Myanmar, China); a few cases have been identified in Panama, Colombia and Brazil.

Risk for Travelers

Unprotected exposure at night

Clinical picture

Abrupt onset of headache, fever, retrobulbar pain, photophobia, rarely vomiting. Depression and encephalitis have been reported. Occasionally a second phase of illness occurs 2 to 12 weeks later. Usually this is mild and self-limited, hardly ever fatal except in local children.

Incubation

3 to 4, occasionally up to 6 days.

Communicability

No person-to-person transmission.

Susceptibility and Resistance

Universal susceptibility, long lasting homologous immunity.

Minimizing Exposure in Travelers

Personal protection measures against sandfly bites at night, e.g. screens with small mesh.

Chemoprophylaxis, Immunoprophylaxis

None

Principles of Therapy

Symptomatic, supportive.

Communicable Control Measures

Destroy sandflies in residential areas.

Additional Readings

Defuentes G et al. Acute meningitis owing to phlebotomus fever Toscana virus imported to France. J Travel Med. 2005;12:295-6.

SCHISTOSOMIASIS

Infectious Agent

Schistosomiasis is caused by a number of species of schistosomes differing in infectivity, clinical manifestations, and geographic location. These include *Schistosoma haematobium*, *S. mansoni*, *S. japonicum*, *S. intercalatum*, and *S. mekongi*, whereas *S. bovis* and *S. mattheei* are rarely the origin of human infections. Several avian schistosomes exist, but in humans they only result in cercarian dermatitis.

Transmission

Ova of the parasites are introduced into stagnant, slow-flowing water through the urine and feces of infected persons in endemic areas. Miracidia are released within a few hours and are picked up by a snail, which acts as intermediate host. They multiply in the snail and transform into cercariae, the form that can infect humans. The cercariae emerge from the snail, attach to the skin of the host, and penetrate within a few minutes. The worms emerge in the liver, as well as in the portal venous system. Adult schistosome worms may live inside a human for decades.

Global Epidemiology

Chronic schistosomiasis is one of the most ubiquitous infectious diseases. There are more than 200 million infected persons around the world, resulting in widespread morbidity and mortality. Schistosomiasis is endemic in Africa (with many reports from the Omo River region in Ethiopia), Asia, South America, and certain Caribbean islands (Figures 39 and 40). Transmission occurs in areas where susceptible snails are found. Even minimal exposure to fresh water in an endemic area poses a risk for the traveler; therefore, bathing, swimming, boating, or rafting are risk activities in these areas. Successful penetration of the skin by cercariae and subsequent infection can take place in as little as 25 minutes. Risk is highest along lake margins and in slow-moving bodies of water, such as irrigation ditches and flooded paddy fields. Individuals may acquire infection in poorly maintained swimming pools or in brackish water near salt-water sources. High

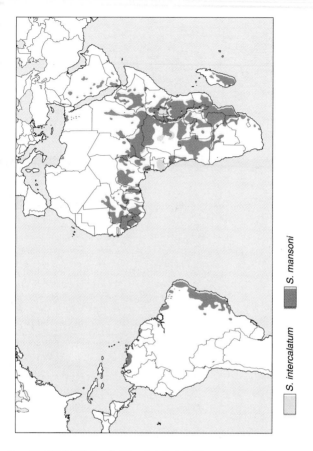

Figure 39 Global distribution of schistosomiasis due to *Schistosoma mansoni* and *Schistosoma intercalatum*

concentrations of cercariae are found during the daytime when there is a greater risk of contracting the disease. Acquisition of infection by drinking water is considered unlikely; the cercariae would be killed by the low pH of the stomach.

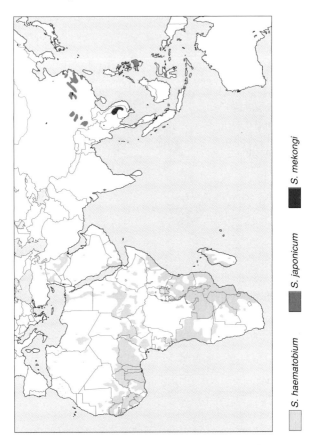

Figure 40   Global distribution of schistosomiasis due to *Schistosoma haematobium, Schistosoma Mekongi,* and *Schistosoma japonicum*

Clinical Picture

The following three syndromes occur in schistosomiasis:

- Cercarial dermatitis, or "swimmer's itch," may follow cutaneous infection with any of the schistosomes, but is most common with avian and other nonhuman schistosomes.

- Acute schistosomiasis (Katayama fever), which is a serum–sickness-like disorder, can occur in previously unexposed persons. Fever, headache, abdominal pain, arthralgias and hepatosplenomegaly are found, often in association with eosinophilia.
- Chronic schistosomiasis is associated with deposition of eggs in tissue and local granuloma formation. Eosinophilia occurs in approximately half of these patients.

Hematuria (typically terminal) accompanied by painful micturition, as well as hematospermia are characteristic of *S. haematobium*. The main clinical manifestation of infection with *S. intercalatum* is rectal bleeding. The final stage is characterized by complications of a more serious nature, involving mainly the bladder, ureters, kidneys, and liver (depending on schistosomes).

Incubation

The incubation period of acute schistosomiasis is 2 to 9 weeks after exposure. Manifestations occurring after a prolonged incubation will develop slowly.

Communicability

Schistosomiasis is not transmitted from person to person.

Susceptibility and Resistance

In the autochthonous population, children become infected when they come in contact with local water sources. In endemic areas, the incidence of infection increases with age, peaking between age 10 and 20. Intensity of infection, rather than incidence, appears to decrease with age thereafter, suggesting that partial immunity occurs with repeated exposure.

Minimizing Exposure in Travelers

The only definitive measure is to avoid contact with water that contains cercariae. If water contact is unavoidable, the use of skin cleansers containing hexachlorophene have been shown to prevent the penetration of cercariae, if applied some time before exposure to infected water. However, for long-term use, this is not recommended. The use of 1% niclosamide lotion to prevent skin penetration of cercariae was found to give insufficient protection. Diethyltoluamide (deet) was recently shown to be effective as a topical agent for preventing skin penetration by *S. mansoni* cercariae, but more data are needed. The use of soap during bathing helps to reduce the risk of infection, which can also be reduced by a vigorous rubdown with a towel straight after exposure to contaminated water. In addition, applying alcohol to exposed skin will help. Cercariae can be killed in bath water by heating to 50 °C (122 °F). Raw water can only be considered free of infective cercariae if stored in drums or tanks for at least 48 hours.

Immunoprophylaxis

Research work on an anti-schistosome vaccine is under way.

Principles of Therapy

Travel history and water contact details are important clues to the diagnosis. Eosinophilia and a history of swimmer's itch should alert the physician. Hematuria is a symptom only of *S. haematobium*. The main diagnostic feature is the presence of eggs in urine or stool or in biopsy specimens (eg, bladder, liver, and rectal snips). The latter method is often used when stool specimens are negative. At the stage of Katayama syndrome, eggs are often not yet evident in stool or urine specimens, but may be seen as lesions at proctoscopy. For *S. haematobium*, eggs are found in urine; for *S. mansoni* and *S. intercalatum*, eggs are found in stools. A new test, based on enzyme-linked immunosorbent assay and immunoblot, appears to be highly sensitive and specific. Sigmoidoscopy, cystoscopy, and proctoscopy are used in the search for lesions of the bowel and bladder. Use ultrasonography to determine calcification of the bladder, ureters, and kidneys in long-standing chronic cases.

Praziquantel, the drug of choice, is effective against all the schistosomes. Malaise, nonspecific gastrointestinal disturbances, headache, and dizziness are the most frequently encountered adverse side effects and are usually mild and transient. The use of praziquantel is not recommended during the first trimester of pregnancy, and use thereafter should occur only if the benefits outweigh the possible risk to the fetus. Oxamniquine is used specifically against *S. mansoni* and can be used to treat cases of

S. mansoni refractory to praziquantel. Anti-schistosomal treatment (praziquantel) is effective if given early in the disease and may prevent further damage by the parasite if given later.

Community Control Measures

Community programs designed to prevent exposure to bodies of fresh water in endemic areas are of some value. Effective control programs are often centered around diminishing the reservoir of the parasite by building of privies, avoiding use of human excreta as a fertilizer, improving sewage disposal, and ensuring widespread chemotherapy of active cases. Molluscicides aimed at reducing the population of the intermediary snail are of limited value.

Additional Readings

Corachan M. Schistosomiasis and international travel. Clin Infect Dis 2002;35:446–50.

Meltzer E et al. Schistosomiasis among travelers. Emerg Infect Dis 2006;12:1696-700.

Outwater AH. Schistosomiasis and US Peace Corps volunteers in Tanzania. J Travel Med 2005;12:265–9.

Schwartz E, et al. Schistosome infection among river rafters on Omo river, Ethiopia. J Travel Med 2005;12:3–8.

Severe Acute Respiratory Syndrome

Infectious Agent

Severe Acute Respiratory Syndrome-associated coronavirus (SARS-CoV)

Transmission

Respiratory droplets spread SARS, with the highest risk from close person-to-person contact and contact with body fluids from the patient. Transmission is also via contact with contaminated objects. Airborne transmission seems to play a minor role, but cannot be excluded. The majority of cases have occurred in hospital workers who have cared for SARS patients and the close family members of these patients.

Global Epidemiology

SARS first appeared in China in November 2002 and spread to Asia in February 2003. Over the next few months, the illness spread to more than two dozen countries in North America, South America, Europe, and Asia before the SARS global outbreak of 2003 was contained. A total of 8,098 people worldwide were diagnosed with SARS during the 2003 outbreak; of these, 774 died. The last case of this outbreak occurred in June 2003. Analysis of the 2003 outbreak indicates that basic public health measures are sufficient to contain a SARS epidemic. A few isolated cases occurred between 2003 and the beginning of 2004; the majority were associated with laboratory incidents. In May 2005, the disease itself was declared eradicated by the the World Health Organization (WHO).

Risk for Travelers

Although international travelers were affected early on in the outbreak and contributed to the global spread, the overall risk of SARS to travelers is small. Travel alerts would again be issued by the WHO to reduce the risk of international spread.

Clinical Picture

Symptoms include fever greater than 100.4 °F (38 °C, measured in axilla), myalgia, headache, sore throat, dry cough, as well as shortness of breath later on. In some but not all cases, these symptoms are followed by hypoxia, pneumonia, and acute respiratory disease syndrome (ARDS), requiring assisted ventilation. Diarrhea rarely occurs. Chest radiograph, in most cases, reveals an atypical pneumonia. Laboratory findings include leukopenia, thrombocytopenia, and mildly elevated transaminases (in particular, elevated lactate dehydrogenase). The case fatality rate is approximately 10 to 15%; the risk of severe complications and death increases with age.

Diagnosis

An enzyme-linked immunosorbent assay test detects antibodies to SARS reliably but only 21 days after the onset of symptoms. An immunofluorescence assay can detect antibodies 10 days after the onset of the disease but is a labor- and time-intensive test. Polymerase chain reaction is very specific, but not sensitive, and can be done on any body fluids.

Incubation

2 to 10 days (usually 3 to 5 days)

Communicability

As soon as symptoms occur, with a peak at 4 to 7 days of illness. No transmission via asymptomatic cases have been reported.

Minimized Exposure in Travelers

Avoid travel to areas that have a current SARS outbreak.

Chemoprophylaxis

None known

Immunoprophylaxis

None available

Self-Treatment Abroad

Ill persons should call ahead to their personal physicians, providing information about where and when they traveled and indicating whether there was contact with someone who had such symptoms.

Principles of Therapy

No specific antiviral therapy known. Steroids or interferon may be beneficial (but this is not proven) in reducing the risk of respiratory distress syndrome that is thought to be most likely due to a hyperimmune response.

Community Control Measures

Carry out barrier nursing practices, including airborne and contact precautions and negative pressure rooms. Provide early isolation of any suspected and probable cases. Do contact tracing. Notify authorities as per national regulations.

Additional Readings

Breugelmans JG, et al. SARS transmission and commercial aircraft. Emerg Infect Dis 2004;10:1502–3.

St. John RK, et al. Border screening for SARS. Emerg Infect Dis 2005;11:6–10.

Vogt TM et al. Risk of Severe Acute Respiratory Syndrome – associated Coronavirus transmission aboard commercial aircraft. J Travel Med 2006;13:268-72.

Wilder-Smith A, et al. Confronting the new challenge in travel medicine: SARS. J Travel Med 2003;10:257–8.

Wilder-Smith A. The severe acute respiratory syndrome: impact on travel and tourism. Travel Med Infect Dis 2005;4;53–60.

Wilder-Smith A, et al. Experience of severe acute respiratory syndrome in Singapore: importation of cases and defense strategies at the airport. J Travel Med 2003;10:259–62.

SEXUALLY TRANSMITTED DISEASES

Infectious Agents

The list of sexually transmitted disease (STD) pathogens is long, and the resulting clinical infectious diseases are varied. In this section, we will consider the more important STD agents, including the following:

- *Neisseria gonorrhoeae* (gonorrhea)
- *Chlamydia trachomatis* (genital chlamydia infection and lymphogranuloma venereum)
- *Haemophilus ducreyi* (chancroid)
- *Calymmatobacterium inguinale* (donovanosis)
- *Treponema pallidum* (syphilis)
- Human papillomavirus (genital warts)
- Herpes simplex virus 1, 2 (herpes anogenitalis)
- Hepatitis B and C (see "Hepatitis B" and "Hepatitis C" above)
- Human immunodeficiency virus (HIV 1, 2; see "Human Immunodeficiency Virus" above)
- Scabies
- Pubic lice ("crab lice")
- *Trichomonas vaginalis*

Transmission occurs when a susceptible person is exposed to an infected person. Tourists may have sexual contact with local persons or with prostitutes, who are at high risk for STD. The STD infections transmitted by blood may also be acquired by contact with non-sterile intravenous needles, infected lancets, or contaminated surgical instruments. Risk of HIV infection is higher in travelers with other STD infections.

Global Epidemiology

Although data are incomplete on the occurrence of STDs in populations, up to 200 million STDs occur yearly throughout the world. About 80% of the infections occur in the developing world. Up to one-third of the world's population has an STD or carry a transmissible STD pathogen. Syphilis, gonorrhea, *C. trachomatis*, and herpes simplex are worldwide pathogens. Chancroid, lymphogranuloma chancroid, lymphogranuloma venereum (LGV) and donovanosis are diseases of the tropic and subtropic regions. Penicillinase-producing *N. gonorrhoeae* (PPNG) are observed worldwide with an increasing frequency.

Risk for Travelers

Tourists may be the source of STDs or may acquire an infective organism during travel. Many seek "sun, sand, and sex" during international travel, having left their inhibitions at home. Alcohol consumption often leads to unprotected intercourse with unfamiliar contacts. Condom use is increasing, but unprotected sex still occurs frequently among international travelers (see also Part 1).

Clinical Picture

Sexually transmitted diseases vary in their clinical presentation, including genital discharge or ulceration, conjunctivitis, uveitis, proctitis, symptoms of pelvic inflammatory disease, hepatitis, skin rash, arthritis, and urethritis. The syphilitic chancre is characteristically non-tender and indurated with a clean base. Significant pain with ulceration is more characteristic of chancroid or herpes genitalis. Genital ulceration beginning as vesicles suggests herpes genitalis. Chancroid ulcers vary in size and have ragged and necrotic borders. Crusted lesions of the genital tract appear as healing genital herpes and scabies. Intensely pruritic genital lesions are seen in scabies. Clinical appearance of specific STDs varies. Laboratory tests are required to make a diagnosis.

Incubation

The various STDs have different incubation periods as follows:

- *N. gonorrhoeae*: 2 to 5 (to 10) days
- *C. trachomatis*: 2 days to 4 weeks
- *H. ducreyi*: 3 to 6 days
- *C. inguinale*: 6 weeks to 1 year
- *T. pallidum*: 3 weeks (10 to 30 days)
- human papillomavirus: 1 month to 1.5 years
- herpes simplex: 4 to 10 days
- HIV 1 and 2: 2 weeks to 10 years

Communicability

Most STD pathogens are fragile and incapable of survival for any significant periods of time outside the infected host, but they are highly communicable through sexual contact or by transfusion of blood products.

Susceptibility and Resistance

Virtually all uninfected persons are susceptible to the wide array of STDs.

Minimizing Exposure in Travelers

Education of travelers in the prevention of STDs is part of standard pretravel counseling. If abstinence from sexual contact during trips is unlikely, condom use must be stressed as an absolute necessity. Travelers should take a supply of condoms with them because they may be of poor quality or unavailable in many destinations (see Part 1).

Although chemoprophylaxis is feasible for a limited number of STDs (eg, gonorrhea), it is not practical or advised.

Immunoprophylaxis

There is no vaccine available for STDs, with the exception of hepatitis B vaccines.

Self-Treatment Abroad

Travelers who develop a symptomatic STD should seek medical attention when symptoms develop. Self-treatment of STDs is not advised.

Principles of Therapy

Ceftriaxone or azithromycin are recommended for gonorrhea, chancroid, and genital chlamydia infections. Doxycycline or azithromycin may be used for *C. trachomatis* infection. Benazathin-penicilline is used to treat early syphilis; acyclovir and derivates are used for herpes, and metronidazole and its derivates are used for *T. vaginalis*. The threat of HIV transmission is reduced by treating STDs, because STDs (particularly, ulcerative processes) facilitate the spread of HIV. (See "Sexually Transmitted Diseases" in Part 4, "Diagnosis and Management of Illness after Return or Immigration")

▌ Community Control Measures

Contact tracing and treating active STD cases are important in reducing the occurrence of STDs, including HIV infection.

Additional Readings

Cabada MM, et al. Sexual behavior of international travelers visiting Peru. Sex Transm Dis 2002;29:510–3.

Center for Disease Control and Prevention. STD treatment guidelines. Clin Infect Dis 2002;35:S135–S224.

Memish ZA, et al. International travel and sexually transmitted diseases. Travel Med Infect Dis 2006;4:86–93.

Richens J. Sexually transmitted infections and HIV among travellers: a review. Travel Med Infect Dis 2006;4:184–95.

Ward PJ, Plourde P. Travel and sexually transmitted infections. J Travel Med 2006;13:300-17.

SMALLPOX

Smallpox has been eradicated, but the virus is stored in an unknown number of laboratories. Smallpox vaccination may be dangerous, both for vacinees and contacts because of risk of generalized vaccinia, eczema vaccinatum, and progressive vaccinia or postvaccinal encephalitis for the vaccinee. Nevertheless, with the threat of bioterrorism, increased interest in smallpox vaccine exists. The vaccine is available in short supply currently. This vaccine is associated with a potentially fatal generalized infection in approximately 1 in 1 million immunized persons. Even with concerns on bioterrorism, this vaccine is currently not recommended for any travelers.

Infectious Agent

Variola virus

Transmission

Normally, transmission occurred by close contact with respiratory discharge and skin lesions of patients or materials that had been contaminated. Airborne spread occurred infrequently (eg, in the German hospital of Meschede).

Global Epidemiology

The last known cases occurred in 1977 in Somalia and in 1978 in a laboratory incident in the United Kingdom.

Risk for Travelers

Currently none

Clinical Picture

It occurs with a sudden onset with fever, malaise, headache, backache, and, occasionally, abdominal pain. After 2 to 4 days, the temperature falls and a rash appears with the following successive stages: macules, papules, vesicles, pustules, and finally scabs that fall off at the end of the third to fourth week. Characteristically, there is a centrifugal distribution with more lesions on the extremities than on the trunk. Fever usually recurs during that period. In the more severe variola major, the coronary flow reserve (CFR) in unvaccinated patients was 20 to 40%, with death mostly occurring in the second week. In variola minor, the CFR usually did not exceed 1%. Two other less frequent clinical presentations, flat (malignant) and hemorrhagic smallpox, are usually fatal.

In differential diagnosis to chickenpox, smallpox has a more clear-cut prodromal phase; the lesions are more simultaneous in stage, are more deeply seated, and are round, hard, confluent or umbilicated. Likewise, the periphery of the extremities, including palmar areas, are more severely affected, compared with the proximal ones.

Incubation

The incubation period can be from 7 to 17 days (most commonly 10 to 12 days to first symptoms).

Minimized Exposure in Travelers

Currently there's no risk—in case of an outbreak, one should follow recommendations issued by international and national advisory groups.

Susceptibility and Resistance

There is universal susceptibility. Permanent immunity usually follows recovery. There is uncertainty about immunity granted by immunization performed 25 or more years ago.

Immunization by Vaccinia Vaccine

Viability: live; various vaccines (different vaccine strains, varying degree of purification) available in different countries, short supply in many countries, particularly in the developing world

Application

Schedule: single dose

Booster: every 3 years was the required routine in international travel

Postexposure prophylaxis: see below

Route: multiple puncture or scratch

Site: deltoid; women in particular often prefer the ventrogluteal region for aesthetic reasons

Availability: worldwide, not marketed; new vaccines under development.

Protection

Onset: 10 days after primary vaccination, 7 days after revaccination

Efficacy: > 95%. CFR of at least primovaccinated persons clearly reduced to 0 to 12%, compared with unvaccinated people. It is unknown whether vaccinia offers cross protection against monkeypox.

Duration: approximately 3 to 5 years, thereafter gradually decreasing

Protective level: protective antibody levels unknown, and no correlation of antibody titers and protection proven; > 95% of primary vaccinees show neutralizing antibody titers of > 1:10.

Adverse Reactions

Accidental autoinoculation (satellite pustules on, for example, face, eye-lid, nose, and mouth), eczema vaccinatum, generalized vaccinia, progressive vaccinia, postvaccinal encephalitis. This is > 10 times more frequent among primary vaccinees and more frequent among infants. Approximately one death in 1 million primary vaccinees.

Vaccinia immune globulin for the treatment of cutaneous, including ocular adverse events is recommended; it is not available on the public market. Cidofovir derivatives in evaluation, not marketed.

Contraindications

Absolute: any kind of immunosuppressed person, including HIV infection, patients with acute or past history of varicella zoster, eczema, atopic dermatitis or similar skin conditions, pregnancy, allergic reaction to a vaccine component.

Vaccination also contraindicated in persons who have household contact with persons with such contraindications.

Relative: any acute illness

Children: age < 18 years in non-emergency situations

Pregnant women: contraindicated, but no routine pregnancy testing recommended

Lactating women: contraindicated

Immunodeficient persons: contraindicated

Interactions

Possibly with varicella vaccine; do not administer simultaneously.

Recommendations for Vaccine Use

Currently not indicated for any travelers (except some military and relief workers dispatched to potential risk areas)

Self-Treatment Abroad and Postexposure Prophylaxis

No self-treatment possible. Postexposure immunization is effective if given within 72 hours (and attenuation of disease possible if given within 7 days) after exposure.

Principles of Therapy

Strict respiratory and contact isolation. Supportive therapy. Treatment of secondary (bacterial) infections. Topical treatment for corneal lesions, cidofovir derivatives under investigation.

Community Control Measures

Notification and further measures as required by national and international regulations.

Additional Readings

Baxby D. Smallpox vaccination techniques. Vaccine 2002;20:2140–9.

Cohen HW. Smallpox vaccinations and adverse events. JAMA 2006;295:1897–8.

Frey SE, et al. Clinical responses to undiluted and diluted smallpox vaccine. N Engl J Med 2002;346:1265–74.

SOIL-TRANSMITTED HELMINTHS

Infectious Agents and Transmission

The soil-transmitted helminths are a group of parasitic nematode worms causing human infection through contact with parasite eggs or larvae. Of particular importance in terms of human infections are roundworms (*Ascaris lumbricoides*), whipworms (*Trichuris trichiura*), hookworms (*Necator americanus* or *Ancylostoma duodenale*) and Strongyloides.

Global Epidemiology

Soil-transmitted helminth infections are widely distributed throughout the tropics and subtropics. Warm temperatures and moisture are essential for larval development in the soil. More than a billion people are infected with at least one species. For Ascaris and Trichuris, the most intense infections are in children aged 5 to 15 years. Although heavy hookworm infections also occur in childhood, frequency and intensity commonly remain high in adulthood, even in elderly people. These infections cause more disability, rather than death. Estimates of annual deaths from soil-transmitted helminth infection vary widely, from 12,000 to as many as 135,000.

Risk to Travelers

The true risk of soil-transmitted helminthic infections in travelers is unknown and depends on destination, activities during travel, living standards and duration of travel. Ascaris and Trichuris are frequently found in stools in children of long-serving expats or missionaries. Children are at higher risk than adult travelers because they may be more often in contact with soil or soil-contaminated objects. Travelers or immigrants with unrecognized Strongyloides who undergo immunosuppressive therapy are at risk of Strongyloides hyperinfection syndrome.

Clinical Picture

All nematode infections can be asymptomatic and only found incidentally on screening. The presence of large numbers of adult ascaris worms in the small intestine can cause abdominal distension and pain. Rare complications are intussusception, volvulus and complete bowel obstruction. Chronic sequelae of chronic ascaris infection is growth stunting and intellectual growth retardation. Trichuris live preferentially in the cecum. Inflammation at the site of attachment from large numbers of whipworms results in colitis. Long-standing colitis produces a clinical disorder that resembles inflammatory bowel disease. Trichuris dysentery syndrome is an even more serious manifestation of heavy whipworm infection, resulting in chronic dysentery and rectal prolapse. The major pathology of hookworm infection results from intestinal blood loss as a result of adult parasite invasion and attachment to the mucosa and submucosa of the small intestine, resulting in iron-deficiency anemia. Severe hookworm infection can result in hypoproteinemia and anasarca.

Prevention

Avoid walking barefoot; wash hands frequently; avoid playing with soil or soil-contaminated objects.

Immunoprophylaxis

Currently none. A hookworm vaccine initiative is under way.

Principles of Therapy

Albendazole 400 mg single dose for ascaris and hookworm, 400 mg for 3 days for heavy Trichuris infections. Mass treatment is performed in endemic areas. For long-term travelers and expats, stool examination every 6 months may be indicated, although there are currently no guidelines to do so. Some expat/missionary families treat their children with single dose of albendazole every 6 to 12 months. Treatment for strongyloidosis: ivermectin.

Additional Readings

Nuesch R, et al. Imported strongyloidosis: a longitudinal analysis of 31 cases. J Travel Med 2005;12:80–4.

Sudarshi S, et al. Clinical presentation and diagnostic sensitivity of laboratory tests for Strongyloides stercoralis in travellers compared with immigrants in a non-endemic country. Trop Med Int Health 2003;8:728–32.

TETANUS

Infectious Agent

Clostridium tetani, the tetanus bacillus, is found in the intestines of animals and humans, where it is harmless.

Transmission

Tetanus spores in soil contaminated with feces may enter the body through wounds. The wounds may have been unnoticed or untreated; in 20% of cases, the source of tetanus entry is unknown.

Global Epidemiology

Tetanus occurs worldwide but is uncommon in the developed nations. In the developing countries, infants and young children are most often affected. In the developed countries, tetanus occurs most often in persons over age 60 who have neglected booster vaccine doses and have lost immunity. The disease is more common in rural areas where contact with animal (mainly horse) excreta is more likely.

Risk for Travelers

Worldwide, there has been only one single case of tetanus reported in a traveler, a person from Germany returning from Spain.

Clinical Picture

Initial symptoms include rigidity in the abdomen and in the region of the injury and painful muscular contractions in the masseter, neck muscles, and later in the trunk muscles. Generalized spasms then occur, followed by risus sardonicus (sardonic smile) and opisthotonos. If untreated, death most often results from spasms of the thoracic muscles. Case fatality rates range from 10 to 20%, depending on the quality of treatment received in intensive care.

Incubation

The incubation period can last from one day to several months (3 to 21 days most commonly), depending on the nature, extent, and location of the wound.

Communicability

There is no direct transmission from person to person.

Susceptibility and Resistance

There is general susceptibility to tetanus. Immunity by tetanus toxoid lasts for at least 10 years after full immunization. Recovery from tetanus does not result in immunity.

Minimized Exposure in Travelers

Immunization should be kept up to date. If, for some reason, this is impossible (perhaps refused), educate the traveler about the necessity of prophylaxis after injury.

Chemoprophylaxis

None

Immunoprophylaxis by Tetanus Toxoid Vaccine

Immunology and Pharmacology

Viability: inactivated

Antigenic form: toxoid of *C. tetani*. Note that, in children, polyvalent vaccines, and, in adults, diphtheria-tetanus vaccines, are preferred to tetanus toxoid alone.

Adjuvants: aluminum phosphate, potassium sulfate or hydroxide

Preservative: 0.01% thimerosal

Allergens/Excipiens: none / not > 0.02% residual-free formaldehyde

Mechanism: induction of protective antitoxin antibodies against tetanus toxin

Application

Schedule: When immunization with tetanus toxoid begins in the first year of life (usually as combined vaccine tri-, tetra, penta- or hexavalent), the primary series consists of three 0.5 mL doses, 4 to 8 weeks apart, followed by a fourth reinforcing 0.5 mL dose 6 to 12 months after the third dose. For children from second year of life, the series begins with two 0.5 mL doses given 4 to 8 weeks apart, and a third 0.5 mL dose given 6 to 12 months later. The same series is followed for adults.

Booster: 0.5 mL after 10 years is routine in most countries, but in the United Kingdom, this is considered not necessary after the age of 20, but a single booster dose is recommended in patients with potentially contaminated wounds.

Postexposure prophylaxis: see below

Route: deeply intramuscularly

Site: deltoid; use anterolateral thigh in infants and small children.

Storage: Store at 2 to 8 °C (35 to 46 °F). Discard frozen vaccine.

Availability: worldwide

Protection

Onset: after third dose

Efficacy: > 99%

Duration: at least 10 years

Protective level: Minimum specific antitoxin levels of ≥ 0.01 units per mL are generally regarded as protective; optimal is ≥ 0.1 units per mL.

Adverse Reactions

Erythema, induration, pain, tenderness, and warmth, plus edema surrounding the injection site occur for several days in 30 to 50% of cases. There may be a palpable nodule at the injection site for several weeks.

Transient low-grade fever, chills, malaise, generalized aches and pains, headaches, and flushing may occur. Temperatures > 38 °C (> 100 °F) following tetanus and diphtheria toxoid (Td) injection are unusual. Patients occasionally experience generalized urticaria or pruritus, tachycardia, anaphylaxis, hypotension, or neurologic complications.

Interaction between the injected antigen and high levels of preexisting tetanus antibody from prior booster doses seems to be the most likely cause of severe Arthus reaction.

Combined Td vaccine causes slightly higher rates of local and systemic adverse reactions than tetanus toxoid vaccine, but the rate of incapacitation is not increased in Td as compared to monovalent tetanus vaccine.

Contraindications

Absolute: persons with a history of serious (particularly neurologic) adverse reactions to the vaccine

Relative: any acute illness. Avoid giving persons with previous severe adverse reactions to the vaccine even emergency doses of tetanus toxoid more frequently than every 10 years. Many of these persons will have generated great quantities of antitoxins during reactions, and levels > 0.01 antitoxin units per mL may persist for decades. Antitoxin levels can be measured.

If the patient's tolerance of tetanus toxoid is in doubt and an emergency booster dose is required, test with a small dose (0.05 to 0.1 mL) subcutaneously. The balance of the full 0.5 mL dose can be given 12 hours later if no reaction occurs. If a marked reaction does occur, further toxoid injections need not be administered at that time, because reducing the dose of tetanus toxoid does not proportionately reduce its effectiveness.

Children: tetanus toxoid is effective and safe for children as young as 6 weeks. Nevertheless, polyvalent vaccines are the preferred immunizing agents for most children until age 7 to 12, depending on national regulations. The preferred immunizing agent for most adults and older children is Td (that is, tetanus toxoid combined with the weaker adult dose of diphtheria toxoid). Increasingly, diphtheria and tetanus toxoids and acellular pertussis vaccine (DTaP) or, if indicated, DTaP-IPV are used.

Pregnant women: category C. Use only if clearly needed. The Td combination is preferred. Recommended in third trimester in developing countries to prevent neonatal tetanus.

Lactating women: it is unknown whether tetanus toxoid or corresponding antibodies are excreted in breast milk. Problems in humans have not been documented.

Immunodeficient persons: persons receiving immunosuppressive therapy or having other immunodeficiencies may experience diminished antibody response to active immunization. For this reason, defer primary tetanus immunization until treatment is discontinued, or inject an additional dose 1 month after immunosuppressive treatment has ceased. Routine immunization of symptomatic and asymptomatic HIV-infected persons is recommended.

Interactions

Like all inactivated vaccines, administering tetanus toxoid to persons receiving immunosuppressant drugs, including high-dose corticosteroids or radiation therapy, may result in an insufficient response to immunization.

No interactions with other travel-related vaccines have been documented.

Recommendations for Vaccine Use

This is a routine immunization worldwide. After completing a primary series, administer a booster dose every 10 years for life (exception: the United Kingdom as explained above), usually together with diphtheria immunization.

▌Self-Treatment Abroad and Postexposure Prophylaxis

Clean all wounds, and immediately flush with soap and water. Apply ethanol (70%) tincture, aqueous solution of iodine, or povidone iodine.

A physician must determine the need for postexposure immunization, taking into account the risk of contamination and the immunization status of the patient (Table 18).

Postexposure treatment depends on the nature of the wound. For clean, minor wounds, patients who have previously received < 3 doses of absorbed tetanus toxoid or whose vaccine status is unknown, give a tetanus-diphtheria vaccine dose with no tetanus immune globulin (TIG). If they have previously received three doses of absorbed tetanus toxoid, give them a tetanus-diphtheria booster dose if > 10 years have elapsed since the last dose of tetanus toxoid (no TIG).

Wounds possibly contaminated with dirt, feces, soil, and saliva, puncture wounds, avulsions; and wounds resulting from crushing, missiles, burns, or frostbite, should be treated as follows:

- If the patient has previously received < 3 doses of absorbed tetanus toxoid or their vaccine status is unknown, give a tetanus-diphtheria vaccine dose, along with TIG 250 IU intramuscularly.

Table 18 Tetanus Prophylaxis in Routine Wound Management.

History of Absorbed Tetanus Toxoid	Clean, Minor Wounds		All Other Wounds*	
	Td†	TIG‡	Td	TIG
Unknown or < 3 doses	Yes	No	Yes	Yes
≥ 3 doses§	No‖	No	No#	No

*Such as, but not limited to, wounds contaminated with dirt, feces, soil, or saliva; puncture wounds; avulsions; and wounds resulting from missiles, crushing, burns, or frostbite.

†For children aged < 7 years the diphtheria and tetanus toxoids and acellular pertussis vaccines (DTaP) or the diphtheria and tetanus toxoids and whole-cell pertussis vaccines (DTP) — or pediatric diphtheria and tetanus toxoids (DT), if pertussis vaccine is contraindicated — is preferred to tetanus toxoid (TT) alone. For persons aged ≥ 7 years, the tetanus and diphtheria toxoids (Td) for adults is preferred to TT alone.

‡TIG = tetanus immune globulin.

‖Yes, if > 10 years since the last dose.

#Yes, if > 5 years since the last dose. More frequent boosters are not needed and can accentuate side effects.

In general, if emergency tetanus prophylaxis is indicated some time between the third primary dose and the booster dose, give a 0.5 mL dose. If given before 6 months have elapsed, count it as a primary dose. If given after 6 months, regard it as a reinforcing dose.

Principles of Therapy

Tetanus immune globulin is used for therapy or, if unavailable, tetanus antitoxin. Metronidazole and active immunization are administered. Supportive care should be given.

Community Control Measures

Notification is required in most countries. No other measures are necessary.

Additional Readings

Broder KR, et al. Preventing tetanus, diphtheria, and pertussis among adolescents: use of tetanus toxoid, reduced diphtheria toxoid and acellular pertussis vaccines recommendations of the Advisory Committee on Immunization Practices (ACIP). MMWR Recomm Rep 2006;55(RR-3):1–34.

Tetanus toxoid for adults — too much of a good thing [editorial]. Lancet 1996;346:1185–6.

Rosenblatt HM et al. Tetanus immunity after diphtheria, tetanus toxoids, and acellular pertussis vaccination in children with clinically stable HIV infection. J Allerg Clin Immunol 2005;116:698-703.

WHO. Tetanus vaccine. Wkly epid Rec 2006;81:198-208.

TICK-BORNE ENCEPHALITIS
(SPRING-SUMMER ENCEPHALITIS)

Infectious Agent

The tick-borne encephalitis (TBE) virus is found in rural Europe; it is closely related to the Russian spring-summer encephalitis virus (also called TBE, Far Eastern subtype) transmitted by other ticks in vast areas of Asian Russia. The vaccine protects against both infections.

Transmission

Tick-borne encephalitis is spread by ticks (Europe, mainly *Ixodes ricinus*; Siberia, mainly *Ixodes persulcatus*), which are most active in forests, fields, or pastures. They climb no higher then 1.5 meters above the ground. Parks in large cities are also increasingly affected. The infection is occasionally acquired from unpasteurized dairy products.

Global Epidemiology

This infection occurs in large parts of rural Europe (Figure 41). Transmission seems to be highest in parts of the Baltic States (including islands in the Baltic Sea), Austria, the Czech Republic, Hungary, and Russia, especially in Siberia. Tick-borne encephalitis rarely occurs at altitudes above 1,300 m or in urban areas. The main period of transmission is April to October but, during warm winters, patients may be infected in almost any month, particularly in the southern endemic regions, such as Northern Italy. Risk of infection is highest in areas favoring the establishment of a virus cycle, such as forests and areas containing shrubs and bushes.

Risk for Travelers

There is almost no risk, unless hiking or camping in forested areas or pastures in endemic areas. Imported cases of TBE have been observed in Australia, Austria, Canada, Denmark, Germany (average age 18 years), Italy, the Netherlands, Norway, Russia, Sweden, the United States, and the United Kingdom. United

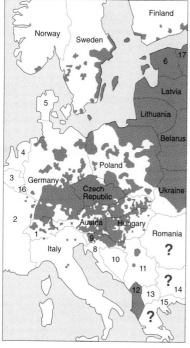

1. Switzerland
2. France
3. Belgium
4. Nertherlands
5. Denmark
6. Estonia
7. Slovakia
8. Croatia
9. Slovenia
10. Bosnia and Herzegovina
11. Serbia and Montenegro
12. Albania
13. Macedonia
14. Bulgaria
15. Greece
16. Luxembourg
17. Russia

▨ TBE cases declared

? TBE cases probable;
no precise documentation of individual
cases of TBE available

Figure 41 Distribution of tickborne encephalitis (TBE) 2006

Nations troops were infected in Bosnia and Kosovo. The risk per
week in Austria is estimated to be 1 per 10,000.

Clinical Picture

In endemic areas, 1 to 2% (and up to 10%) of ticks harbor the
TBE virus. Infection is symptomatic in 10% of patients, who
develop flu-like symptoms, with a second phase of febrile illness
developing in 10% of those cases. This second phase is associated with encephalitis, which may result in paralysis with

subsequent sequelae or death. The above rates mean that, after a tick-bite in an endemic area, only 0.1% at maximum will develop neurologic symptoms. Prognosis is worse with increasing age.

Incubation

The incubation period ranges from 2 to 28 days (usually 10), followed by an interval with no symptoms for 4 to 10 days.

Communicability

No person-to-person transmission occurs. Theoretical concerns exist for breast-feeding and blood transfusions.

Susceptibility and Resistance

Inapparent infections are common, particularly in children, among whom the overt disease is rare. Long-term homologous immunity follows infection.

Minimized Exposure in Travelers

Travelers should wear clothing that covers as much skin as possible when walking in endemic areas. The use of repellants significantly reduces the risk of tick bites. These measures result only in partial protection. Whenever a tick is detected, it should be removed as soon as possible (see below).

Chemoprophylaxis

None

Immunoprophylaxis by TBE Vaccine

Immunology and Pharmacology

Viability: inactivated
Antigenic form: purified whole virus
Adjuvants: aluminum hydroxide
Preservative: thimerosal 0.01%
Allergens/Excipiens: none (EncepurN) or human albumin 0.5 mg per 0.5 mL (FSME-Immun) / formaldehyde <0.01 mg per 0.5 mL, traces of antibiotics

Mechanism: induction of active immunity against the causative virus

Application

Schedule: three 0.5 mL doses at 0, 1 to 3, and 9 to 12 months (conventional schedule). Accelerated schedules are registered for EncepurN adults/children (day 0 to 7 to 21 days and first booster after 12 to 18 months), and for FSME-Immun, where the second dose can be given as soon as 2 weeks after the first dose. To achieve immunity before the beginning of tick activity, the first two doses should be given during the winter months. When departure to an endemic region is imminent, administer a specific immune globulin in a single dose to offer protection for at least 1 month. Currently, however, the use of immune globulin is no longer recommended by experts, due to concerns about an enhancement effect.

Booster: recommended 3 years after the primary series or last booster

Route: IM

Site: deltoid

Storage: Store at 2 to 8 °C (35 to 46 °F). Discard frozen vaccine.

Availability: available in many European countries as EncepurN (adult or children; Novartis (formerly Chiron) Vaccine), or FSME-Immun Inject (Baxter)

Protection

Onset: following the second injection

Efficacy: over 90% of vaccine recipients are protected against TBE for 1 year after the second dose. Efficacy increases to 98% for the year following the third dose. The TBE vaccine is also effective against Eastern (Russian/Asian) subtype strains; the determining protein E is at least 94% congruent with the European strain.

Duration: at least 3 years, probably considerably longer. The official Swiss recommendations now include booster doses only every 10 years.

Protective level: unknown

Adverse Reactions

Erythema and swelling around the injection site may occur, as well as swelling of regional lymph glands. Systemic reaction such as fatigue, limb pain, headache, fever > 38 °C (100 °F), vomiting, or temporary rash occasionally occur. Rarely, neuritis is seen.

Contraindications

Absolute: persons with a history of serious, adverse reactions to the vaccine

Relative: any acute illness

Children: none. Usually unnecessary in first year of life.

Pregnant women: category C. Use only if clearly needed.

Lactating women: It is unknown whether the vaccine or corresponding antibodies are excreted in breast milk. Problems in humans have not been documented.

Immunodeficient persons: Persons receiving immunosuppressive therapy or having other immunodeficiencies may experience diminished antibody response to active immunization.

Interactions

Like all inactivated vaccines, TBE vaccine administered to persons receiving immunosuppressant drugs, including high-dose corticosteroids, or radiation therapy may result in an insufficient response to immunization.

Interactions with other travel-related vaccines have not been documented.

Recommendations for Vaccine Use

This vaccine is recommended for travelers (particularly adults and adolescents) who are planning outdoor activities in rural areas of endemic regions.

▌ Self-Treatment Abroad

Remove the tick as soon as possible by grasping it with a forceps as close to the skin as possible and pulling slowly, constantly, and straight, taking care to remove the tick whole and to avoid leaving mouthparts behind. Avoid using oil, varnish, or other substances to suffocate the tick; this may prompt ejection of more infectious material into the body. Flat forceps that squeeze the tick to vomit into the human skin also are a disadvantage. Mouthpieces still seen in the skin are usually no indication for surgical removal because, for the most part, no local infection occurs. For borreliosis see specific chapter.

Postexposure prophylaxis with tick-borne immune globulin is no longer considered beneficial, even if given within 48 hours.

Principles of Therapy

Supportive

Additional Readings

Jensenius M, et al. Threats to international travellers posed by tick-borne diseases. Travel Med Infect Dis 2006;4:4–13.

Pitches DW. Removal of ticks. Eurosurveillance 2006;11:196–8.

Rendi-Wagner P. Risk and prevention of tick-borne encephalitis in travelers. J Travel Med 2004;11:307–12.

TRAVELERS' DIARRHEA

Infectious Agents

Travelers' diarrhea is caused by a number of microbial pathogens, of which bacterial agents are most common. Enterotoxigenic *Escherichia coli* (ETEC) and enteroaggregative *E. coli* (EAEC) are the most important in the developing world causing between 20 and 50% of diarrhea cases in high-risk areas (Figure 42, Table 20).

The invasive bacterial pathogens, *Salmonella, Shigella*, and *Campylobacter jejuni*, account for 5 to 30% of cases contracted in high-risk areas. Invasive *E. coli* occasionally causes travelers' diarrhea. When ETEC rates drop in Mexico and Morocco during the drier seasons, *C. jejuni* becomes more important. In Thailand, *C. jejuni* and Aeromonas are major causes of travelers' diarrhea. *Plesiomonas shigelloides*, non-cholera vibrios, and, rarely, *Vibrio cholerae* 01 (the cause of cholera) causes diarrhea generally associated with seafood consumption. Noroviruses (and to a lesser degree rotaviruses) are important causes of gastroenteritis in all populations, including travelers. The parasitic pathogens are not common causes of travelers' diarrhea, although they are found more often among travelers to Nepal (especially Cyclospora), St. Petersburg (Giardia and Cryptosporidium), and to mountainous areas of North America (Giardia). *Entamoeba histolytica* is a rare cause of travelers' diarrhea, but occurs especially among those who live close to the local population, such as volunteers and missionaries. Parasitic agents are suspected in returning travelers with persistent diarrhea because most cases of bacterial and viral infection are self-limiting or respond to antibacterial therapy.

Transmission

Food and, to a lesser degree, water are the principal sources of enteric infection for travelers in high-risk areas. Food and beverages are categorized based on potential for contamination by diarrhea-causing microbes. The most dangerous food items are those containing moisture and those served at room temperature or that have been kept that way for some time. The safest foods and beverages are those served steaming hot. Most diarrhea-causing enteropathogens are inactivated at temperatures at or above

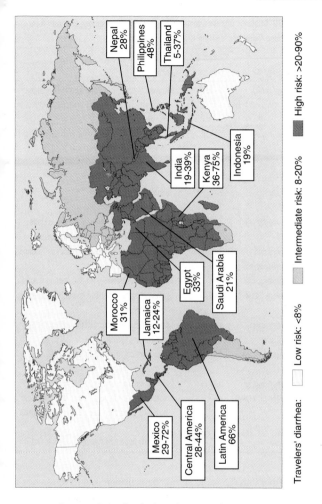

Figure 42   Risk countries for traveler's diarrhea and proportion of enterotoxigenic
E. coli (ETEC)

60 °C. Other generally safe foods are those served without moisture (e.g. bread), with high sugar content including syrups, jellies,
jam and honey, fruit that has been peeled and fruit juices with no
added liquid. Bottled carbonated beverages are considered safe.

Table 20 Etiologic Agents Causing Travelers' Diarrhea among Persons from Developed Countries Visiting High-Risk Areas

Etiologic Agent	Frequency –Range (%)	Comment
Enterotoxigenic *Escherichia coli* (ETEC)	5–50	The most common travelers' diarrhea pathogen worldwide; seasonal pattern in some semitropical regions
Enteroaggregative *Escherichia coli* (EAEC)	10–20	Common cause of symptomatic and asymptomatic infection in travelers
Enteroinvasive *Escherichia coli* (EIEC)	0–6	Variable importance
Salmonella spp	2–7	Variable importance
Shigella spp	2–15	Variable importance
Campylobacter jejuni	3–50	Variable importance; seasonal pattern in some semitropical regions: important in Thailand
Aeromonas and *Plesiomonas*	3–15	Important in some tropical areas such as Thailand
Vibrio cholerae 01	.005	Rare cause of potentially life threatening diarrhea
Non-cholera *Vibrios*	0–3	Occasional cause of seafood associated diarrhea in coastal areas
Noroviruses and Rotaviruses	5–20	Common cause of gastroenteritis with vomiting as the primary clinical symptom
Giardia lamblia	0–5	Common among travelers to Russia or to recreational waters in proximity to wildlife
Cryptosporidium	0–5	Common among travelers to Russia
Entomoeba histolytica	<1	Amoebiasis occurs in persons who are living close to a local population living under poor hygienic conditions
Cyclospora	0–5	Particularly important among travelers to Nepal

Ice cubes and tap water should be considered to have low-level contamination, whether in a hotel or elsewhere. Rinsing toothbrush and mouth with tap water in most urban areas is probably safe, but drinking tap water not first boiled is not advised.

Global Epidemiology

Diarrhea often occurs in international travelers. The frequency of the resultant illness depends on the countries of origin and destination (Table 21). The world may be divided into three levels of

Table 21 Risk of Acquiring Diarrhea among Travelers According to Host Country and Country Visited

Country of Origin	Country to be Visited		
	Low	Intermediate	High
Low	2–4%	10–20%	20–90%
Intermediate	2–4%	Uncertain	8–18%
High	2–4%	N/A	8–18%

risk for diarrhea based on degree of hygiene. The low-risk areas include Northern, Western, and now many parts of Southern Europe, the United States and Canada, the more hygienic Caribbean islands, Australia, New Zealand, and Japan. High-risk areas include Latin America, most of Southern Asia, and North, West, and East Africa. Intermediate or moderate-risk areas include some of the northern Mediterranean countries and the Middle East (although Turkey was found to be high-risk), Jamaica, China, and Russia, the other countries of the former Soviet Union, and South Africa.

Enteric infection and diarrheal diseases are the most commonly reported medical complaint among travelers from the developed countries to tropical and semitropical areas. The incidence of diarrhea among persons from low-risk areas visiting other low-risk areas is approximately 2 to 4%, 10 to 20 for travel to intermediate-risk areas, and 20 to 40% for travel to high-risk areas. In select groups (eg, Nile cruises), the rate may be as high as 90%. The 2 to 4% rate above for persons visiting low-risk areas also applies to travelers from high or intermediate-risk areas.

These background rates of illness probably relate to dependence on public eating establishments for most travelers, stress, and differences in behavior (eg, increased consumption of alcohol). These rates are based on published studies, which are few in number except for travel from low-risk to high- and intermediate-risk regions.

Clinical Picture

Enteric infections vary widely in severity, from subclinical or self-limiting and mild diarrhea to cholera-like, potentially fatal, diarrhea accompanied by dehydration, febrile dysentery, or enteric (typhoid-like) fever. Travelers' diarrhea typically develops during the first week after arrival. The illness may be divided into three categories based on severity, each with different recommendations for treatment. In mild diarrhea, normal activities can be carried out. In moderate diarrhea, activities are limited, but the person is able to function. In severe diarrhea, the person is incapacitated—usually confined to bed.

The specific clinical enteric syndromes and etiology of enteric infection in international travelers vary widely as shown in Table 22.

The symptoms, to some extent, suggest the etiology. When vomiting is the primary symptom, the patient has gastroenteritis secondary to ingestion of preformed toxins in foods or to viral agents.

The preformed toxins are produced by *Staphylococcus aureus* or *Bacillus cereus*. The most important viral pathogens in travelers' diarrhea are the noroviruses. Watery diarrhea, with or without vomiting, is seen with any of the known bacterial, viral, or parasitic enteropathogens. Fever and passage of bloody stools, frequently containing mucus, indicate dysenteric illness often due to either *Shigella* or *Campylobacter*. Other enteric pathogens that less frequently cause dysenteric disease in the traveler include invasive *E. coli*, *Salmonella*, *Aeromonas*, non-cholera vibrios, and *Entamoeba histolytica*.

Table 22 Clinical Syndromes Caused by Enteric Pathogens

Clinical Enteric Syndrome	Etiologic Agent to Consider
Gastroenteritis with vomiting as the predominant symptom	Noroviruses and to a lesser extent rotaviruses or preformed toxins of *Staphylococcus aureus* or *Bacillus cereus*
Watery diarrhea, with or without vomiting	Any bacterial, viral or protozoal pathogen
Febrile dysentery (passage of bloody stools)	*Shigella* spp or *Campylobacter jejuni* likely; other possibilities include invasive *Escherichia coli*, *Salmonella* spp, Aeromonas spp, non-cholera *Vibrios*, *Entamoeba histolytica*
Persistent diarrhea (duration ≥ 14 days)	Parasitic agents, (*Giardia, Cryptosporidium, Cyclospora, Microsporidia*), Bacterial enteropathogens, small bowel bacterial overgrowth syndrome, lactase deficiency, Brainerd diarrhea, post-infectious irritable bowel syndrome
Typhoid (enteric) fever	*Salmonella typhi, Salmonella paratyphi*, other *Salmonella* spp

Between 2–10% of travelers' diarrhea lasts longer than 2 weeks. This persistent diarrhea may be caused by a bacterial enteropathogen, by a parasitic pathogen such as *Giardia, Cryptosporidium, Cyclospora,* or *Microsporidium,* by small bowel bacterial overgrowth, by lactase deficiency, by an idiopathic form of chronic diarrhea classified as Brainerd diarrhea or post-infectious irritable bowel syndrome. Typhoid fever is unusual in travelers.

Susceptibility and Resistance

Persons from low-risk areas are particularly susceptible to enteric infection in moderate- and high-risk areas. Persons from intermediate- and high-risk areas visiting other high-risk areas experience lower rates of illness, compared with persons from low-risk areas. This suggests that they have had prior exposure to the prevalent microbes.

Risk factors for acquiring travelers' diarrhea are multiple (Table 23). Young children who eat at the table and young adults with large appetites appear to be at higher risk than adults. Young infants who eat only carefully prepared formula or who are breastfed will be at reduced risk. Illness in infants may occur with crawling in a contaminated environment and by frequently putting their hands in their mouths. Adventure travelers and those living close to the local population (eg, Peace Corps volunteers and mis-

Table 23 Established Risk Factors Predisposing to Travelers' Diarrhea

Risk Factor	Comment
Age	Rates are highest for young infants (toddlers) exposed to contaminated environment and young children eating from the table and adolescents with large appetites.
Type of travel	Adventure travelers and persons living close to the local population (eg, missionaries, Peace Corps Volunteers) are at greater risk
Beverage and food restrictions	Persons who do not exercise care in the food and beverages they consume are likely to have higher rates of diarrhea
Genetics	Certain persons are more susceptible to illness based on genetic factors
Prior travel to high-risk regions	Previous travel to high-risk areas within the prior 6 months is associated with a reduced rate of travelers' diarrhea
Hypochlorhydria and Achlorhydria	Low gastric acidity, whether induced by prior surgery or proton pump inhibitor, predisposes to travelers' diarrhea

sionaries) have higher rates of illness compared with those staying in the better hotels. Certain persons appear to show variable rates of enteric infection based on genetic factors. Host genetic polymorphism in mediators of gut inflammation has recently been identified with increased susceptibility to travelers' diarrhea. Some strains of animals have an absence of receptors for attachment of ETEC, the principal cause of travelers' diarrhea, while others do not. Similar genetic differences probably exist in human populations. Persons with blood type O are predisposed to cholera and may experience more severe disease.

Stomach acidity is an important defense against enteric infectious disease agents, particularly bacterial enteropathogens. Persons with hypochlorhydria or achlorhydria based on genetic or nutritional factors, those who have had prior gastric surgery, or those taking proton pump inhibitors such as omeprazole are at greater risk of acquiring travelers' diarrhea, although the increase in risk is only of moderate level. Nocturnal use of H2 receptor antagonists appears to be a lower risk factor for develeopment of diarrhea than regular use of proton pump inhibitors. Travel to high-risk areas within 6 months after traveling to the same, or another, high-risk area seems to afford some protection against the illness. This suggests that prior exposure to prevalent agents results in protective immunity.

Means of Preventing Diarrhea in International Travelers

Travelers consuming low-risk foods and beverages may reduce their risk of contracting travelers' diarrhea (see Figure 8).

Chemoprophylaxis

The pros and cons of chemoprophylaxis are outlined in Table 24. Bismuth subsalicylate (BSS) is 65% effective in eliminating travelers' diarrhea, probably through the antimicrobial effects of bismuth. BSS causes minor side effects, including blackening of the tongue and stools and mild tinnitus in a small percentage of users. There are no major side effects of BSS when used as a prophylactic agent, although it is not recommended for use in patients with mucosal disease, such as that seen in advanced AIDS, or inflammatory bowel disease, where bismuth absorption may lead to bismuth encephalopathy.

Table 24 Protection, Minor and Major Side Effects of Conventional Therapy for Resultant Diarrhea in Patients Using or Not Using Chemoprophylaxis to Prevent Travelers' Diarrhea

Use of Chemoprophylaxis	Protection Rate	Number Ill per 100	Minor Side Effects	Major Side Effects	Treatment of Diarrhea
None	0%	40	0%	0%	Conventional*
Bismuth subsalicylate	65%	14	Common†	0%	Conventional*
Quinolone (for adults)	90%	4	3%‡	.01§	Azithromycin
Rifaximin	70–77%	8–12	None	None	Quinolone or Azithromycin

*Antibacterial agent plus loperamide (see Table 28)

†Black tongues, black stools, tinnitus

‡Skin rash, vaginal yeast infection, insomnia, irritability, headache

§Anaphylaxis, antibiotic-associated colitis, aplastic anemia, superinfection

Antibacterial agents, including fluoroquinolones and rifaximin are more effective and convenient prophylactic agents than BSS, providing between 70 and 90% protection. The systemically absorbed drugs occasionally produce minimal, but objectionable, side effects, including insomnia, irritability, headache, skin rash, or fungal vaginitis. In rare instances (estimated to occur < 0.01), travelers taking a fluoroquinolone as a prophylactic (< 0.01%) may experience a major side effect. The authors recommend the poorly absorbed rifamycin, rifaximin as the preferred antibacterial drug for prophylaxis in view of efficacy against diarrheagenic E. coli and its safety profile. Studies are needed to determine the value of rifaximin in preventing invasive forms of diarrhea (e.g. diarrhea caused by strains of *Shigella*, *Salmonella*, and *Campylobacter*).

Many authorities recommend against routine chemoprophylaxis for travelers' diarrhea prevention because self-treatment is so successful. Preventive medication may be considered, however, if the traveler is on a tight schedule and cannot afford an illness lasting 6 to 10 hours, (eg, politicians, musicians, athletes and lecturers), for those who have had travelers' diarrhea in previous trips (suggesting an increased susceptibility), or when the traveler has a predisposing condition such as immunodeficiency (AIDS), advanced malignancy, organ transplantation, inflam-

**Table 25 Recommended Approach to Chemoprophylaxis for Travelers'
According to Indication for Disease Prevention**

Patient Category	Prophylaxis Recommended
Most travelers to high-risk areas	Prophylaxis offered as one option
Traveler requests prophylaxis	Rifaximin prophylaxis
Travelers with underlying medical problem or have been ill in previous trips	Rifaximin is first choice
Travelers' itinerary will not allow a 6- to 10-hour illness	Rifaximin is first choice; quinolones, second choice
Trips to high-risk regions longer than 3 weeks	Prophylaxis is not recommended

matory bowel disease, regular use of proton pump inhibitors of
gastric acid, or insulin-dependent diabetes mellitus.
Chemoprophylaxis is reasonable to use in those travelers who
request this approach. Table 25 outlines the recommended approach
for prophylaxis for travelers according to category.

Chemoprophylaxis dosage is shown in Table 26. For BSS, two
tablets are taken with meals and at bedtime (8 tablets daily). For
adults opting for quinolone treatment, norfloxacin 400 mg,
ciprofloxacin 500 mg, or levofloxacin 500 mg are taken once a
day. The recommended dose of rifaximin is 200 mg (one tablet)
once or twice a day (taken with major daily meals). In each case,
travelers begin the drug the first day they are in the high-risk area
and continue the drug for approximately 1 to 2 days after returning. Chemoprophylaxis with an absorbed drug is not advised for

**Table 26 Prophylactic Regimens Preventing Travelers' Diarrhea for Trips
of 14 Days or Less**

Drug Used in Prophylaxis	Dosing Regimen
Bismuth subsalicylate	Two 265 mg tablets chewed well with meals and at bedtime (eight tablets/d) during stay in high risk area and for 2 days after leaving area
Rifaximin	One 200 mg tablet once or twice each day with major meals
Norfloxacin (NF), ciprofloxacin (CF), levofloxacin (LF)	NF 400 mg, CF 500 mg, or LF 500 mg once a day during stay in high risk area and for 2 days after leaving area

trips longer than 14–21 days in duration to high-risk areas, owing to the cost of the drug in prolonged prophylaxis, increased risk of adverse reactions, and interference with natural immunity. Although untested for periods longer than 2 weeks, it is our impression that rifaximin can be used for trips up to 3 weeks, in view of safety. Chemoprophylaxis is not advised for persons remaining at risk for more than 3 weeks.

Table 27 Available Enteric Vaccines and Those in the Planning Stages

Enteric Vaccine	Status

Enterotoxigenic *Escherichia coli*
  rCTB-CFA ETEC
  LT/ST Toxoids
  Attenuated *E. coli*
  CFSs/Attenuated *S. typhi* or Shigella
  LT patch vaccine given transcutaneously
	The rCTB-CFA ETEC vaccine has been field test resulting in short-term immunity.
	The LT patch vaccine is currently being field tested in Mexico and Guatemala.

Vibrio cholerae 01 and 0139
  rCTB-WC (01)
  BS-WC 01/0139
  Various live attenuated orally administered vaccines and lipopolysaccharide antigens
	These vaccine candidates are in advanced field testing. CVD 103 HgR and rCTB/WC accines are both marketed in some countries

Campylobacter jejuni	These vaccine candidates are in early development

Salmonella typhi
  Oral Live Ty21a Vaccine,
  Vi Antigen Vaccine
	The two vaccines are commercially available and 70% protective against typhoid fever

Shigella spp *Shigella* antigens in an avirulent carrier bacterium or attenuated *Shigella* mutants, O-polysaccharide-carrier protein conjugate or ribosomal vaccine	These vaccine candidates are in early development
Rotavirus Attenuated animal or reassortant animal-human or reassortant human vaccine strain	Preparations are either licensed or near licensure in most countries

BS = binding subunit; CVD = Center for Vaccine Development; rCTB = recombinant B subunit of cholera toxin; CFA = colonization factor antigen, attachment fimbriae of ETEC strains; CFS = ; LT = heat labile enterotoxin; ST = heat stable enterotoxin; Ty21a = orally adminstered attenuated typhoid fever strain; Vi = virulence antigen; WC = whole cell.

▌ Immunoprophylaxis

Vaccines are being developed to help prevent travelers' diarrhea. For this approach to be widely recommended, it may require a multivalent preparation directed against the most important pathogens. Poor hygienic standards in high-risk destinations remain a constant problem. That natural immunity tends to develop as persons remain in these areas makes prospects for vaccines promising. The organisms being targeted include ETEC, *V. cholerae* 01, *C. jejuni*, *Salmonella typhi*, *Shigella* sp, and rotavirus (Table 27).

The risk of cholera is so low for most travelers that vaccination is of doubtful value. An oral cholera vaccine, Dukoral from SBL Vaccines is available in some countries (see "Cholera"). Dukoral is a recombinant cholera binding toxin subunit of cholera toxin (rCBT) plus whole *V. cholerae* cells (WC) given in two oral doses. Dukoral has some efficacy against LT-producing ETEC strains causing diarrhea and, in some areas, is marketed as a "travelers' diarrhea vaccine." If we assume that a destination has a 60% incidence rate of diarrhea and that ETEC may cause a third of the cases, this corresponds to an overall 20% ETEC diarrhea incidence. If we continue to assume that 50% have an ST-only toxin, whereby the vaccine is ineffective, we have a remaining 10% incidence in pathogens wherein the vaccine may be effective. Dukoral showed protective efficacy of 60% against the LT-producing ETEC; thus, this vaccine would prevent approximately 5% of all travelers' diarrhea. However, it would benefit 6% of all travelers, which is more than any other vaccine. There is also great interest in developing safe and more effective vaccines against *S. typhi.* Immunity against *C. jejuni* occurs with age. Potential vaccine candidates against the organism are currently being investigated by several laboratories. Efforts are also under way to develop an effective vaccine against prevalent serotypes of *Shigella.*

Vaccines against rotavirus gastroenteritis are available or will be available soon in many countries. This would be an important initiative, considering the role of rotavirus in causing fatal disease among infants in the developing countries. A role of rotavirus vaccine in travel health has not yet been defined but the vaccine should be recommended for unimmunized infants and young children who will be residing in countries with high rates of rotavirus gastroenteritis.

Table 28 Self-Therapy of Travelers' Diarrhea

Therapeutic Agent	Dosage
Bismuth subsalicylate	Two 262 mg tablets chewed well or if liquid 2 tablespoons taken every ½ hour for 8 doses. May be repeated on day 2
Loperamide*	4 mg (2 tablets) initially followed by 2 mg (1 tablet) after each unformed stool passed, not to exceed 8 mg (4 tablets) per day for a maximum of 48 hours
Quinolone*: norfloxacin (NF), ciprofloxacin (CF), or levofloxacin (LF)	NF 400 mg bid, CF 500 mg bid, or 750 mg qd for 1 to 3 days, depending on response
Azithromycin*	500 mg qd for 1 to 3 days or 1,000 mg in a single dose
Rifaximin*	200 mg tid or 400 mg bid for 3 days

*Loperamide can be give with one of the antibacterial if the patient does not have fever and is not passing bloody stools.

Self-Treatment Abroad

All travel medicine experts recommend giving future travelers to high-risk areas, antidiarrheal medication to treat the illness if it occurs (Table 28). The two types of empiric therapy for adults are

- symptomatic treatment with either bismuth subsalicylate or loperamide
- antibacterial treatment

Table 29 Management of Travelers' Diarrhea Based on Clinical Symptoms*

Mild diarrhea (1 or 2 unformed stool passed per 24 hours and normal activities are continued)	Moderate (activities limited) to severe diarrhea (patient disabled)	
	Fever (38.5°C body temperature) or passage of bloody stools	Other cases
No other therapy or symptomatic therapy (see Table 28)	Antimicrobial therapy (see Table 28)	Antimicrobial plus loperamide therapy (see Table 28)

*All patients should receive oral fluids and electrolytes such as diluted fruit juice, soft drinks, or soups and broth with saltine crackers.

Designating the severity of illness determines self-therapy (Table 29). It is appropriate to take symptomatic therapy for milder forms of illness and give antibacterial therapy for diarrhea that is severe enough to lead to a change in trip schedule. All persons should take antibacterial drugs if they show any signs of bacterial invasion of the mucosa (fever or passage of bloody stool). With the emergence of ciprofloxacin-resistant *Campylobacter* in many parts of the world, new drugs have been evaluated to treat this illness. Azithromycin is an absorbed drug active against invasive and non-invasive forms of diarrhea. Rifaximin is effective in treating non-invasive forms of bacterial diarrhea of travelers not associated with fever or dysentery. Nonabsorbed (<0.4%) rifaximin is recommended as the drug of choice for travelers' diarrhea without fever or dysentery. A pediatric suspension form of rifaximin is available in some countries. The drug should be safe in pregnancy but it is not approved for use in pregnancy or in women who are breastfeeding.

Particularly in infants, children, and elderly travelers, it is paramount to avoid dehydration by administering oral rehydration therapy (ORT) (Table 30). ORT is effective because glucose-coupled sodium results in absorption of water by the small intestine during the course of infection. Although ORT is highly effective for combating dehydration and its consequences, it does not diminish the amount or duration of diarrhea, which

Table 30 Oral Rehydration Solutions and Oral Beverages

Product	Na mEq/L	K mEq/L	Base HCO3	mOSM/L*
ORS (WHO)	90	20	30	310
Pedalyte	45	20	30	270
CeraLyte-50, -70, -90	50–90	20	30	250–275
Cola†	2	0.1	13	550
Juice	3	20	0	700
Broth	250	5	0	250
Gatorade	20	3	3	330
Tea	0	0	0	5

ORS = oral rehydrate solution.

leads to a lack of confidence in the treatment, particularly in mothers and in rushed travelers. More recently developed reduced osmolarity- and amylase-resistant starch ORTs have advantages over glucose-based brands in speeding recovery.

The amount of ORT administered within 4 to 6 hours is 5% of body weight in mild dehydration, 6 to 9% in moderate dehydration, and 10% in severe dehydration. Administer oral rehydration in small quantities at regular intervals. Also, give plain water and food to minimize the monotony and the nausea or vomiting induced by ORS. After rehydration, the ongoing losses through stool or vomiting are corrected, and maintenance solutions with smaller amounts of sodium (40 to 90 mEq per liter) can be used (eg, Infalyte, Lytren, Pedialyte, Resol, CeraLyte). Intravenous fluid and electrolyte therapy is administered only in those with protracted vomiting, with signs of dehydration either reappearing or worsening, or in unconsciousness.

Although normal aciduric bacteria in the human intestine inhibit the growth of certain bacterial pathogens, *Lactobacillus*, *Bifidobacterium*, *Saccharomyces boulardii*, and *Streptococcus faecium* have shown limited or no beneficial effect in the treatment of acute diarrhea. Charcoal, kaolin, and other agents can bind and inactivate bacterial toxins, but results of clinical use have been disappointing. Moreover, some of these agents may interfere with the absorption of critical drugs also given to travelers.

Reducing food consumption is frequently observed due to anorexia. However, except for milk and dairy products in the initial 24 to 48 hours, food should not be deliberately withheld during the diarrheal episode, because calories and macronutrients are still absorbed and play an important role in enterocyte renewal. Moreover, children who ate some food showed better results and sustained weight gain better than those children who did not eat. After recovery, encourage extra nourishment.

Additional Readings

DuPont HL, et al. Prevention and treatment of traveler's diarrhea. N Engl J Med 1993;328:1821–7.

DuPont HL, et al. A randomized, double-blind, placebo-controlled trial of rifaximin to prevent travelers' diarrhea. Ann Intern Med 2005;142:805–12.

DuPont HL, et al. E. Treatment of travelers' diarrhea: randomized trial comparing rifaximin, rifaximin plus loperamide, and loperamide alone. Clin Gastroenterol Hepatol. 2007;5:451–6.

DuPont HL. Azithromycin for the self-treatment of traveler's diarrhea. Clin Infect Dis. 2007;44:347-9.

Ericsson CD, et al. Loperamide plus azithromycin more effectively treats travelers' diarrhea in Mexico than azithromycin alone. J Travel Med 2007, in press.

Glenn GM, et al. Safety and Immunogenicity of an enterottoxigenic Escherichia coli Vaccine Patch Containing Heat-Labile Toxin: Use of Skin Pretreatment to Disrupt the Stratum Corneum. Infect Immun. 2007;75:216–70.

Gorbach SL. How to hit the runs for fifty million travelers at risk. Ann Intern Med 2005;142:861–2.

Riddle MS, et al. Incidence, etiology, and impact of diarrhea among long-term travelers (US military and similar populations): a systematic review. Am J Trop Med Hyg 2006;74:891–900.

Steffen R, et al. Epidemiology of travelers' diarrhea. J Travel Med 2004;11:231–7.

Tribble DR, et al. Traveler's diarrhea in Thailand: randomized, double-blind trial comparing single-dose and 3-day azithromycin-based regimens with a 3-day levofloxacin regimen. Clin Infect Dis. 2007;44:338-46.

Trypanosomiasis, American (Chagas Disease)

Trypanosomiasis American (Chagas Disease)

Infectious Agent: *Trypanosoma cruzi*

Transmission

Bloodsucking reduviid insects, having fed on infected humans or animals, spread the infection to a susceptible host.

Global Epidemiology

The organism and associated insect vector are widely distributed, from Mexico and Central America as far south as central Argentina and Chile (Figure 43). The vector is characteristically found in cracks and holes in poorly constructed housing. For this reason, the disease is a public health problem among the rural poor living in substandard conditions.

Risk For Travelers

Currently none.

Risk to Travelers

International visitors may become infected when they live under similar conditions, as may be the case for medical volunteers or missionaries. Infection may be acquired from a chronically infected blood donor during a blood transfusion. The typical traveler to endemic areas does not become exposed to the insect vector and parasite.

Clinical Picture

In acute disease, a local inflammatory lesion (chagoma) may be seen at the site of entry of the parasite < 1 week following the insect bite. Periorbital swelling may be seen if the infection occurs by the conjunctival route. Further symptoms include fever, generalized adenopathy, skin rash, and hepatosplenomegaly. Myocarditis and meningoencephalitis may also occur in the acute phase. Symptoms subside within several weeks in most cases.

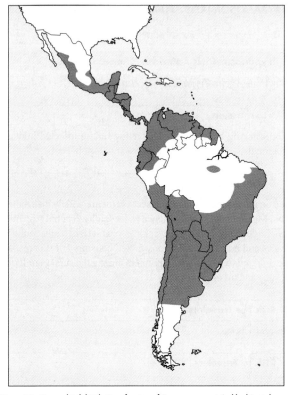

Figure 43   Geographical distribution of vectors of *Typanosoma cruzi*. Goddard J. et al. Kissing Bugs and Chagas Disease. Infect Med 1999, adapted

Chronic infection may cause arrhythmias, cardiomegaly, or right-sided congestive heart failure. Mega-disease of the esophagus or colon is a secondary manifestation of chronic infection.

Diagnosis is made by identifying motile trypanosomes upon direct microscopic examination of anticoagulated blood or from a buffy coat preparation. Serologic techniques and xenodiagnosis techniques may be used for acute infection. Chronic Chagas' disease is diagnosed by serologic procedures.

Treatment

Nifurtimox or benznidazole. Chronic heart disease is treated with conventional supportive and antiarrhythmic drugs. Mega-gastrointestinal disease may benefit from surgical interventions.

Control

Chagas' disease is one of the diseases targeted for elimination. Adequate housing, public education about the disease, home use of insecticides, and serologic testing of blood in endemic areas will help prevent spread of the infection.

TRYPANOSOMIASIS, AFRICAN (AFRICAN SLEEPING SICKNESS)

African Trypanosomiasis (African Sleeping Sickness)

Infectious Agent: Trypanosoma brucei rhodesiense (seen in East Africa from Ethiopia to eastern Uganda and south to Botswana) or *T. brucei gambiense* (seen in West and Central Africa) (Figure 44).

Transmission

The organism is spread to humans by the bite of the tsetse fly. Although the usual repellants are ineffective against this fly, ethylhexamedial (Rutgers 612) is effective.

Risk to Travelers

Travelers to East Africa on safari or on hunting or fishing trips are at low risk, but several cases have been imported, mainly to Europe.

Clinical Picture

The Gambian or West African form is a chronic illness involving the central nervous system. Several days after receiving a tsetse fly bite, a nodule or chancre appears with erythema and swelling. Clinical symptoms present in 1 to 2 weeks and consist of fever, headache, weakness, and adenopathy. After months to years, meningoencephalitis may develop. The East African form is a more rapidly progressive disease with acute neurologic symptoms and, occasionally, cardiac failure. Early onset of fever, headache, and malaise without adenopathy is followed by altered mental status. Without treatment, the East African form may lead to death. Diagnosis is made based on clinical suspicion, likelihood of exposure to insect vector, and demonstration of trypanosomes in blood, bone marrow, centrifuged cerebrospinal fluid, or other biologic tissue. Central nervous system disease is confirmed by lumbar puncture. Pleocytosis and increased cerebrospinal fluid protein, as well as the presence of trypanosomes in the spinal fluid, indicate central nervous system involvement. Serologic tests are available.

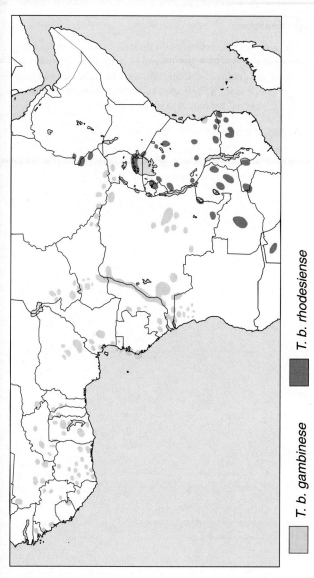

T. b. rhodesiense

T. b. gambinese

Figure 44   Geographical distribution of trypanosomiasis foci in Africa (WHO, 1989)

▌ Treatment

The customary treatment for the disease, suramin, does not penetrate the blood-brain barrier and is inadequate treatment for neurologic disease. Suramin administered early (before neurologic involvement) is an effective treatment. Melarsoprol is required once the central nervous system is involved.

Additional Readings

Barrett MP, et al. The trypanosomiases. Lancet 2003;362:1469–80.
Jelinek T, et al. Cluster of African trypanosomiasis in travelers to Tanzanian national parks. Emerg Infect Dis 2002;8:634–5.

TUBERCULOSIS

Infectious Agent

Mycobacterium tuberculosis, and occasionally *Mycobacterium africanum*, *Mycobacterium bovis*, and other mycobacteria are the infectious agents responsible for tuberculosis (TB).

Transmission

Bacteria are spread primarily by inhalation of aerosolized infectious droplet nuclei from patients with active pulmonary or laryngeal TB.

Global Epidemiology

Tuberculosis is a major global health problem (Figure 45). The World Health Organization currently estimates that one-third of the world's population has been infected with *M. tuberculosis*. More than 7.5 million cases of active TB occurred globally in 1990, with most of the burden in developing countries. In Africa, there is a co-epidemic between human immunodeficiency virus (HIV) and TB. In developed countries, the resurgence of TB is mainly due to the HIV epidemic and immigrants. TB is also increasingly an urban problem where many live in crowded, substandard housing.

Risk for Travelers

The risk for the general traveler is low. Recent evidence shows, however, that TB may be transmitted during a prolonged flight or during extended train and bus travel. The risk of TB may increase with extended exposure in endemic countries (specifically, in aid workers or refugee workers). Data on the incidence of latent tuberculosis infection are scarce, but one Dutch study showed that the incidence among Dutch travelers to TB-endemic countries for more than 3 months was 1.9%. During the annual hajj to Saudi Arabia, more than 2 million pilgrims from all over the world congregate over an extended period of time, often from developing countries endemic for TB. Data show that, during this pilgrimage, the most common cause of hospitalized pilgrims with pneumonia is TB.

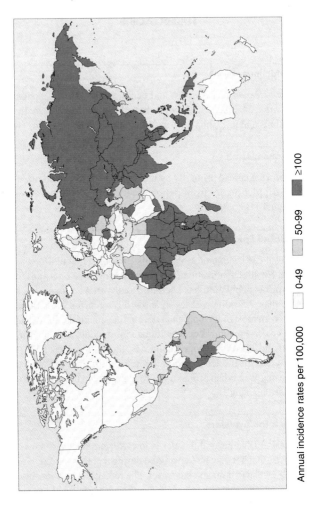

Figure 45   Estimated incidence rates of tuberculosis in 2000 (WHO 2001)

Clinical Picture

There are many clinical forms of TB. The initial infection usually remains unnoticed, but with a tuberculin test, purified protein derivative (PPD) sensitivity appears within a few weeks. After a latency lasting months, years, or even decades (less in those infected by HIV), there is a risk of reactivation to pulmonary or extrapulmonary tuberculosis, and nearly every organ is potentially involved in the latter. With early and adequate treatment, the prognosis is good.

Incubation

The incubation period, from exposure to the infective agent until development of a significant tuberculin reaction or primary infection, is 4 to 12 weeks.

Communicability

Communicability persists for as long as tubercle bacilli are being discharged in the sputum, up to several weeks following initiation of effective chemotherapy. In the past, 12 months was the mean exposure time to become infected, whereas now, a few hours in an airplane seems sufficient, most likely due to restricted ventilation and a dry environment, which result in a negligible settling tendency of droplet nuclei.

Susceptibility and Resistance

Risk of infection is related to degree of exposure and previous contact with *M. tuberculosis*. Genetic and other host factors do not appear to influence susceptibility. Risk of developing the disease varies with age, with highest risk in children age < 3 years and lowest risk in later childhood, and increasing risk again in the elderly population. There is a marked increase in tuberculosis among those with HIV infection and other types of cellular immunosuppression. *Mycobacterium tuberculosis* infection induces a degree of resistance, but reinfection can occur, particularly with changes in host immunity. Reactivation of long-latent infection can occur.

Immunoprophylaxis by BCG Vaccine

The current tuberculosis vaccines are prepared from the Bacille Calmette-Guérin (BCG) strain of *M. bovis*.

Immunology and Pharmacology

Viability: live, attenuated
Antigenic form: whole bacterium
Adjuvants: none
Preservative: none
Allergens/Excipiens: lactose/none
Mechanism: induction of cell-mediated immunity

Application

Schedule/Dosage: different recommendations for different countries

- 0.1 mL intradermally, or
- percutaneous in infants and children, using BCG with 10 times higher strength. Drop 0.2 to 0.3 mL (children age < 1 year, one-half dose) onto cleansed surface of skin, tense skin, and administer percutaneously with instrument provided (eg, multiple puncture disc). No dressing is required, but keep the site dry for 24 hours. In countries with high endemicity, the repeat vaccination is administered after > 3 months if the person remains negative to a 5-TU tuberculin skin test. In other countries, no control test is recommended.

Booster: no routine boosters recommended in persons who had a positive tuberculin test (using PPD)
Route: percutaneous, ID for some products in some countries
Site: deltoid region
Storage: Store powder at 2 to 8 °C (35 to 46 °F). Protect from light. Lyophilized material can be frozen.
Availability: worldwide

Protection

Onset: tuberculin skin test conversion within 8 to 14 weeks, however, this does not correlate with protection
Efficacy: 0 to 80%, with lower rates closer to the equator. The BCG vaccine probably confers protection against serious forms of tuberculosis, such as meningeal or miliary forms in infants up to 1 year of age, but most experts consider BCG ineffective in older children or adults. It probably does not prevent infection.
Duration: long-lasting, although tuberculin reactivity gradually diminishes
Protective level: not available

Normal and Adverse Reactions

Normal reactions consist of a small, red papule appearing at the vaccination site within 2 to 6 weeks. It may reach a diameter of 3 mm within 4 to 6 weeks, after which it will scale and slowly disappear, leaving a small scar. In persons prone to keloid formation, a larger scar may persist. Note that in > 90% of vaccinees, tuberculin reactivity is induced.

Severe or prolonged ulceration occurs in 1 to 10% of cases. Self-inoculation at other body sites may occur.

Mild systemic reactions may include flu-like symptoms, fever, fatigue, anorexia, myalgia, or neuralgia, usually lasting a few days. Lymphadenitis may persist for several weeks. Abdominal pain, diarrhea, anemia, leukopenia, coagulopathy, and pneumonitis have been reported following TB vaccination.

Anaphylaxis, osteomyelitis (1 per million), disseminated BCG (0.1 to 1 per million), and death have also followed vaccination.

Contraindications

Absolute: immunodeficiency, history of hypersensitivity or other serious adverse reactions, positive PPD skin test

Relative: any acute illness

Infants and children: safely used

Pregnant women: it is unknown whether BCG–vaccine-induced antibodies cross the placenta. Avoid use.

Lactating women: it is unknown whether BCG–vaccine-induced antibodies are excreted in breast milk. Problems in humans have not been documented.

Immunodeficient persons: avoid use. Do not immunize HIV-positive, asymptomatic persons.

Interactions

Immunosuppressant drugs and radiation therapy may result in an insufficient response to immunization or in disseminated BCG infection. Simultaneous application of BCG vaccine with oral polio vaccine is safe and immunogenic. No published data exist on concurrent use with other vaccines.

Recommendations for Vaccine Use and Tuberculin Testing

There is no agreement on the indication of BCG. The World Health Organization recommends it "for children and young adults expected to make an extended stay in an area of high tuberculosis endemicity." The Center for Disease Control and Prevention does not recommend vaccination; rather, it suggests tuberculin skin testing (preferably with a two-step approach, with two tuberculin tests performed 1 to 3 weeks apart to minimize the likelihood of interpreting a boosted reaction as a true conversion because of recent infection) before departure, if there will be prolonged exposure to potentially infective patients. Those who test tuberculin-negative should have a repeat test 3 months after return, whereas those who test positive are unlikely to become infected. If necessary (eg, tuberculin test conversion), tuberculosis can be successfully treated.

Live virus vaccines may interfere with tuberculin testing results; perform both on the same day or at least 4 weeks apart. An HIV-positive person may have an impaired response to this test; thus, the travel health professional should inquire about possible HIV infection.

Self-Treatment Abroad

None. Medical consultation is required for assessment, followed by treatment, if necessary.

Principles of Therapy

Antimicrobial therapy. Those who are diagnosed to have developed recent latent TB infection benefit from a course of preventive therapy (ie, isoniazid alone for 6 months or rifampin and pyrazinamide for 2 months).

Community Control Measures

Notification is mandatory in many countries. Treating active cases of tuberculosis decreases the reservoir of *M. tuberculosis*. Conduct active case finding among contacts, and isolate patients with sputum-positive pulmonary tuberculosis. Quarantine is not required. Consider preventive treatment of close contacts.

Additional Readings

Cobelens FG, et al. Association of tuberculin sensitivity in Dutch adults with history of travel to areas of high incidence of tuberculosis. Clin Infect Dis 2001;33:300–4.

Cobelens FG, et al. Risk of infection with *Mycobacterium tuberculosis* in travellers to areas of high tuberculosis endemicity. Lancet 2000;356:461–5.

Larsen NM, et al. Risk of tuberculin skin test conversion among health care workers: occupational versus community exposure and infection. Clin Infect Dis 2002;35:796–801.

Rieder HL. Risk of travel-associated tuberculosis. Clin Infect Dis 2001;33:1393–6.

von Reyn CF, et al. New vaccines for the prevention of tuberculosis. Clin Infect Dis 2002;35:465–74.

von Reyn CF. Routine childhood Bacille Calmette Guérin immunization and HIV infection. Clin Infect Dis 2006;42:559–61.

Wilder-Smith A, et al. High risk of *Mycobacterium tuberculosis* infection during the Hajj pilgrimage. Trop Med Int Health 2005;10:336–9.

TULAREMIA

Francisella tularensis can infect humans through the skin, mucous membranes, gastrointestinal tract, and lungs. Inoculated organisms spread to the regional lymph nodes, multiply further, and may then disseminate to organs throughout the body. Through inhalation of the bacteria, as few as 10 organisms can lead to hemorrhagic inflammation of the respiratory tract, progressing to bronchopneumonia. Pleural involvement occurs commonly. Clinical presentation may be ulceroglandular, oculoglandular, glandular, oropharyngeal pneumonic, or septic depending on the portal of entry. A pulse-temperature dissociation is common. Bioterrorism leading to a cluster of cases should be considered when multiple persons develop a severe respiratory illness with unusual epidemiologic and clinical features (eg, atypical or unresponsive pneumonia, pleuritis, hilar adenopathy, or lymphatic disease).

Tularemia would be an unusual cause of illness in an international traveler. However, it should be considered in any person who has undefined and atypical pneumonia, particularly if it occurs in a hunter or trapper who handles infected animal carcasses. It occasionally occurs in a cluster of exposed individuals.

The diagnosis is not easily made. The organism may be identified by direct examination of secretions, exudates, or in biopsied tissue by fluorescence studies or immunochemical strains. *F. tularensis* may be grown from body tissues and blood cultures. Treat adults with gentamicin 5 mg/kg/ intramuscularly (IM) or intravenously (IV) once daily for 10 to 14 days. Doxycycline 100 mg IV or orally (PO) twice daily, or ciprofloxacin 400 mg IV or 500 mg PO given twice daily are effective alternatives. For children, gentamicin is given in a dose of 2.5 mg/kg IM or IV three times daily for 14 days.

Additional Readings

Ellis J, et al. Tularemia. Clin Microbiol Rev 2002;15:631–46.

TYPHOID FEVER

The Greek word "typhos" means fog or mist. When bacteriologic assessment was not yet available, various acute diseases characterized by fever and confusion were named "typhus," including enteric fever (applied not only to typhoid but also to paratyphoid fevers), relapsing fever, epidemic or classic typhus, and brucellosis.

Infectious Agent

Typhoid fever is caused by *Salmonella typhi*, whereas the clinically similar paratyphoid fevers and enteric fevers, including paratyphoid A, B, and C, *S. choleraesuis*, and *Salmonella enteritidis* serotype *dublin*, are caused occasionally by other *Salmonella* species. These often take a milder course. Part of the Enterobacteriaceae family, the genus *Salmonella* includes flagellated, non–spore-bearing gram-negative bacilli, which usually can ferment glucose, but not urea, lactose, or saccharose. There are various subspecies within a species, differentiated by DNA structure and biochemical properties. These are divided into serotypes (also called serovars), based on their somatic (O) and flagellar (H) antigens. A cell wall lipopolysaccharide virulence (Vi) antigen, often associated with virulence, is found in *Salmonella typhi*, *S. enteritidis* serotype *hirschfeldii* (also called *Salmonella paratyphi* C), and, occasionally, in other enterobacterial organisms. On the basis of antigen characteristics, Kauffmann and White have classified more than 2,000 serotypes of nontyphoid *S. enteritidis*. *Salmonella typhi* belongs to group D, having O-antigens 9, 12, Vi, and H-antigen d. At present, more than 100 types can be distinguished by phage typing.

Boiling destroys *S. typhi* immediately by removing the thermolabile Vi antigen.

Transmission

Salmonella typhi is unique among the *Salmonella* species in having humans as its only natural hosts and reservoir. Characteristically, food or beverages contaminated with feces from an *S. typhi* carrier are ingested. Direct fecal-oral contact may result in infection, although less commonly. The risk increases when sewage seeps into wells, or river water is used without appropriate treatment. Fruit watered with contaminated river water, vegetables fertilized by night-soil, milk and milk products contaminated by workers' hands, and, in some countries, shellfish harvested from contaminated coastal waters, have all been associated with typhoid. Canned food and bottled water are usually safe but have been contaminated through faulty processes. Typhoid fever occasionally results from laboratory contamination when workers are not sufficiently careful.

Epidemics originating from water contamination are particularly explosive, partly because a water source may serve a large population and partly because water dilutes gastric acid, which inactivates pathogenic agents. Additionally, water and beverages remain in the stomach only very briefly. Transmission by food, however, is associated with larger inocula and higher attack rates. It should be noted that typhoid fever often has a high incidence in high socioeconomic neighborhoods, where salads or other uncooked dishes are eaten more often, either at home or in restaurants.

Global Epidemiology

The incidence of typhoid fever increased with urbanization before the advent of modern sanitation. Epidemics have often occurred because of war (eg, Berlin from 1945 to 1946) but have rarely broken out after natural catastrophes.

It is estimated that, in 2000, the worldwide annual incidence of typhoid was 16.6 million cases, with 580,000 deaths. Typhoid fever is endemic in all the developing countries, where children age 5 to 19 years are the most affected. Typhoid incidence dropped markedly during the 1990s in parts of South America, where sanitary facilities were developed and sewage was properly restored after the cholera epidemic.

Some low endemicity remains in southern and eastern Europe. Elsewhere in Europe and in North America, Australia, and New Zealand, typhoid fever is now almost exclusively an imported infection. Figure 46 lists the annual incidence of selected regions.

Typhoid rates are related to the quality of sewage disposal and water treatment in a given area and the number of typhoid carriers in that area. Water quality improvements reduce typhoid incidence but not dysentery; the latter is a low inoculum disease, more frequently a result of person-to-person contact than contamination of water supply. Secondary spread of *S. typhi* is unusual,

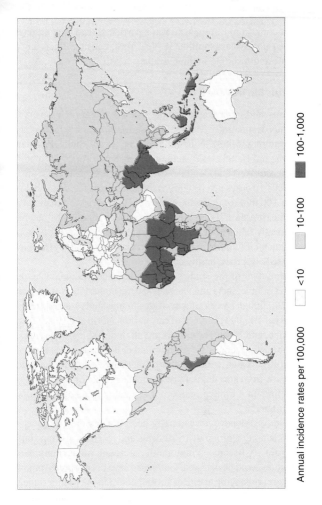

Annual incidence rates per 100,000

■ 100–1,000

▨ 10–100

▨ <10

□

Figure 46   Annual incidence of typhoid fever in various parts of the world (CDC 1999)

but sporadic infections occur in the developed countries as a result of unrecognized chronic excreters of *S. typhi* contaminating the food they prepare. This most often happens in households but may also occur in public restaurants. "Typhoid Mary," an immigrant cook from Europe who was a carrier, spread typhoid fever among upper-class families in New York, causing illness in 54 people and resulting in three deaths.

Risk for Travelers

Various studies have assessed the risk of typhoid for travelers to various destinations. Most studies show particularly high attack rates among visitors to the Indian subcontinent (India, Pakistan, Nepal, and Bangladesh), some parts of South America (mainly Peru), and West and Central Africa. The attack rate in these areas exceeds 10 cases per 100,000 visitors, whereas the rate is below 1 per 100,000 for many frequently visited tourist destinations in Southeast Asia and East Africa. In southern Europe, the rate has drastically fallen in the past decades; almost exclusively, persons visiting their families in their native villages (eg, in Italy) are now affected—tourists, hardly ever.

Only two of the studies also include data on incidence per period of time. India and Pakistan had the highest rates at 10 cases per 100,000 per week of stay. Rates in one study ranged from 2 to 10 per 100,000 per week of stay in Iran, North and West Africa, Mexico, and Haiti. These rates are all underestimates because a number of infections are not reported or diagnosed as being successfully treated with antibiotics or treated abroad. The latter appears, from anecdotes, to be particularly true for young people traveling on a limited budget for several months on the Indian subcontinent.

Outbreaks have occasionally been documented, such as in 1991, among a group of 15 students and teachers visiting Haiti, wherein six became symptomatic, although no asymptomatic infection could be detected. Outbreaks have been reported among tour groups staying at one or several hotels in the Mediterranean (eg, on the Greek island of Kos in 1983). To our knowledge, no typhoid outbreaks due to airline catering have been documented since the 1970s.

Clinical Picture

Clinical features range from not apparent to fatal, depending on the number of ingested organisms. In healthy volunteers, 109 viable bacteria induced the disease in 95% of them, whereas 103 viable bacteria only rarely did so. That single cases typically occur in families suggests exposure to low doses in nature. The Vi–antigen-positive strains cause illness more frequently than do non-Vi variants. The Vi envelope antigen protects the organism from antibodies directed at the complex cell wall O antigen, allowing the organism to escape opsonization and phagocytosis. According to seroepidemiologic studies, at least seven subclinical infections occur for every clinical case.

Typhoid fever shows an insidious onset with rising intermittent fever, headache, nonproductive cough, malaise, lassitude, insomnia, nightmares, and anorexia. Constipation occurs more often than diarrhea in adults and older children.

In the second week of untreated illness, the patient has a sustained fever and looks toxic. Often, a relative bradycardia, dicrotic pulse, and hepatosplenomegaly in a distended abdomen are found.

Hepatomegaly can be documented in one-third of cases, and jaundice will be found in one-third of these. Respiratory symptoms may predominate early in typhoid fever, and patchy pneumonia may occasionally be documented. In some patients, the illness resembles a primary pulmonary process. Patients frequently have abdominal complaints, including constipation, diarrhea, pain, and ileus or abdominal tenderness. Segmental ileus is frequently found in acute typhoid. Dilated loops of small bowel filled with air and fluid may be felt by deep palpation of the abdomen.

Rose spots that are 2 to 4 mm in diameter (pink papules that fade on pressure) may be observed on the trunk of Caucasian patients in 25 to 50% of cases.

The third week of untreated typhoid is characterized by further aggravation, with persisting high fever, a toxic clinical picture, and a delirious, confused state. The patient becomes weak and has rapid breathing and a feeble pulse. The abdomen is distended and the bowel sounds are decreased or absent. Diarrhea resembling pea soup is common.

Ulceration of Peyer's patches resulting in intestinal hemorrhage or perforation with peritonitis will begin in the second week of illness, particularly in untreated cases. Gut perforation is the most serious complication of typhoid fever and occurs in approximately 2% of cases. It is unrelated to clinical severity of the illness. Intestinal hemorrhage occurs in approximately 4% of patients, accompanied by edema of Peyer's patches with subsequent necrosis. The bleeding may be massive and includes hematochezia or melena. Corticosteroids do not predispose the patient to hemorrhage. Provided that medical evaluation and, on rare occasions, blood transfusions are available, hemorrhage does not worsen the overall prognosis for typhoid fever.

Toxemia, myocarditis, and pneumonia resulting from typhoid fever may also lead to death. Other complications include hepatitis, cholecystitis, meningitis, polyneuritis, osteomyelitis, disseminated intravascular coagulation, hemolytic-uremic syndrome, glomerulitis, acute pancreatitis, thrombocytopenia, Reiter's syndrome, and polymyositis.

If left untreated, the usual duration for a case of average severity is 4 weeks, with the fourth week showing general improvement. Gastrointestinal complications may still occur. Relapses occur in 5 to 12% of untreated cases, which were slightly more common (10 to 20%) following antibiotic treatment in the pre-quinolone era. Relapse usually takes place about 1 week after therapy is discontinued but has been observed as late as 70 days thereafter. The severity of relapses is inversely related to the severity of primary illness but is usually milder and of shorter duration than the initial illness. Rarely, second and third relapses occur.

The case fatality rate in the pre-antibiotic era was 10 to 20% but has been reduced to less than 1% with appropriate therapy, particularly in a well-nourished population. The case fatality rate is higher in older patients; their symptoms are often less characteristic, and diagnosis may be delayed.

Incubation

The usual incubation period for typhoid fever is 1 to 2 weeks, with a range of 3 days to 3 months following ingestion of contaminated food or liquids. The incubation period is inversely related to the ingested bacterial dose.

Communicability

Bacilli appear in the excreta usually from the first week until convalescence. About 10% of untreated typhoid fever patients discharge bacilli for 3 months after the onset of symptoms, and 2 to 5% become chronic carriers. Carriers are typically women with gall bladder disease, who excrete up to 1,011 organisms/gram in their stools. Organisms are found in gall bladder stones or scarred foci in the intrahepatic biliary system. Persisting urinary carriage is rare except in patients with coexistent urinary tract pathology, such as schistosomiasis. Non-typhoid *Salmonella* carriers rarely carry the disease as long as 1 year.

Susceptibility and Resistance

Children are at higher risk for typhoid fever than are adults, because they are prone to fecal-oral infections and have a less effective gastric acid barrier. Like other salmonellae, *S. typhi* is relatively sensitive to the action of gastric acid. Hypochlorhydria resulting from age, disease, gastric surgery, or medication may mean that a lower dose of pathogenic agents is necessary to cause symptomatic infection. Normal bacterial flora of the intestine have a protective effect, and antibiotics depleting them may have an effect on the inoculum necessary to cause symptoms.

Relative immunity following recovery from typhoid fever is inadequate to protect against subsequent ingestion of large numbers of *S. typhi*.

Helicobacter pylori infection is associated with increased risk of typhoid fever.

Diagnosis

Typhoid fever should be considered a possible diagnosis in any case of fever of unknown origin accompanied by bradycardia and leukopenia. Nonspecific laboratory findings may include initial leukocytosis, followed by leukopenia with neutropenia eosinopenia, normocytic anemia, thrombocytopenia, slightly elevated hepatic transaminases, and mild proteinuria.

According to the Center for Disease Control and Prevention (CDC), a confirmed case of typhoid shows "a clinically compatible illness that is laboratory confirmed," whereas a probable case shows a "clinically compatible illness that is epidemiologically linked to a confirmed case in an outbreak." The laboratory criterion referred to for establishment of a diagnosis is "isolation of *S. typhi* from blood, stool, or other clinical specimen."

Diagnosis therefore depends on isolation of the typhoid organism. Blood cultures are usually performed and are positive in 80% of untreated patients during the first week. This rate declines rapidly over the course of the illness. Culture of bone marrow aspirate has been shown to give a recovery rate of 90 to 95%, because it is less influenced by antecedent antimicrobial therapy than are blood cultures. *Salmonella typhi* may also be isolated from rose spots (60% positive) and much less frequently from stools and urine. Isolation from stool and urine provides strong evidence of typhoid fever only when there is a characteristic clinical picture, because the individual being tested may be a chronic carrier.

The traditional Widal's test measures antibodies against H and O antigens of *S. typhi*. It provides some support for the diagnosis of typhoid if there is a fourfold rise in the titer of antibody to the O antigen. H antibodies appear shortly after O antibodies but persist longer than just a few months. Thus, rising or high O antibody titers generally indicate acute infection, whereas a raised H antibody helps identify the type of enteric fever. Widal's test, however, can be misleading. Raised antibodies may result from typhoid immunization, or earlier infection with salmonellae or other gram-negative bacteria sharing common antigens. High Vi capsular antibody suggests a carrier state, but high rates of false positives and false negatives can exist. According to the CDC, serologic evidence alone is insufficient for diagnosis.

Minimized Exposure in Travelers

Safe drinking water and sanitary disposal of human feces and urine are essential for prevention of typhoid fever. Adequate hand-washing facilities are required, particularly for handlers of food. Sufficient toilet paper supplies, insect screens, and use of insecticides will all help minimize risk. Sanitary improvements in many parts of the developing world have been hampered, however, by economic conditions and civil unrest.

When travelers are uncertain about sanitary practices—and they should be almost anywhere in the developing world—they should select only freshly cooked food that is served at temperatures of at least 60 °C. Fruit that can be peeled by the traveler, bread, and cookies are safe, as well as hot tea and coffee, freshly pressed fruit juice, and carbonated bottled water. Otherwise, water can be boiled or chemically treated. Many travelers, unfortunately, often do not take such precautions.

Chemoprophylaxis

Although no chemoprophylaxis is specifically recommended for typhoid fever, those using quinolones for preventing travelers' diarrhea would often be protected from *S. typhi* infection. Such chemoprophylaxis of travelers' diarrhea is, however, recommended only for special-risk groups (see Table 21).

Immunoprophylaxis by Typhoid Vaccines

Two different typhoid vaccines are now widely available. The oral and the parenteral Vi-vaccines are clearly superior to the disappearing parenteral TAB vaccine with respect to tolerance (Table 27) although, according to a recent meta-analysis, the TAB vaccine may be more effective if two doses are given.

Oral Typhoid Vaccine (Ty21a)

Immunology and Pharmacology

Viability: live, attenuated bacteria

Antigenic form: whole bacterium, 2 to 6 × 109 colony forming units (CFU) Ty21a gal E mutant strain of *S. typhi*

Adjuvants: none

Preservative: none

Allergens/Excipiens: 100 to 180 mg lactose per capsule / each capsule contains 26 to 130 mg sucrose, 1.4 to 7 mg amino acid mixture, 3.6 to 4.4 ng magnesium stearate, and ascorbic acid

Buffer: was only in the liquid form Vivotif L, which is currently not marketed anywhere

Mechanism: induction of specific protective antibodies directed against *S. typhi* lipopolysaccharide. This bacterial strain is restricted in its ability to produce complete lipopolysaccharide, which impairs its ability to cause disease but not its ability to induce an immune response.

Application

Schedule: one capsule orally on days 1, 3, 5, and in the United States and Canada, additionally on day 7

Booster: same as primary vaccination described above, recommended every year in Europe (unless continuously exposed to *S. typhi*), every 5 years in the United States and Canada, based on field trials in endemic countries

Route: oral

Storage: Store at 2 to 8 °C (35 to 46 °F) prior to use and between doses. If frozen, thaw the capsules before administering. Product can tolerate 48 hours at 25 °C (77 °F). Advise travelers to store the vaccine in refrigerator until use.

Availability: Available in many countries as Vivotif (Berna Biotech) and Typhoral L (Novartis/Chiron).

Protection

Onset: 2 weeks after third dose (Europe), 1 week after fourth dose (United States and Canada)

Efficacy: 70% with a range of 33 to 94% in populations continuously exposed to *S. typhi*. Unknown in nonimmunes.

Duration: 1 year in European travelers, 5 years in United States and Canadian travelers (see schedule and booster). Every 3 to 7 years for residents of endemic countries

Protective level: unknown

Adverse Reactions

Diarrhea in 0.1 to 5% of vaccinees, usually mild; fever in 1 to 2% with no dirrence to placebo

Contraindications

Absolute: persons with immunodeficiency and children age < 2 years

Relative: persons with acute illness, diarrhea, vomiting, and users of antimicrobial agents and antimalarials (see "Interactions" below)

Children: The lower age limit for use of Ty21a capsules varies between countries, but they are generally not recommended below the age of 6 years as they might be unable to swallow the capsules

Pregnant women: category C. Use typhoid vaccine only if clearly needed (ie, if disease risks exceed vaccination risks). It is unknown whether Ty21a or induced antibodies cross the placenta. Generally, most immunoglobulin (Ig) G passage across the placenta occurs during the third trimester.

Lactating women: It is unknown whether Ty21a or induced antibodies are excreted in breast milk. Problems in humans have not been documented.

Immunodeficient persons: Do not give Ty21a capsules to immunocompromised persons, including persons with congenital or acquired immune deficiencies, whether because of genetics, disease, or drug or radiation therapy, regardless of possible benefits from vaccination. This product contains live bacteria. Avoid use in human immunodeficiency virus-positive persons. Rather, use the parenteral, inactivated typhoid vaccine in these patients.

Interactions

Concomitant application of antimicrobials, antimalarials (mefloquine, pyrimethamine/sulfadoxine) results in reduced antibody response. Simultaneous application of Ty21a vaccine with oral polio vaccine is probably safe and immunogenic, although various sources advise against simultaneous use. There is no indication of interactions with other travel vaccines.

Parenteral Vi Polysaccharide Typhoid Vaccine

Immunology and Pharmacology

Viability: inactivated

Antigenic form: Vi polysaccharide from *S. typhi*

Adjuvants: none

Preservative: 0.5% phenol

Allergens/Excipiens: veal / agar, bactopeptone

Storage: Store at 2 to 8 °C (35 to 46 °F). Do not freeze. Can tolerate 10 days at room temperature

Mechanism: induction of specific protective antibodies

Availability: available in most countries as Typhim Vi (Sanofi Pasteur Merieux Connaught). Typherix (Glaxo SmithKline Biologicals) has been introduced in many countries. Conjugate typhoid vaccines have been successfully tested; however, they have not been marketed yet.

Application

Schedule: single 0.5 mL dose

Booster: after 2 years in the United States and 3 years in Europe

Route: intramuscularly

Site: deltoid region

Protection

Onset: optimal after 2 weeks

Efficacy: 70% with a range of 55 to 75% in populations continuously exposed to *S. typhi*. Unknown in nonimmunes. *S. typhi* strains lacking Vi antigen have been documented in India and in other countries.

Duration: 2 to 3 years

Protective level: unknown

Adverse Reactions

Local reactions are usually mild and transient. Erythema occurs in 4 to 11% of vaccinees, induration in 5 to 18%. Systemic reactions include fever in < 1 to 5% of vaccinees, malaise, myalgia, nausea, headache, and lymphadenopathy. Occasionally, hypotension and urticaria have been reported.

Contraindications

Absolute: persons with a previous serious reaction to the vaccine

Relative: any acute illness

Children: age < 2 years

Pregnant women: category C. It is unknown whether typhoid vaccine or induced antibodies cross the placenta. Generally, most IgG passage across the placenta occurs during the third trimester. Use typhoid vaccine only if clearly indicated.

Lactating women: It is unknown whether typhoid vaccine or corresponding antibodies are excreted in breast milk. Problems in humans have not been documented.

Immunodeficient persons: Persons receiving immunosuppressive therapy or having other immunodeficiencies may experience diminished antibody response to active immunization.

Interactions

Immunosuppressant drugs and radiation therapy may cause an insufficient response to immunization.

Administer subcutaneously to patients receiving anticoagulants.

Salmonella typhi Vi conjugate vaccine

The currently licensed typhoid vaccines confer only about 70% immunity, do not protect young children, and are not used for routine vaccination. A newly devised conjugate of the capsular polysaccharide of *Salmonella typhi*, Vi, bound to nontoxic recombinant *Pseudomonas aeruginosa* exotoxin A (rEPA), has enhanced immunogenicity in adults and in children. It is shown to be safe and immunogenic and has more than 90% efficacy in children 2 to 5 years old. The antibody responses and the efficacy suggest that this vaccine should be at least as protective in persons who are more than 5 years old. The conjugate vaccine should offer several advantages over the other licensed typhoid vaccines.

Recommendations For Ty21a Or Vi Polysaccharide Vaccine Use

Typhoid vaccination is mostly recommended for those traveling to the developing countries, those who may be at risk, and, in some countries, to food handlers. Activities placing travelers at risk include the following:

- Exposure of at least 1 month
- Travel to remote areas and consumption of local food
- Consumption of food and beverages purchased from street vendors
- Travel of any duration to any destination in South Asia (India and neighboring countries), North (except Tunisia), Central or West Africa

Self-Treatment Abroad

None. Medical assessment and therapy are required.

Principles of Therapy

To prevent secondary spread, take strict enteric precautions with respect to hospitalized patients. Chloramphenicol (the standard treatment in the developing world), amoxicillin or, for children, trimethoprim-sulfamethoxazole, have all shown similar efficacy, each given for 2 weeks. More recently, quinolones and, to a lesser extent, third-generation cephalosporins, the latter particularly for children, have been used as first-line strategies wherever multiresistant typhoid fever repeatedly occurs, such as on the Indian subcontinent and in the Arabian peninsula. In view of increasing resistance and the potential fatality of typhoid fever treated with ineffective drugs, test all isolates for antimicrobial susceptibility. Oral medication is preferred if the patient can swallow. Standard therapy for adults consists of ciprofloxacin 750 mg or ofloxacin 300 to 400 mg, given twice daily for 7 to 10 days. Short-course quinolone therapy has been effective but is currently not recommended.

Short-term, high-dose corticosteroid (usually dexamethasone) treatment reduces mortality and is routinely given to severely ill patients, particularly when there is central nervous system involvement. Supportive care should be provided according to the clinical picture.

Carriers often suffer from chronic cholecystitis, frequently with cholelithiasis. Cholecystectomy is usually indicated in these cases, although the procedure does not always eradicate infection, due to the intrahepatic location of the organisms. Oral quinolones have successfully eliminated carriage in over 75% of cases. Norfloxacin 400 mg bid or ciprofloxacin 750 mg for 28 days is the standard therapy for typhoid carriers.

Community Control Measures

Notification is mandatory in many countries. Quarantine is not required. Follow enteric precautions, and immunize contacts exposed to carriers. The source of infection and contacts (eg, travel groups) should be actively sought out.

Additional Readings

Bhan MK, et al. Typhoid and paratyphoid fever. Lancet 2005;366:749–62.

Caumes E, et al. Typhoid and paratyphoid fever: a 10-year retrospective study of 41 cases in a Parisian hospital. J Travel Med 2001;8:293–7.

Cobelens FG, et al. Typhoid fever in group travelers: opportunity for studying vaccine efficacy. J Travel Med 2000;7:19–24.

Mai NL, et al. Persistent efficacy of Vi conjugate vaccine against typhoid fever in young children. NEJM 2003;349:1390–1.

Reller ME et al. Sexual transmission of typhoid fever: a multistate outbreak among men who have sex with men. Clin Infect Dis 2003;37:141-4.

VARIANT CREUTZFELDT-JAKOB DISEASE

Creutzfeldt-Jakob disease (CJD) is a rare, but always fatal neuro-logical disorder. The presumed cause are prions (proteinaceous infectious particles). Other than the classical forms of the disease, the variant form (vCJD) most likely reflects a transmission from bovine spongiform encephalopathy (BSE) to humans. Worldwide, the total cumulative number of diagnosed vCJD cases was 138 by September 2002. The disease occurred in eight countries (United Kingdom, 127 cases, France, 6, Ireland, 1, Italy, 1, China [Hong Kong], 1, Canada, 1, and the United States, 1). Some of the indi-viduals who were diagnosed outside the United Kingdom might have been infected during their residency in the United Kingdom.

The vCJD illness starts mostly with psychiatric features, fol-lowed by other neurologic symptoms. Disease duration is usually between 9 and 18 months. The mean age of vCJD patients is 27 years, and the incubation time is considered to be years or decades. There is no known case of human-to-human transmission of vCJD, but transmission via surgical instruments or via blood transfu-sion is theoretically conceivable. No chemo- or immunoprophylaxis or other treatment is available.

The risk of becoming infected cannot be excluded in coun-tries where indigenous or imported BSE-risk material may be included in consumer products. The Center for Disease Control and Prevention (CDC) has estimated 1 case per 10 billion serv-ings in the United Kingdom. To further reduce this risk, the European Union (EU) countries and Switzerland have been imple-menting a range of protective measures to prevent transmission.

Additional individual measures, such as avoiding beef and beef products, are not recommended by EU experts. In contrast, the CDC advises in Europe "to consider either 1) avoiding beef and beef products altogether or 2) selecting beef or beef products, such as solid pieces of muscle meat (vs. brain or beef products, such as burgers and sausages), that might have a reduced opportunity for contamination with tissues that might harbor the BSE agent." Milk and dairy products are not considered risky food and beverage items.

Additional Readings

Belay ED, et al. Variant Creutzfeldt-Jakob disease death, United States. Emerg Infect Dis 2005;11:1351–4.

McKnight C. Clinical implications of bovine spongiform encephalopa-thy. Clin Infect Dis 2001;32:1726–31.

VIRAL HEMORRHAGIC FEVERS, OTHER

Hemorrhagic fever, the syndrome of fever and bleeding diathesis, is caused by a virus from one of four families of hemorrhagic fever viruses (HFVs): Flaviviridae (dengue, yellow fever, Omsk hemorrhagic fever, Kyasanur Forest disease); Bunyaviridae (Crimean-Congo hemorrhagic fever, Rift Valley fever, hantavirus and other viruses that cause hemorrhagic fever with renal syndrome); Arenaviridae (Lassa and new world Arenaviridae); or Filoviridae (Ebola or Marburg viruses). It typically occurs following contact from an infected animal or arthropod vector.

HFVs are small ribonucleic acid (RNA) viruses with lipid envelopes that reside in animal hosts or arthropod vectors. The reservoir in nature for filoviruses is unknown. Persons in endemic areas are infected incidentally by a biting arthropod that is infected or from an aerosol from contaminated rodent urine or animal carcass. Clinical illness caused by HFVs are nonspecific, including a severe illness with fever (> 38.3 °C) and at least two hemorrhagic manifestations: hemorrhagic rash, epistaxis, hematemesis, or melena, or bright red blood in stools and hemoptysis. Patients characteristically have myalgias, skin rash, and encephalitis. The common laboratory findings are thrombocytopenia and reduced levels of coagulation factors. The various HFVs do not look clinically unique. The incubation period ranges from 2 to 21 days. When HFV infection is suspected, the patient is provided supportive treatment (fluids and electrolytes, mechanical ventilation, dialysis, and antiseizure medication), and ribavirin may be initiated and HFV-specific precautions observed.

To prevent HFVs among travelers to areas where these viral infections are endemic, the following measures should routinely be employed: yellow fever vaccine; mosquito-avoidance measures; and tick-avoidance measures (protective clothing, pants tucked into socks and shoes or boots, tick repellent, and body searches for ticks) for backpackers and hikers. Fortunately, the non-dengue hemorrhagic fevers are rarely acquired by travelers. Expatriates living in endemic areas remain at greater risk, particularly following contact with body fluids of a person or an animal potentially infected with an HFV.

Additional Readings

Isaacson M. Viral hemorrhagic fever hazards for travelers in Africa. Clin Infect Dis 2001;33:1707–12.

Ryan ET, et al. Illness after international travel. N Engl J Med 2002;347:505–16.

West Nile Virus

West Nile Virus (WNV) infection was first reported in Uganda in 1937, with subsequent spread to Europe, Asia, Africa, and the Middle East. It first appeared in the United States in 1999 and became widespread in 2002. The culex, or night-biting mosquito, is the main vector, but the day- and night-biting Asian tiger mosquito has been shown in the United States to be an important vector.

Several cases in travelers have been reported, e.g. in Canada and Germany. During a known epidemic of WNV infection, travelers to the region should exert optimal antimosquito measures to prevent exposure. This includes multi-daily application of insect repellent on skin surfaces, use of permethrin on clothing, staying indoors at night, and using mosquito-avoidance methods in the places where persons are staying (eg, screens and bed nets).

Most WNV infections are mild or clinically inapparent, with about 20% of those infected developing a mild illness (West Nile fever). Approximately 1 in 150 infections result in severe neurologic disease. The most significant risk factor for severe disease is advanced age. Encephalitis is more common than meningitis. The incubation period is 3 to 14 days, and symptoms generally last 3 to 6 days. The diagnosis is made on strong index of suspicion, in the face of a known outbreak and by specific laboratory tests. Suspect adults age > 50 years who develop unexplained encephalitis or meningitis in the summer or early fall as having WNV infection. The death rate of the disease is about 10% of those with clinical illness.

The diagnosis is confirmed by detecting immunoglobulin M antibody using enzyme-linked immunosorbent assay to WNV in serum or cerebral spinal fluid collected within 8 days of the illness (cross-reacts with flaviviruses: yellow fever, Japanese encephalitis, dengue). Treatment is supportive, often involving hospitalization. Ribavirin in high doses and interferon-α have activity against the virus in vitro, yet they haven't been shown to be as effective as steroids.

Additional Readings

Charles PE. Imported West Nile virus infection in Europe. Emerg Infect Dis 2003;9:750.

Meeuse JJ, et al. Patient with West Nile fever in the Netherlands. Ned Tijdschr Geneeskd 2001;145:2084–6.

Petersen LR, et al. West Nile virus: a primer for the clinician. Ann Intern Med 2002;137:173–9.

YELLOW FEVER

Infectious Agent

Yellow fever (YF) is an arboviral infection of the Flaviviridae family, genus *Flavivirus*.

Transmission

YF is transmitted primarily by the bite of the infected Aedes aegypti mosquito and, in the forests of South America, mainly by mosquitoes of genus *Haemagogus* and *Sabethes*. Bites may occur throughout the day, with risk highest at sunrise and in late afternoon. These mosquitoes may be found at altitudes as high as 2,500 m.

Global Epidemiology

There is both a sylvatic, jungle cycle involving mosquitoes and nonhuman primates and an urban cycle involving Aedes aegypti mosquitoes and humans. Urban and jungle YF occur only in parts of Africa and South America (Figure 47). There is no YF in Asia, but the presence of Aedes causes concern that it may someday be imported. Jungle YF is an enzootic infection among nonhuman primates in South American forests, occasionally transmitted to humans between January and March. In Africa, transmission occurs during the late rainy and early dry season in savannah habitats. Epidemics may flare up after long intervals. Kenya, for example, was free of reported YF from 1942 to 1992. It is true, however, that there is much underreporting, particularly of oligosymptomatic cases. The World Health Organization (WHO) estimates that 300,000 YF infections cause 20,000 deaths yearly; however, only 2,570 cases in Africa and 629 in South America were notified to WHO in the 2000 to 2004 period. The WHO Weekly Epidemiological Record regularly reports on the infected provinces and districts, although virus activity may extend beyond officially reported infective zones.

Compulsory or recommended vaccination makes cases of YF rare in travelers. There was only one case of YF, despite vaccination, in 20 years (reported in a Spanish traveler). From 1979 to 1981, four unimmunized hunters and travelers, including one

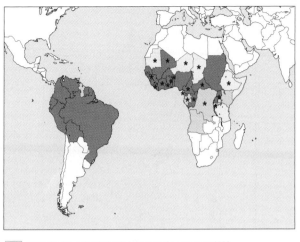

countries ith   potential risk, no reported cases ate r 1980

countries noti in g YF 1980-1999

countries noti in g YF since 2000

*   countries with required yellow fever vaccination (transit requirements not indicated)

Figure 47   Yellow fever (YF) endemic countries (reported cases, underreporting common)
Note: no YF in Asia, Europe and North America

long-term resident, acquired YF in West Africa; three of them died. From 1996 to 2001, several unimmunized tourists from the United States and Europe acquired YF, most likely during an excursion in the Manaus region of Brazil or during stays in Venezuela, on the Ivory Coast, and in The Gambia. The absence of reported cases among the local population in an endemic area provides no assurance that YF will not be acquired by unimmunized travelers.

Clinical Picture

Severity varies from inapparent or flu-like symptoms to severe hepatitis and hemorrhagic fever. Onset is sudden, with fever, headache, muscle pain, and vomiting, followed in 10 to 20% of cases by worsening jaundice. Patients often show hemorrhagic symptoms and liver and renal failure after a very brief remission. The case fatality rate in jaundiced patients is 30 to 50%.

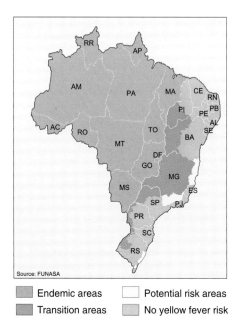

Figure 48   Yellow fever in Brazil 2003

YF can be communicated from patients to mosquitoes for 5 days from shortly before the onset of fever. There is no communicability from person to person or through soiled articles.

Susceptibility and Resistance

Recovery from YF results in lasting immunity. Transient passive immunity occurs for up to 6 months in infants born to immune mothers.

Minimized Exposure in Travelers

Personal protection measures against mosquito bites should be employed throughout the day.

Chemoprophylaxis

None

Immunoprophylaxis with Yellow Fever Vaccine

Immunology and Pharmacology

Viability: live, attenuated 17D (also known as Rockefeller, Asibi) strain, free of avian leukosis, 17DD is used in Brazil (99.9% homologous).

Antigenic form: whole virus, 1000 LD50 (mouse units, lyophilized)

Adjuvants: none

Preservative: none

Allergens/Excipiens: residual egg protein, neomycin, and polymyxin. YF vaccine has more egg protein per dose than do other egg-cultured vaccines. US Pharmacopeia (USP) requirement—must not contain human serum

Mechanism: induction of protective neutralizing antibodies

Application

Schedule: single injection (0.5 mL) at least 10 days before departure, in accordance with current International Health Regulations (IHR)

Booster: every 10 years in accordance with current IHR. Every 15 years is sufficient for protection.

Route: subcutaneously

Site: over deltoid

Storage: depends on the vaccine. For some, –30 to 5 ˚C (–22 to 41 ˚F), preferably < 0 ˚C (32 ˚F). For others, such as Stamaril, 2 to 8 ˚C (35 to 46 ˚F). Check with manufacturer's instructions. Use the vaccine within 1 to 2 hours when reconstituted, depending on the product.

Availability: available worldwide as Stamaril, Amaril or YF-Vax (Sanofi Pasteur); in contrast Arilvax is no longer available, and Flavimun (Berna Biotech, basing on the RKI strain) expecting to be available in some countries in 2007.

Protection

Onset: 7 days, with an upper limit of 10 days set by current IHR

Efficacy: essentially 100%. There was one case of YF in an allegedly immunized traveler from Spain.

Duration: 10 years according to IHR; > 15 years, effectively

Protective level: unknown

Adverse Reactions

About 10% of recipients may experience fever or malaise following immunization, usually appearing 7 to 14 days after administration, with 0.2% being incapacitated. Anaphylaxis may occur. In the 1992 to 2005 period, the scientific community became aware of 37 reports of yellow fever vaccine (YEL)-associated viscerotropic disease (YEL-AVD) cases and four reports of YEL-associated neurotropic disease (YEL-AND) worldwide, changing our understanding of the risks of the vaccine. Among the 37 YEL-AVD, 18 were fatal: 5 among the 7 fatal cases in the United States were more than 60 years old; by contrast, all 6 fatal cases in Brazil were at most 22 years old, and no clear age related pattern was observed elsewhere. There were 722 adverse event reports after YEL was submitted to the United States Vaccine Adverse Event Reporting System in 1990 to 2002. The reporting rates of serious adverse events were significantly higher among vaccinees aged ≥60 years than among those 19 to 29 years of age (reporting rate ratio = 5.9, 95% CI 1.6–22.2). Yellow–fever-associated neurotropic disease (previously "postvaccinal encephalitis") has been estimated to occur in 0.5 to 4 per 1,000 very young infants and in fewer than 1 in 8 million vaccinees over age 9 months. Viscerotropic disease (previously "febrile multiple organ system failure") yields a reported incidence of 2.5 in 1 million doses distributed.

Contraindications

Absolute: history of hypersensitivity to vaccine, allergy to egg proteins

Relative: any acute illness (see "Immunodeficient persons" below)

Children: Do not administer to infants age < 6 (preferably < 12) months, unless travel to a high-risk area is unavoidable and the child is at risk of infection.

Pregnant women: Avoid unless travel to a high-risk area is unavoidable. It is unknown whether 17D YF virus or corresponding antibodies cross the placenta. Generally, most immunoglobulin G passage across the placenta occurs during the third trimester. After vaccination campaigns conducted during epidemics, no specific problems had been associated with yellow fever vaccination performed during pregnancy.

Lactating women: It is unknown whether 17D YF virus or corresponding antibodies are excreted in breast milk. Problems in humans have not been documented.

Immunodeficient persons: Avoid using in immunodeficient persons, including persons with congenital or acquired immune deficiencies, whether these are due to genetics, disease, or drug or radiation therapy. The vaccine contains live viruses. Avoid use in asymptomatic human immunodeficiency virus (HIV)-positive persons unless the CD4 cell count is > 400 and travel will take place in a current endemic area. Note that poor antibody response has been documented in children infected with HIV. It is unknown whether this increases risk of contracting YF.

Interactions

As with all live viral vaccines, administration to patients receiving immunosuppressant drugs, including steroids, or radiation may predispose patients to disseminated infections or provide insufficient response to immunization.

Concurrent vaccination against hepatitis B and YF reduced the antibody titer expected from YF vaccine in one study. There, it was recommended to separate these vaccinations by 1 month, if possible, but this is hardly ever feasible.

YF vaccination may lead to false positive HIV serologic tests when particularly sensitive assays (eg, PERT) are used. This is related to EAV-0, an avian retrovirus in residual egg proteins.

Vaccination Recommendations

Various countries require proof of YF vaccination administered at an approved vaccination center and documented in the International Certificate of Vaccination (see Figures 11 and 48, Appendix B) as a condition of entry. Although many countries require such proof only from travelers arriving from infected or potentially endemic areas, others require it from all travelers, sometimes even from those in transit. Documented YF vaccination is valid for 10 years starting 10 days after vaccination.

Travelers with contraindications to YF vaccination should obtain a waiver to the above requirements. Additional waivers of requirements obtained from embassies or consulates of the countries in which the traveler will visit may be useful, because health authorities have occasionally refused medical waivers.

So far, whether required or not, this vaccination was recommended for all travel outside urban areas in YF endemic zones (see Figure 48). When the risk of yellow fever in unvaccinated travelers is compared to the risk of severe adverse events, this recommendation becomes questionable (at least in endemic situations) and particularly where no cases have been reported for decades (Table). In the German package inserts, there is a new warning to immunize travelers above the age of 60 years, but the analysis described above demonstrates that all age ranges are at risk of adverse events.

Laboratory personnel who might be exposed to virulent yellow fever virus or to concentrated preparations of the 17D vaccine strain by direct or indirect contact or by aerosols should also be vaccinated.

Self-Treatment Abroad

None

Table 31 Risk of yellow fever vs risk of vaccine at various destinations (Monath and Cetron 2002, Khromava et al. 2005, Monath TP et al. 2005)

Destination	Yellow fever infection in unvaccinated persons		Yellow fever vaccine, serious adverse event (SAE)		
	Incidence per 100,000/wk	Death per 100,000/wk	YEL-ADV / -AND* per 100,000		Fatal SAE* per 100,000
Age group			1-99 y	60y	60y
Africa					
- endemic	23.8	12	0.7		
- epidemic	357	179		5.3	2
South America			(1.6**)		
- endemic	2.4	1.2			
- epidemic	35.7	17.9			

YEL-ADV = yellow fever vaccine associated viscerotropic disease

YEL-AND = yellow fever vaccine associated neurotropic disease

* = all cases occurred in primary yellow fever vaccinees

** = including other severe adverse reactions

▌ Community Control Measures

Case reporting is universally required by IHR. Isolate the patient, and follow adequate blood and body fluid precautions. Contacts should receive immunization promptly, wherever there is mosquito activity.

Additional Readings

Center for Disease Control and Prevention. Fatal yellow fever in a traveler returning from Amazonas, Brazil, 2002. JAMA 2002;287:2499–500.

Cetron MS, et al. Yellow fever vaccine. Recommendations of the Advisory Committee on Immunization Practices (ACIP), 2002. MMWR Recomm Rep 2002;51(RR–17):1–11.

Colebunders R, et al. A Belgian traveler who acquired yellow fever in the Gambia. Clin Infect Dis 2002;35:113–6.

Khromava AY, et al. Yellow fever vaccine: an updated assessment of advanced age as a risk factor for serious adverse events. Vaccine 2005;23:3256–63.

McMahon AW et al. Neurologic disease associated with 17D-204 yellow fever vaccination: a report of 15 cases. Vaccine 2007;25:1727–34.

Monath TP, Cetron MS. Prevention of yellow fever in persons traveling to the tropics. Clin Infect Dis 2002;34:1369–78.

Suzano CES et al. The effects of yellow fever immunization (17DD) inadvertently used in early pregnancy during mass campaign in Brazil. Vaccine 2006;24:1421-6.

Vellozzi C et al. Yellow fever vaccine-associated viscerotropic disease (YEL-AVD) and corticosteroid therapy: eleven United States cases, 1996-2004. Am J Trop Med Hyg 2006;75:333-6.

WHO. Yellow fever situation in Africa and South America, 2005. Wkly epidem Rec 2006;81:317-24.

PART 3

NONINFECTIOUS HEALTH RISKS AND THEIR PREVENTION

ACCIDENTS

Risk Assessment for Travelers

Accident rates among World Bank consultants (Figure 6) with varying degrees of experience in international travel demonstrate that inexperienced travelers are more at risk. Compared with their non-traveling counterparts, those with one trip had 1.8 more accidents, those with two to three trips had 1.76 more accidents, and those with four trips had 1.68 more accidents. Inexperienced travelers are unaware of differences in infrastructure and customs, particularly in the developing countries, and are therefore more likely to encounter problems.

Motor Vehicle Injuries

Motor vehicle accidents are the leading cause of death from injury among travelers. In particular, high rates of fatal traffic accidents are reported in many developing countries—as much as 84 times higher than in the industrialized world. Differences are attributable to the extent that rules are observed, that equipment is maintained, that roads are under construction, and that people avoid driving while intoxicated. The consequences of accidents stemming from the above causes are particularly serious in the developing countries. The lack of seat belts results in more serious injuries; poor infrastructure results in inadequate and delayed medical evacuation, and the limited capabilities of regional emergency medical services reduce the chances of survival and quick recovery.

Travelers who rent motorcycles or mopeds are particularly at risk. Among Peace Corps volunteers, 33% of all motor vehicle crash deaths resulted from this mode of transportation. Typical resort destinations such as Bermuda show an accident rate two to five times higher for this mode of transport among tourists older than age 40 years, compared with locals of the same age group. At many destinations, helmets are not mandatory, which greatly increases the risk of serious head injury.

Surface Sport and Incidental Injuries

Travelers are frequently injured in sporting activities such as hiking or mountaineering. Senior travelers are prone to falling on hotel premises during the evening or at night because of impaired night vision and because they are in an unfamiliar environment. Balcony falls resulting in spinal cord injury repeatedly occur in countries where the minimum height for balcony guards is lower than at home. These accidents usually occur within the first few days of a vacation, and alcohol plays a part.

Water Sport Injuries

Water sports accidents are very common among travelers. Drowning is a frequent cause of death among travelers of all ages. Unknown currents are often responsible (eg, Kuta Beach in Bali). Many adult drowning victims are under the influence of alcohol. Increased confidence, impaired risk awareness of hypothermia, hypoglycemia, nausea, and vomiting are associated with swimming while intoxicated. In the Dead Sea, serum electrolyte elevation has been associated with repeated near-drowning incidents, possibly owing to the large solute load victims are exposed to.

Surfing has an injury rate of 3.5 per 1,000 surfing days, mainly lacerations and soft-tissue injuries and, occasionally, back, shoulder, and head injuries. Lacerations from rocks, coral, glass, and metal are common in beach sports.

Criminal Injuries

Terrorism and assaults are epidemiologically of less concern than traffic and water sport accidents, although they generate more media attention. The terrorist attack against tourists in 1997 in Luxor, Egypt, with over 50 victims, reduced tourism in that country to virtually nil. The same occurred after the Kuta Beach attacks on Bali in 2002 and 2005, and to a limited degree after September 11, 2001, in New York. By contrast, attacks resulting in no or low casualties in foreigners, such as in Madrid in 2004 or in Mumbai in 2006, have minimal impact on international traffic. Cheap packages may gradually bring tourists back after such incidents; however, the threat may still be there. Many countries now have warning systems in place against terrorist attacks.

Minimized Exposure in Travelers

To avoid traffic accidents, the traveler should avoid the following:

- Moped or motorcycle rental (wear a helmet when activity undertaken; the risk reduction of head injury is 72%)
- Nighttime off-road driving
- Excessive alcohol consumption
- Renting unsafe cars—worn tires, no seat belts
- Careless driving
- Unsafe equipment

Prevention of surface sport and incidental injuries varies with the sport. Senior travelers should familiarize themselves with the layout of their hotel or residence during the day, if possible.

Swimmers must respect yellow or red flags on the beach that indicates swimming is dangerous or not allowed. They should ask the local people about river or sea currents.

To avoid assaults, it is wise to avoid walks or travel in unsafe areas alone at night. Avoid traps such as offers to change money at attractive rates. One should not wear expensive jewelry or show large amounts of money, and expatriates should not drive expensive cars or have a predictable routine.

Additional Readings

Liu B, et al. Helmets for preventing injury in motorcycle riders. Cochrane Database Syst Rev 2004;(2):CD004333.

McInnes RJ, et al. Unintentional injury during foreign travel. J Travel Med 2002;9:297–307.

World Health Organization. Available at: http://www.who.int/world-health-day/2004/infomaterials/wordl_report/eu/ (accessed).

Wilks J. International tourists, motor vehicles and road safety. J Travel Med 1999;6:115–21.

Wilks J, Coory M. Overseas visitors admitted to Queensland hospitals for water-related injuries. Med J Aust 2000;173:244–6.

Wilson N, Thomson G. Death from international terrorism compared with road crash deaths in OECD countries. Inj Prev 2006;11:332–3.

ALTITUDE

Risk Assessment for Travelers

The partial pressure of oxygen decreases as a function of barometric pressure at high altitude, which can lead to hypoxia. The following conditions may be expected with increased altitude:

- High altitude, 1,500 to 3,500 m (4,900 to 11,500 ft)—decreased exercise performance, increased ventilation
- Very high altitude, 3,500 to 5,500 m (11,500 to 18,000 ft)—hypoxia, altitude sickness
- Extreme altitude, > 5,500 m (18,000 ft)—severe hypoxia, hypocapnia, progressive deterioration

High (and, especially, very high) altitude may lead to acute mountain sickness or its complications (Figure 49).

There are genetic, individual differences in susceptibility. Individuals without acclimatization, those living at low altitudes, and, possibly, younger people are at greatest risk. Respiratory infection, strenuous exertion, and group trekking are additional risk factors, the latter because of in-group competition and the fear of being left behind. The influence of alcohol is uncertain.

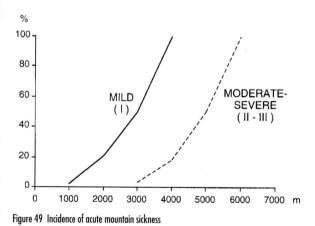

Figure 49 Incidence of acute mountain sickness

Clinical Picture

Acute hypoxia sets in after a rapid ascent or accidental decompression in an aircraft. Victims become dizzy, faint, and may become unconscious unless oxygen is given.

Acute mountain sickness (AMS) may develop within 1 to 6 hours of being at high altitudes. It is characterized by bifrontal headache followed by anorexia, nausea and vomiting, and insomnia, accompanied by fatigue and lassitude. Patients are often irritable and wish to be left alone. Acute mountain sickness closely resembles an alcohol hangover.

Periodic sleep breathing with apneic phases sometimes exceeding 10 seconds may occur, but this is not associated with the severity of AMS.

Life-threatening complications of AMS include high altitude pulmonary edema, cerebral, peripheral, and retinal edema, and thromboembolic problems. Stupor, coma, and death may occur within 8 to 24 hours after the onset of ataxia and changes in mental status.

Minimized Exposure in Travelers

Make travelers aware of the problems that may be associated with ascent to high altitudes. They should know that AMS may occur and that this may cause complications requiring immediate measures, particularly rapid descent.

Acclimatization for two to three nights at 2,500 to 3,000 m (8,000 to 10,000 ft) helps prevent AMS. One should avoid flying or driving directly to higher altitudes. If this is impossible (eg, flight to La Paz, Bolivia, in the Andes Mountains), avoid overexertion, large meals, and alcohol. The ideal rate of ascent varies with the individual.

Vacationers often claim a lack of time for acclimatization. It may be better to limit one's ambitions in such circumstances.

Chemoprophylaxis

The usual drug of choice is acetazolamide. While a meta-analysis concluded that dosage should exceed 500 mg per day, the usual adult dosage is 250 mg per 24 hours, divided in two doses, commencing 24 hours before the ascent and continuing up to and including the first 2 days at maximum altitude. Prophylaxis can then be discontinued, but therapy with the same agent may be undertaken if symptoms develop. Many world experts agree that higher doses (500 mg daily) are not useful. The effectiveness of such prophylaxis in reducing the symptoms of AMS is 75%. Side effects include tingling in the fingertips, increased urination, and the sensation that carbonated beverages taste flat. Vomiting, drowsiness, and itching occasionally occur. Acetazolamide is a sulfa drug; allergic reactions, however, are rare.

Alternate chemoprophylaxis regimens are dexamethasone, 4 mg every 12 hours starting the first day of ascent and continuing for the first 2 days at altitude. However, this results in more adverse events than with acetazolamide; specifically, stomach upset may result. Nifedipine is usually reserved for therapy, but like salmeterol, it may be considered for persons with a previous history of AMS who have not responded to other agents. *Gingko biloba*, as often as not, was no more effective than placebo, but sildenafil citrate (Viagra) may have some beneficial effects.

Chemoprophylaxis of AMS and its complications is indicated for those with a past history of AMS, unavoidable rapid ascent to > 3,000 m (10,000 ft), or a request for such medication.

Management On-Site

The fundamental principle of management of mild AMS is rest and acetazolamide, and, in severe AMS, it is descent (walking or by helicopter). Treat headache, the most frequent symptom of mild AMS, with mild analgesics (aspirin, 320 mg every 4 hours, acetaminophen with or without codeine) but these may be ineffective in moderate AMS. Nausea and vomiting are best treated with prochlorperazine, 5 to 10 mg intramuscularly because this also augments the hypoxic ventilatory response. Use short-acting benzodiazepines to prevent frequent wakening but only in healthy subjects; they may cause respiratory depression and decrease oxygenation. Dexamethasone 4 mg every 6 hours is indicated in more severe cases; sildenafil may be beneficial in pulmonary edema.

The therapeutic steps indicated in the various stages of AMS and its complications are shown in Table 29. The crucial principles to avoid death are:

- Learn to recognize and admit symptoms
- Avoid ascending with symptoms
- Descend if symptoms worsen
- Avoid leaving someone alone, even if the person requests others to do so

Table 32 **Management of Acute Mountain Sickness (AMS) and its Complications**

Mild AMS (headache, nausea, some vomiting, slight breatlessness, insomnia)

    Analgesics: Aspirin 650 mg or acetaminophen 500–1000 mg, possibly with codein

    Antiemetic: Perchlorperazin 5–10 mg IM (augments also hypoxic ventilatory response)

    Against frequent wakening: Triazolam 0.25 mg or temazepam 15 mg or other short

        acting benzodiazepine; not to be used in more severe AMS because of respiratory

        depression

    Acclimatization can be improved by acetazolamide 125 mg twice daily

    Stop ascent, or descend if easily possible

Moderate AMS (headache resistent to analgesics as above, vomiting, dyspnea, lassitude to

    the extent of the patient requiring assistance)

    Immediate descent

    Low flow oxygen if available

    Acetazolamide 125–250 mg twice daily

    Dexamethasone 4 mg every 6 hours PO, IM, or IV

    Hyperbaric therapy

Severe AMS with cerebral or pulmonary edema: early recognition is paramount!

    Evacuation or at least immediate descent

    Minimize exertion, keep warm

    Oxygen 2–4 L/min

    Dexamethasone 8 mg, then 4 mg every 6 hours PO, IM, or IV

    Nifedipine 10 mg PO in pulmonary edema, or 30 mg every 6 hours if no oxygen or

        descent possible

    Furosemide 20–40 mg every 12 hours (potential hypovolemia, incapacitation!)

    Hyperbaric therapy if descent is impossible

Additional Readings

Basnyat B, et al. Azetazolamide in the prevention of acute mountain sickness. High Alt Med Biol 2006;7:17–27.

Chow T, et al. Ginko biloba and acetazolamide prophylaxis for acute mountain sickness. Arch Intern Med 2006;166:296–301.

Hackett PH, Roach RC. High-altitude illness. N Engl J Med 2001;345:107–14.

Richalet JP, et al. Sildenafil inhibits altitude-induced hypoxemia and pulmonary hypertension. Am J Respir Crit Care Med 2005;171:275–81.

Sartori C, et al. Salmeterol for the prevention of high-altitude pulmonary edema. N Engl J Med 2002;346:1631–6.

www.ismmed.org

ANIMAL BITES AND STINGS

Risk Assessment for Travelers

The incidence of animal bites in human travelers is unknown. Several thousand people are killed yearly by mammalian bites and roughly 60,000 by snakebites. Approximately 100 shark attacks occur yearly in coastal areas. Destination and activity determine the nature of the bite or sting. In addition to mainly soft tissue injuries, bites and stings may transmit infectious diseases, including vector-borne diseases. The bites from venomous animals can be life-threatening, and such species are found in most climates and natural settings.

Although the risk of being seriously injured by native wildlife is low, the probability of a vacation being ruined by mosquitoes, fleas, ticks, bees, or wasps is high. Awareness, protective clothing, and insect repellents should always be used (see Part 1), and those with a history of allergic reactions should carry their emergency kit. Local information and advice concerning wildlife in the area should always be taken seriously.

Snakes

Venomous snakebite occurrence is highest where dense human and venomous snake populations coexist. This is the case in Southeast Asia, sub-Saharan Africa, and the tropical parts of the Americas. In the state of Maharashtra, India, alone, more than 1,000 people die each year from snakebites; in the United States, there are 45,000 bites yearly, with approximately 10 deaths. Concentration of human and snake populations may result from flooding, with subsequent snakebite epidemics. Snakebites are a negligible hazard for tourists engaged in sightseeing or recreation. The risk for those involved in agriculture, engineering projects, or scientific or humanitarian fieldwork is higher but still small. Venomous snakes are widely distributed worldwide up to altitudes of 2,500 m, except Iceland, Ireland, most islands of the western Mediterranean, most Pacific islands (including Hawaii, New Caledonia and New Zealand), Chile and Madagascar. Most snakebites occur after provocation, usually when the snake is trodden on, mainly at night. Some species enter dwellings at night and bite people while they sleep.

Scorpions and Spiders

Scorpions are widespread and found in tropic, subtropic, and desert areas. Scorpion bites are a public health concern; mortality is caused mainly by lack of available intensive care support and antivenom.

Spider species have a fairly well-defined geographic distribution, although some, such as the black widow, are cosmopolitan. Spiders like the brown recluse or black widow are not naturally aggressive toward humans and bite only when threatened or trapped. In contrast, the funnel-web spiders of Australia are aggressive and armed with potent venom, making them the most dangerous spiders in the world.

Aquatic Animals

Marine creatures hazardous to humans are found predominantly in tropical oceans. They may envenomate, bite, or puncture.

The coelenterates are a diverse group of invertebrates that includes fire corals, jellyfish, and sea anemones, which are venomous and potentially dangerous to humans. Severity of envenomation is related to species and season, amount of venom released, and size and age of the victim. Seabather's eruption, a papulous, itchy dermatitis on the skin area covered by the swim- or wetsuit, is attributed to the nematocysts of Cnidaria (jelly-fish, Portuguese man-of-war, sea anemones). Swimmer's itch is a painful dermatitis caused by algae (*Lyngbya majuscola*) present in rivers, lakes, pools, and oceans. The box jellyfish, found in the shallow waters off Australia's northern coast, is reputed to be the most venomous sea creature, with death occurring within 2 minutes of the sting.

The risk of shark attack is unlikely, provided that travelers keep a discreet distance, and avoid waters that are known to be frequented by sharks.

Clinical Picture

Mammalian Bites

Tearing, cutting, and crushing injuries may occur in animal bites. Considering the power and weight of many animals, internal organ damage, deep arterial and nerve damage, or multiple fractures are possible, if attacked. For this reason, we advise a complete evaluation in all but the most trivial and isolated of bite injuries.

Snake Bites

Many snakes are not venomous, and even venomous snakes often do not inject venom when they bite. The complexity and diversity of snake venoms are reflected in the wide range of signs and symptoms. The venom's multiple protein and peptide biotoxins produce diverse pathophysiologic effects in humans, such as local tissue and microvascular damage leading to tissue necrosis and hemorrhage. The components best understood are the neurotoxins, found in most elapid and sea snake venoms. These may induce paresthesia, weakness, and paralysis, including that of the respiratory muscles. Venom contacting the eyes from any of the spitting cobras does not produce systemic symptoms but does cause severe eye damage, possibly followed by blindness, if untreated. Almost all snake venoms affect blood coagulation which can result in hemorrhage with hemodynamic consequences, including hypotension and shock. Coagulopathy is a characteristic finding after snake envenomation. Myotoxins cause muscle damage with outpouring of potassium and myoglobin, followed by severe renal and cardiac problems.

Scorpion venom is most often a neurotoxin, causing local pain and paresthesia and occasionally somatic skeletal neuromuscular dysfunction and seizures. Other complications include nausea, vomiting, hypertension, tachycardia, and respiratory distress.

Spider venom often serves as a digestive juice, containing various proteolytic substances and often a neurotoxic component to immobilize the victim. In humans, the latter causes severe pain, muscle spasm with nerve dysfunction or hemolysis, and cell necrosis, depending on the species. Spiders such as tarantulas may cause severe irritation of the human skin by hair containing toxins.

Aquatic Animals

Jellyfish envenomation results primarily in skin irritations. There is an immediate stinging sensation, accompanied by pain, pruritus, and paresthesia with visible "tentacle prints." These symptoms may progress over several days to local necrosis, ulceration, and secondary infection compounded in severe cases by systemic reactions, including neurologic, cardiovascular, respiratory, and anaphylactic disorders. These may be life-threatening for the victim.

Sea urchins or star fish cause immediate pain with edema and possible systemic reactions because of their venom. The embedded spines are difficult to extract and frequently cause secondary infection. Stings by poisonous fish, such as lion fish, scorpion fish, stone fish, or sting rays, may cause various severe systemic disorders and even death.

Minimized Exposure in Travelers

Make travelers aware of the dangers posed by the local fauna.

Mammalian Bites

Animals rarely attack people without provocation, with the exception of some large carnivores and animals infected by rabies. Travelers should consider restrained or captured animals high risk. Most wild animals have a strong sense of territoriality, and intrusion can trigger an attack, particularly when the nest or the young are being protected.

Avoid eye contact with dogs; it will be interpreted as a threat or challenge. Running away often provokes a chase. When a dog is about to attack, the best reaction is to freeze and turn sideways, leaning away from the dog.

Animal attack is often best avoided by avoiding contact. Upon entering bear country, one should make enough noise to let the bear know a person is present; constant conversation along the trail is usually sufficient. If fresh signs are seen, the bear may be in the vicinity. Advise hikers to take an alternative route.

Snake Bites

Snakes are generally afraid of humans, and if given the opportunity, they will quickly retreat. Unless confronted at very close range, snakes are unlikely to strike. However, one should avoid known snake habitats, which are generally areas where they seek protection. Hands or feet should not be placed where snakes may be hiding (cracks in rock), and it is better not to sit on logs or rock piles that may be harboring a snake. Hikers should stay on paths and, if entering an overgrown area, should check questionable obstacles with a stick before proceeding. Adequate protective clothing, especially leather boots and long trousers, should be worn. Extra caution is necessary at night, when most venomous snakes are active.

Scorpions and Spiders

Scorpions and spiders are usually nocturnal and are more active during the warmer season. Scorpion stings always occur under accidental circumstances, more often at night, and particularly when the weather is stormy. Stings occur in houses, tents, palm, cane, or banana plantations or gardens during agricultural work, or on trips. The parts of the body most frequently stung are the limbs or occasionally the head and neck of sleeping persons. The latter case is more frequent in infants and young children. Scorpions have their "domiciles" in infested areas under stones, rocks, logs, loose bark of trees and around human habitations in gardens, old lumber, boxes, garages, washhouses, sacks, porches, chicken houses, under wash clothes, and in old shoes, mattresses, clothes or piles of newspapers stored in dark places. In infested areas, scorpions may be eradicated or their numbers much reduced by the use of insecticides. The following precautions may be of value for travelers or residents in areas harboring dangerous scorpions:

- Do not walk with bare feet during the night. Always wear a shoe or, better, a half-boot covering your ankle.
- Don't keep old clothes, mattresses, newspapers, and other "rubbish" in your house, because they provide a good domicile for scorpions.
- When camping outdoors, keep your garbage in closed bags; garbage attracts cockroaches and other insects, which in turn attract scorpions preying on them.
- Always check your shoes before putting your feet in.
- Houses in infested areas should have a step of at least 20 cm high that is made of glazed bricks or paint all around to prevent scorpions climbing in from outside.
- Use insecticides in suspected areas when a scorpion is seen or caught.

Aquatic Animals

Aside from wearing protective clothing such as a "stinger suit" and using a mask or goggles, there is little that swimmers can do to protect themselves from jellyfish stings. If jellyfish are sighted, swimmers should stay at a distance because the tentacles trail. Even dead jellyfish on the beach can inflict serious stings. Follow advice from local authorities. Partial prophylaxis of seabather's eruption may be provided by washing with soap and water after swimming. Footgear should be worn when walking in shallow waters, especially near tropical reefs. When walking in sandy areas known to be frequented by stingrays, to frighten them off, it is wise to shuffle. Divers should educate themselves on appropriate behavior toward dangerous or unknown sea creatures. Fingers should not be placed in holes or cracks where sea animals may reside.

Chemoprophylaxis

None.

Management Abroad

The local health professionals are usually experienced with regional animal bites and wounds and should be consulted immediately. It should be noted that some therapies (for instance, against jellyfish) may be successful in one place but not in another.

Mammalian Bites

Initiate local treatment of wounds immediately (see "Rabies" in Part 2, "Infectious Health Risks and Their Prevention"). Early cleansing reduces the risk of bacterial infection and effectively kills rabies and other pathogenic agents. Move the patient to a hospital as soon as possible where further treatment, including tetanus prophylaxis, can be administered.

Snake Bites

Although snake venom poisoning is a medical emergency, the traveler should avoid panic with its additional stress reaction. The victim should retreat from the snake's range, which is approximately the length of the snake. Killing the snake can be dangerous and may produce another victim. Even the decapitated head of a snake can bite with envenomation for up to 60 minutes.

Immobilize the bitten extremity to diminish local tissue necrosis and to delay systemic absorption of the venom. Reduce physical activity to a minimum for the same reason. Evacuate the patient to the nearest hospital as quickly, as comfortably, and as passively as possible. This may require transporting the victim on an improvised stretcher. The solitary victim should walk slowly with periodic resting. If prolonged evacuation time is expected, a pressure bandage may be applied to the bitten extremity to occlude lymphatic and venous but not arterial circulation. A tight arterial tourniquet above the elbow or knee is justified only in bites by dangerous neurotoxic elapids, sea snakes, and Australian snakes to delay the development of respiratory paralysis. Release the tourniquet for 15 seconds every 30 minutes, and do not apply it for more than 2 hours. To maintain renal flow and control intravascular volume, frequent drinking of at least 2 liters of water per 24 hours is recommended. Incisions in the wound are not effective and may result in various complications with no proven benefit. Suction devices to extract venom from the wound cause additional trauma and are not recommended. Avoid the use of antivenom in the field, due to the potential risk of anaphylactic reactions. In fact, administer antivenom treatment only in a professional setting.

Scorpions and Spiders

Treatment in the field is supportive. Local pain can be controlled with ice applied for 30 minutes every hour keeping cloth between the ice and skin. Oral analgesics are useful. The victim should be taken to a medical facility as soon as possible for treatment, especially if symptoms worsen. Antivenom administration is controversial as it is incomplete and can cause allergic reactions.

In the case of a venomous spider bite, the affected limb may be immobilized and pressure wrapped to minimize lymphatic return before adequate medical treatment is received. Within intensive care facilities, victims often can be treated symptomatically. Antivenom may be applied, depending on the spider species and the severity of clinical signs.

Aquatic Animals

Persons stung by jellyfish should leave the water, and they should immediately rinse the affected skin with sea water, not freshwater. A vinegar solution or alcohol (40 to 70%) should then be continuously applied for 30 minutes to inactivate the toxin; this will, in most cases, relieve the pain. Remaining tentacles should then be scraped from the skin. Local anesthetics may be used, but systemic signs are best managed by the nearest medical facility. Administer antivenom as soon as possible following envenomation by the box jellyfish.

The wound from a sea urchin, stingray, or stone fish sting should be soaked in non-scalding hot water (45 °C or 113 °F) as soon as possible for 30 to 90 minutes to attenuate the thermolabile components of the venom. Surgical exploration is required to remove remaining spines, and systemic symptoms must be treated appropriately. Stonefish antivenom is recommended for serious stings from stone fish or other species of scorpion fish.

Treatment of sea snakebites is similar to that for terrestrial snakebites. Polyvalent or specific sea snake antivenom is available.

Table 33 Treatment after Injuries due to Marine Hazards

Hazard	Measures (sequential)
Sponges	Gently dry skin / remove spicules with adhesive tape / vinegar
Coelenterates	Remove cysts by rinsing with sea water (early fresh water would increase envenomation!) / forceful stream of fresh water to dislodge tentacles / remove tentacles with forceps / vinegar or baking soda if unavailable / close observation of children and elderly
Seabather's eruption	Soap and water scrub / papain, powdered or dissolved / for pruritus eruption calamine lotion with 1% menthol
Sea urchins	Nonscalding hot water / remove pedicellariae by applying shaving foam, gentle razor scraping / remove spines if possible, they often brake
Starfish	Nonscalding hot water / remove foreign material / irrigate wound
Bristleworms	Remove spines: dry skin / adhesive tape or facial peel
Cone shells	Pressure immobilization
Octopus	Pressure immobilization
Stingrays	Irrigate with sea water / remove foreign material / nonscalding hot water / anesthetics, surgery often needed / prophylactic antibiotics
Scorpionfish, Lionfish and Stonefish	Nonscalding hot water / debridement / anesthetic / antibiotics
Sea Snakes	Similar to terrestrial snakes: immobilization, etc.

DETAILS:

- vinegar/5% acetic acid: apply for 10–30 minutes four times per day
- nonscalding hot water: up to 45°C or 113°F for 30–90 minutes
- antibiotics: third generation cephalosporins, ciprofloxacin, aminoglycoside, co-trimoxazole

(adapted from Klein JR, Auerbach PS. Textbook of travel medicine and health, 2nd edition. Hamilton, ON: BC Decker, 2003)

Table 33 summarizes the treatments for injuries caused by a selection of aquatic animals.

Additional Readings

Barbier HM, Diaz JH. Prevention and treatment of toxic seafood diseases in travelers. J Travel Med 2003;10:29–37.

Durrheim DN, Leggat PA. Risk to tourists posed by wild mammals in South Africa. J Travel Med 1999;6:172–9.

Fenner PJ. Dangers in the ocean: the traveler and marine envenomation. J Travel Med 1998;5:135–41,213–6.

Ismail M, Memish ZA. Venomous snakes of Saudi Arabia and the Middle East: a keynote for travellers. Intern J Antimicrob Agents 2003;21:164–9.

Woolgar JD, et al. Shark attack: review of 86 consecutive cases. J Trauma 2001;50: 887–91.

ANTARCTIC AND ARCTIC TRAVEL

Increasing numbers of seaborne tourists are visiting Antarctica, and Arctic Expeditions are increasingly en vogue. Long-term assignment in the Antarctic poses specific occupational health problems. Health risks and requirements for transient visitors differ from those of over-winter expeditioners who often must rely on telemedicine.

Dehydration on a heated, air-conditioned ship in a dry, windy, and cold climate is a real risk, and high water intake is paramount. Although hypothermia may be a concern, the reality of hyperthermia from overdressing and physical exertion is more a daily reality. Upper respiratory tract infections are the most frequent problems during such a cruise. Accidents from slipping on ice or loose rocks, sustaining sprains and bruises, are another problem on land visits.

Arctic and Antarctic tourists should be fit. Further, influenza immunization may be of benefit for these costly voyages. For personnel stationed in these regions, this is even more relevant, and psychological fitness is paramount.

Additional Readings

Cooke FJ, et al. A study of the incidence of accidents occurring during an arctic expedition. J Travel Med 2000;7:205–7.

Kupper TE. Drugs and drug administration in extreme environments. J Travel Med 2006;13:35–47.

Provic P. Health aspects of Antarctic tourism. J Travel Med 1998;5:210–2.

DEEP VEIN THROMBOSIS AND
PULMONARY EMBOLISM

There is an increased risk of venous thrombosis after air travel (see "Essentials of Aviation Medicine" in Part 1, "Basics"), but the underlying mechanism is unclear. The "economy class syndrome" is a misnomer; in fact, the problem may occur in air passengers traveling in classes where more space is offered, and it has been reported in bus ("coach syndrome"), train, and car travel. Deep vein thrombosis (DVT) is due to venous stasis. There is general agreement that additional studies are needed to quantify the risk and to determine specific recommendations for prevention.

Risk Assessment for Travelers

The estimates on the risk of developing DVT after a long-distance flight usually vary between 0.01 and 0.4 per 1,000 in the general population, but in up to 10% of long-haul travelers, symptomless DVT may be demonstrated. Most case control studies result in significant odds ratios of 2.3 to 4.0. The frequency among those who travel more than 5,000 km is 150 times as high as the frequency in those who traveled less.

The seven cabin-related risk factors are:

- Immobilized sitting
- Compression of the popliteal vein on the edge of the seat ("coach position")
- Duration of flight
- Low humidity
- Diuretic effect of alcohol
- Insufficient fluid intake
- Hypoxia, resulting in two- to eightfold activated coagulation

Some 70 to 90% of DVT in travelers has been associated with at least one of eight patient-related risk factors:

- History of previous DVT
- Presence of chronic disease or malignancy
- History of smoking
- Obesity

- Thrombophilic disorders such as familial thrombophilia, factor V Leiden mutation, and deficiencies of natural anticoagulants, such as antithrombin, protein C, and protein S
- Female gender, particularly when on hormone therapy or pregnant
- Recent injury or surgery, particularly of the lower limb
- Age over 60 years

Clinical Picture

DVT: usually painful swelling, mostly of lower limb, often cyanotic

Pulmonary embolism: various symptoms from shortness of breath to sudden death

For details, see internal medicine textbooks.

Minimized Exposure in Travelers

Provide the following general advice to all passengers: occasionally walk around and exercise the calf muscles while seated by flexing and rotating the ankles; drink plenty of fluids, avoiding alcohol and coffee.

Recommend that passengers of the intermediate risk group with one or a few risk factors wear compression stockings.

Advise high-risk travelers (eg, those with previous DVT, known thrombophilia, recent orthopedic or other major surgery, previous stroke, malignancy, or pregnancy) additionally to get low-molecular-weight heparin (LMWH) for each long-range flight (> 4 hours) as close to boarding the plane as possible.

Chemoprophylaxis

Use LMWH for high-risk groups. In view of the short half-life, apply this briefly before the flight; instruct intelligent travelers to administer this themselves prior to boarding. Some may choose to inject themselves in an airport toilet; in large airports, medical facilities may give the subcutaneous injection. Those visiting developing countries may often need a special certificate for carrying injections. The usual dose is approximately 2,850 U/L nadroparine calcium (eg, Fraxiparin 0.3 mL) or 40 mg enoxaparine (eg, Clexane 0.4 mL), if necessary, to be repeated after 12 to 24 hours. It must be kept in mind that LMWH is not free of adverse events: rarely (probably < 0.1%) thrombocytopenia type II may occur, particularly when repeat doses are needed, a weekly thrombocyte count may be indicated. Allergic reactions to heparin have also been described.

The role of oral throbin inhibitors (e.g. pentasaccharides) has not yet been determined. Aspirin is not to be recommended; it has little effect on veins and results in more than 10% of mild gastrointestinal effects.

Management Abroad

State-of-the-art procedures.

Additional Readings

Ansari MT et al. The association between seated immobility and local lower-limb venous coagulability in healthy adult volunteers: a simulation of prolonged travel immobility. Blood Coagul Fibrinolysis. 2006,17.335–41.

Aryal KR and Al-Khaffaf H. Venous thromboembolic complications following air travel: what's the quantitative risk? A literature review. Eur J Vasc Endovasc Surg. 2006;31:187–99.

Cesarone MR, et al. Prevention of venous thrombosis in long-haul flights with Flite Tabs: the LONFLIT-FLITE randomized, controlled trial. Angiology. 2003;54:531–9.

Clarke M, et al. Compression stockings for preventing deep vein thrombosis in airline passengers. Cochrane Database Syst Rev 2006;(2):CD004002.

Eklof B. Air travel related venous thromboembolism—an existing problem that can be prevented? Cardiovasc Surg 2002;10:95–7.

Schreijer AJM, et al. Activation of coagulation system during air travel. Lancet 2006; 367:832–8.

Scurr JH, et al. Frequency and prevention of symptomless deep-vein thrombosis in long-haul flights: a randomized trial. Lancet 2001;357:1485–9.

DERMATOLOGIC PROBLEMS

Risk Assessment for Travelers and Clinical Picture

Exposure to light may induce photoallergic and phototoxic reactions, polymorphous light eruption, hydroa vacciniforme, solar urticaria, or phytophotodermatitis.

Phototoxic Reactions

Phototoxic dermatitis occurs when drug use and sun exposure are combined. The drug molecules absorb energy, which is transmitted to tissue and alters the skin. Phototoxic dermatitis occurs on skin exposed to the sun. Unlike photoallergic dermatitis, prior sensitization is not required. Phototoxic dermatitis can occur in any individual, depending on exposure to sunlight and the dose of medication taken. Symptoms are a sunburn type of reaction with erythema in the areas exposed to the sun. Erythema occurs in 5 to 20 hours and worsens within 48 to 96 hours. Sunburn may persist in a netted pattern; that is, erythematous and tinged with blue. Nails may also be involved (photo-onycholysis). Drugs most frequently causing phototoxic reactions include tetracycline, sulfonamides, phenothiazines, non-steroidal anti-rheumatic drugs (NSAR), amiodarone, captopril, furosemide, and psoralen.

Phototoxic contact reactions are primarily due to topical agents found in plants such as lime, orange, celery, parsnip, fig, and anise, and in fragrances containing bergamot oil. Furocoumarins in plants may cause erythema, blistering, or bullae on exposed areas (phytophotodermatitis or dermatitis bullosa striata pratensis). Coal tar may cause phototoxic dermatitis with residual hyperpigmentation. Some drugs can provoke both phototoxic and photoallergic reaction, which raises confusion in the use of these terms; "photosensitive" is a more appropriate generic term.

Photoallergic dermatitis is an eczematous skin reaction that is caused by concurrent use of a photosensitizing substance and exposure to sunlight. Drugs inducing photoallergy include chloroquine, chlorothiazides, carbamazepine, tolbutamide, chlorpromazine, promazine, amitriptyline, chlorthalidone, indomethacin, piroxicam, and many others. Topical inducers of photoallergy are bithionol, sulfathiazole, salicylanilides, carbanilides, hexachlorophene, and aminobenzoic acid (PABA).

Clinical symptoms are similar to those of contact dermatitis. Papulovesicular eczematous or exudative dermatitis occurs within 24 to 48 hours, mostly on areas exposed to the sun but also elsewhere on the body.

Polymorphous Light Eruption

Polymorphous light eruption (PLE), or "sun allergy," occurs mainly when unadapted skin is exposed to strong sunlight. The term PLE describes a group of heterogenous, idiopathic, acquired photodermatoses. They are characterized by delayed abnormal reaction to ultraviolet radiation. The various skin lesions, which may appear, include erythematous macules, papules, plaques, and vesicles, each of which is monomorphous.

See below for sunburn and tumors following chronic ultraviolet (UV) B exposure.

Dermatologic Side Effects of Prophylactic Medication

Malaria chemoprophylaxis may result in cutaneous adverse reactions, the most severe being erythema multiforme, Stevens-Johnson syndrome, and toxic epidermal necrolysis reported mainly after use of the sulfadoxine-pyrimethamine combination drug Fansidar. The incidence ranges from 1 in 5,000 to 1 in 80,000. Chloroquine and mefloquine are also associated with severe cutaneous adverse reactions.

The antibiotics recommended for prophylaxis of traveler's diarrhea, such as sulfamethoxazole, trimethoprim, doxycycline, or quinolones, may also cause adverse dermatologic reactions.

Minimized Exposure in Travelers

Agents used in malaria chemoprophylaxis initiated 1 week prior to departure may be altered, if adverse events occur. Travelers should be instructed to contact a doctor abroad if moderate to severe skin reactions occur.

Henna tattoos may contain para-phenylenediamine (PPD) which may result in dramatic and long-lasting allergic reactions—obviously abstention from such tattoos abroad (PPD is illegal in industrialized countries) is the only recommendation.

Travelers to the tropics should avoid excessive exposure to the sun. Persons prone to phototoxic or photoallergic reactions should avoid any type of ultraviolet light irradiation and agents that have previously caused phototoxic or photoallergic reactions.

Travelers can evade frostbite by wearing warm, dry clothing. Further, they should avoid smoking and consumption of alcohol; this may result in vasoconstriction and vasodilatation.

Frequent showers and wearing cotton clothing will help to elude skin infection in tropical climates. Persons with hyperhidrosis may profit from aluminum chloride solutions or they can use baby powder.

Applying sunscreens with a high sun protection factor (at least SPF 20) will prevent herpes infection. In addition, kissing people with herpes labialis should be avoided.

Wearing sandals, which helps keep feet dry and clean, may help avoid fungus infection of the feet.

Chemoprophylaxis

Several reports indicate chloroquine, 200 mg base daily, may be partially effective in preventing polymorphous light eruption. However, travelers should try sun blocks first. PUVA (photochemotherapy) or UVB are highly effective, but it has to be performed before the sunny season or before taking a trip to a sunny region. Canthaxanthine, a β-carotene, may be of value for patients with abnormal reaction to ultraviolet A and visible light (PLE, erythropoietic protoporphyria); however, this agent may cause retinal deposits. Antimalarials and carotenes do not protect against sunburn, because their spectrum of absorption is not within the UVB zone.

Management Abroad

Phototoxic reactions are treated by stopping the drug, by avoiding sunlight, and by applying therapy similar to that used in sunburn. Topical or systemic corticosteroids can help.

Make travelers aware that wounds tend to become severely infected in a warm and humid climate. Disinfection and regular wound dressing are essential. Telemedicine may be useful.

Additional Readings

Caumes E, et al. Dermatoses associated with travel to Burkina Faso and diagnosed with means of teledermatology. Br J Dermatol 2004;50:312–6.

James WD. Imported skin diseases in dermatology. J Dermatol 2001;28:663–6.

DIVING

Scuba diving requires physical and emotional aptitude. Usually, divers need to present a certificate stating that they are fit to dive, at least for the training course. Such medical evaluation should contain examinations for factors listed in Table 34.

Risk Assessment For Travelers

Scuba diving accidents are described in the specialized literature. The main risks involved are decompression sickness, air embolism, panic, and disorientation (eg, in caves). Despite the large number of scuba divers, fatal incidents are comparatively rare due to the rigorous training courses and regulations implemented world-wide by various international organizations.

Divers frequently experience sinus problems and external otitis following repeated dives. Diving without equipment may be risky, because previous hyperventilation can reduce blood carbon dioxide levels, causing diminished breathing stimulus, hypoxia, and unconsciousness. The low partial pressure of the diver's remaining oxygen may fall below a critical point upon surfacing, which may lead to unconsciousness and drowning.

Snorkeling poses few risks except for lacerations and serious sunburn. Snorkeling at depths greater than 50 cm may lead to pulmonary edema.

Clinical Picture

Decompression sickness occurs when a diver surfaces too quickly, causing gases in the blood that would normally be excreted through the lungs to effervesce. This may lead to a wide range of clinical conditions. Decompression problems must be considered in any presenting symptoms after a dive.

Barotrauma may occur when the compression on gases in the middle ear, paranasal sinuses, and teeth, cannot be properly equalized. Even a slight imbalance may result in alternobaric vertigo in a diver, which can be particularly problematic if the water is turbid or dark.

The risk of hypothermia is often underestimated during and following a dive. It is not only uncomfortable but can cause colds and their complications.

Table 34 Evaluation of the Aptitude for Diving: The Most Frequent Problems*

Evaluation	Risks	Contraindications
Ear / Nose / Throat		
Ear wax, other obstruction of ear canal	Rupture of tympanic membrane	(Treatment before aptitude is granted)
Ear canal with exostosis, – atresia	Barotrauma of middle ear	Occlusion
External otitis	Barotrauma in case of occlusion	If tympanic membrane not visualized
Perforation of tympanic membrane	Disorientation, vomiting	Perforation
Scarring of tympanic membrane	Rupture of tympanic membrane	Large, thin scars
Hearing loss	Aggravation, deafness	Unilateral deafness
Septal deviation	Barotrauma of middle ear and sinuses	Negative Valsalva's maneuver
Rhinitis, sinusitis	Barotrauma of middle ear and sinuses	Negative Valsalva's maneuver
Eustachian tube blockage	Barotrauma of middle ear	Negative Valsalva's maneuver
Vertigo	Disorientation, vomiting	Most cases, depending on history
Disorders of lips, mouth, and tongue	Poor bite on regulator mouthpiece	Depending on function
Eyes		
Conjunctivitis	Superinfection	If persistent
Cataract surgery, recent	Wound dehiscence (cornea is slow to heal)	At least 12 months
Loss of one eye, absolute hemianopia	Difficulties in orientation	4 months
Visual field defects	Poor contact with buddies	Depending on case, experience
Errors of refraction, reduced visual acuity	Inability to check instruments, disorientation	Hyperopia with > 4 D correction required
Bronchopulmonary		
Asthma	Rupture of alveoli and pneumothorax, exhaustion	$FEV_1/VC < 0.7$
Acute bronchitis	Rupture of alveoli, aspiration due to cough	Acute bronchitis
Pneumothorax	Recurrence, tension pneumothorax, air embolism	At least 3 months

Table 34 **(continued)**

Evaluation	Risks	Contraindications
Cardiovascular		
Ischemic heart disease	(Re-)infarction, arrhythmia, syncope	Angina, even treated
Arrhythmia	Dyspnea, exhaustion, syncope	Depending on case
Hypertension	None, if well controlled	Uncontrolled hypertension
Hypotension	None	None
Nervous system		
Seizure disorder	Seizure, loss of consciousness, drowning	< 5 y free from seizures and off medication
History of decompression sickness (DCS)	Recurrence	Panic reactions
Psychiatry		
Hyperventilation syndrome	Muscle spasms, vasoconstriction, loss of consciousness	Recurrent episodes
Panic reactions	Uncontrolled reactions, emergency ascent, DCS	Panic reactions
Personality disorders, psychosis	Uncontrolled reactions, may endanger team members	Usual, depending on case
Drug dependence (drug abuse incl. alcoholism)	As above, additionally withdrawal symptoms	Usual, depending on case
Various		
Endocrine disorders, eg, diabetes	Impaired consciousness	Depending on case
Peptic ulcer disease, gastroesophageal reflux	Dyspepsia, nausea	Acute ulcer, subjective symptoms
Intestinal adhesions	Intestinal barotrauma	Recurrent symptoms
Hernia	Incarceration, aggravation when lifting weight	Should be repaired before diving
Urolithiasis, cholelithiasis (gallstones)	Colic may cause panic reaction, emergency ascent	Subacute, depending on case
Benign prostatic hyperplasia	Acute urinary retention	Recurrent urinary retention
Arthrosis and other rheumatic disorders	Impaired control of body, poor physical fitness, pain	Depending on case

Table 34 (continued)

Evaluation	Risks	Contraindications
Obesity	DCS due to impaired metabolism of lipid-rich tissues	Persons with BMI ≥ 30 to be warned of DCS, if BMI > 35 critically assess for exercise tolerance
Pregnancy	Congenital abnormalities, miscarriage, DCS	Discourage travel
Medication	Side effects	Depending on case

*For rare conditions see specialized literature.

Minimized Problems in Travelers

The basic rules of diving safety formulated by various international scuba diving organizations (eg, PADI, Divers Alert Network [DAN]) must be strictly adhered to. Abstinence from alcohol and drugs is essential. The risk of external otitis may be reduced by rinsing the external ear canal with clean water following a dive. (See also Part 1.)

Exclude candidates with medical conditions contraindicated in diving (eg, asthma, diabetes, epilepsy, patent foramen ovale) through the initial medical examination. If in doubt, a specialist experienced in diving can be consulted. Apparently, many experienced scuba divers continue to dive despite medical conditions.

Chemoprophylaxis

There is no recommended chemoprophylaxis. Some divers use pseudoephedrine hydrochloride, two 3 mg tablets, 30 minutes before a dive to facilitate pressure equalization, although there is some concern about reverse blockage. Contraindications include hypertension, heart disease, diabetes, and thyroid disease. There may be some side effects such as dizziness or nervousness.

Management Abroad

Follow the advice of the local emergency service. For serious problems, contact the DAN at +1-919-684-8111, or visit the Web site at <http://www.diversalertnetwork.org>.

Additional Readings

Harrison D, et al. Controversies in the medical clearance of recreational scuba divers. Curr sports Med Rep 2005;4:275–81.

Taylor DM, et al. Experienced, recreational scuba divers in Australia continue to dive despite medical contraindications. Wilderness Environ Med 2002;13:187–93.

In-Flight Incidents

Risk Assessment for Travelers and Clinical Picture

In-flight medical events are documented in 1 per 11,000 to 40,000 passengers. The rate may be higher, because not all incidents are reported. Up to 70% are managed by the cabin crew, sometimes with telemedicine type advice from the ground by specialized institutions (eg, MedAire). Varying equipment and drugs are in the in-flight kit, which can be extensive and now often includes a defibrillator or cardiac monitors allowing transmission of the data to ground-based advisory services.

The most common medical events are cardiac (10 to 20%), vasovagal (4 to 22%), gastrointestinal (8 to 28%), neurologic (8 to 12%), respiratory (5 to 8%), and traumatic (3 to 14%). Simple fainting is probably most common.

Minimized Exposure in Travelers—The Doctor's Mission, Medicolegal Protection

Passengers with preexisting conditions need to be fit to fly as described in Part 1, "Essentials of Aviation Medicine." Doctors who volunteer to help should remember the following:

- The basic rule is "first, do no harm."
- The goal of the intervention is to stabilize the condition of the ill passenger.
- They should accept the offer of telemedicine options whenever possible.
- Their role is to assist the flight crew, not to take control.
- Fear of liability should not prompt reluctance to offer assistance.

To diminish the risk of medicolegal consequences, health professionals volunteering to help should:

- identify themselves and state their qualifications;
- obtain consent for intervention from the patient, except for incapacitated passengers, or the family;
- obtain a complete history, including used medication, possibly with an interpreter;

- examine the patient as needed;
- inform the patient, family, and flight crew on the evaluation and suggested management;
- practice within the limits of their capacities;
- establish communications with ground-based medical professionals for additional recommendations and transferal of the patient;
- if a serious condition exists, request a flight diversion to the nearest appropriate airport;
- establish a full written report on assessment, management, and communications

Chemoprophylaxis

Usually none; tranquilizers may be considered in patients with anxiety.

Additional Readings

Dowdall N. "Is there a doctor on the aircraft?" Top 10 inflight medical emergencies. B M J 2000;321:1336–7.

Gendreau MA, DeJohn C. Responding to medical events during commercial airline flights. N Engl J Med 2002;346:1067–73.

Van Gerwen LJ, et al. Behavioral and cognitive group treatment for fear of flying. J Behav Ther Exp Psychiatry 2006 [epub]

JET LAG

Jet lag occurs when long flights across several time zones result in dissociation between environmental time cues and the body's internal clock.

Risk Assessment for Travelers

Surveys have shown that up to 94% of long-distance travelers suffer from jet lag and that 45% consider their symptoms severely bothersome. The severity of the symptoms depends on the number of time zones crossed, the flight direction and travel schedule, and individual characteristics such as age, chronotype, and motivation. Jet lag and the resulting impairment of physical and mental performance may have serious consequences, especially for pilots, business people, athletes, and military personnel. Studies in pilots have shown performance efficiency to decrease by 8.5% after an eastbound flight across eight time zones. Athletes may experience changes in their performance rhythm, and anaerobic power and dynamic strength may be affected for 3 to 4 days. There is also evidence that chronic jet lag may lead to cognitive deficits, possibly in working memory.

Clinical Picture

Jet lag is characterized by sleep disturbances, daytime fatigue, reduced mental and physical performance, irritability, gastrointestinal problems, and generalized malaise.

Without specific jet lag countermeasures, it takes 4 to 6 days after a transmeridian flight to establish a normal sleep pattern, and it takes approximately 4 days before travelers do not experience daytime fatigue. The resynchronization of endogenous circadian rhythms, including those of body temperature, melatonin, and cortisol, requires even more time. With a time change of 8 hours, for instance, it can take up to 15 days after an eastbound flight and up to 12 days after a westbound flight for complete readjustment.

To minimize the effects of jet lag, various nonpharmacologic countermeasures have been proposed, although only a few have been scientifically validated.

The use of timed bright light is a promising method; the light-dark cycle is the most important factor controlling the body clock. Bright light in the early morning (5 am to 11 am) causes a phase advance in body rhythms, whereas it causes a phase delay in body rhythms in late evening (10 pm to 4 am). Under laboratory conditions, light is very effective in phase shifting, whereas it is impractical after a transmeridian flight, because portable light sources are generally cumbersome and natural light conditions are difficult to control. However, as a supplement to other jet lag treatments (eg, melatonin), seeking or avoiding light at specific times after an intercontinental flight may help minimize jet lag symptoms. After crossing up to nine time zones in a westward direction, exposure to the natural light-dark cycle will be sufficient to promote adjustment to the new time zone; no specific light-dark regimen is necessary. After eastbound flights, avoid morning light (eg, by wearing dark sunglasses) to prevent a phase shift in the wrong direction. Avoid evening light after trips crossing more than nine time zones in either direction.

Jet lag diets have been proposed based on the fact that carbohydrates induce sleep by facilitating serotonin synthesis, and that proteins promote alertness by stimulating the synthesis of catecholamines. The effectiveness of this diet is controversial, and it seems likely that it is the exact timing of the meals rather than their composition that hastens resynchronization.

Exercise has been shown to be effective in phase-shifting and synchronizing circadian rhythms in rodents. Preliminary studies in humans support the hypothesis that increased physical activity during the habitual rest period alters body rhythms. Because little is known about the optimum time and the amount of exercise required to counteract jet lag, no specific recommendations can be made.

The following behavioral recommendations may provide assistance:

- Get a good night's sleep before the trip.
- During night flights, try to sleep. If the day is prolonged by westbound travel, you may take brief naps to reduce sleep loss; avoid prolonged sleep periods, however, for they will counteract adjustment to the new time zone.
- Adopt local time and routines immediately upon arrival (eg, timing of meals, going to bed).

- Allow plenty of time to sleep and rest in your new location before commencing work or touring activities.

Pharmacologic Prophylaxis and Treatment

Pharmacologic treatment approaches for jet lag symptoms attempt to enhance daytime alertness, promote sleep, and resynchronize the body's clock.

Caffeine is the most commonly used stimulant and has been shown to antagonize alertness and performance decrements, resulting from prolonged wakefulness, jet lag, or sleep inertia. Typical doses used in performance studies range from 200 to 600 mg. Amphetamines are very potent stimulants but unsuitable for routine use, owing to potentially severe side effects and the potential for abuse. Modafinil, a newer psychostimulant, is considered safer than amphetamines. Clinically, this agent is used to treat narcolepsy and other disorders associated with excessive daytime sleepiness. Little is known, however, about chronic use and tolerance of alertness-enhancing drugs, and further investigation is required to optimize the dosage regimen.

Short-acting benzodiazepines, such as temazepam, triazolam, and lorazepam, have been used to induce sleep during and minimize sleep loss after transmeridian flights. Although they have been effective in alleviating sleep problems, there are concerns about their safety. Several studies have reported residual effects, including amnesia. Use of these sleep aids must therefore be carefully considered for those who will be performing complex psychomotor or intellectual tasks on the following day (eg, pilots). Zolpidem, an imidazopyridine, has successfully been used to treat sleep disturbances associated with jet lag; it has a short half-life (2.5 hours), and an absence of active metabolites, as well as residual effects. Amnesia, however, has been reported, particularly with concurrent alcohol consumption.

Timed administration of melatonin is the most promising method of alleviating jet lag. Melatonin is a pineal hormone produced mainly during the dark phase of the day. The presence of specific melatonin receptors in the suprachiasmatic nucleus, where the body clock is located, indicates that melatonin directly modulates the circadian clock. Exogenous melatonin can shift the endogenous circadian system according to a phase-response curve; melatonin given in the afternoon advances the body clock, and melatonin administered in the early morning delays the circadian system. Based on the phase-response curve of melatonin, elaborate treatment schedules have been developed, taking into account flight direction and number of time zones crossed. These treatment regimens typically require daily adjustments of the melatonin administration times. However, a simplified regimen that includes administering melatonin at bedtime, irrespective of flight direction and number of time zones crossed, has also proven effective. This regimen combines the acute sleep-inducing and the chronobiotic effects of melatonin. In summary, travelers should take 3 to 5 mg of melatonin at bedtime (local time), after both east- and westbound flights, starting the first evening after arrival and continuing for 4 to 6 days. When traveling on an eastbound night flight, take one dose of melatonin in the late afternoon to advance the biologic clock and facilitate sleep during the flight. This may, however, reduce alertness prior to the flight, for instance, while driving to the airport. For westbound flights, no preflight or in-flight dose is recommended.

Additional Readings

Herxheimer A, Petrie KJ. Melatonin for preventing and treating jet lag. [update in Cochrane Database Syst Rev 2002;2:CD001520; 12076414.]. Cochrane Database Syst Rev 2001;(1):CD001520.

Reilly T, et al. Jet lag and air travel: implications for performance. Clin Sports Med 2005;24:367–80.

Revell VL, et al. Advancing human circadian rhythmus with afternoon melatonin and morning intermittent bright eight. J Clin Endocrinol Metab 2006;91:54–59.

MOTION SICKNESS

Risk for Travelers

Motion sickness may occur in all modes of transportation. It arises from a variety of physical stimuli, mainly changes in acceleration patterns, resulting in a "sensory conflict" between inputs about body movements and what is expected. Motion sickness has become rare in large aircraft except in the case of severe turbulence. In contrast, almost everyone can be affected on a rough sea voyage if no preventive medication is used. Motion sickness is rare before the age of 2 years and the maximum incidence is reached by the age of 12 years; the rate then decreases with age. Women are three times more susceptible than men, with the highest risk from 3 days before to 5 days after the onset of menstruation. Predisposing factors are fatigue, alcohol, a variety of drugs, history of migraine, bad odors (eg, vomit), and emotional conditions, with anxiety leading to a higher risk, especially in air travel. Acclimatization, as for example in crew members, reduces the tendency to experience motion sickness but self-selection may also play a role. There seems to be no association between seasickness and cabin location. The front seat of a car or a seat over the wing in the aircraft cabin are more stable—to reduce the risk of motion sickness persons prone to suffer should request such seating.

Clinical Picture and Impact

The symptoms include pallor, gasping, malaise, drowsiness, lassitude, cold sweats, salivation, abdominal discomfort, nausea, culminating in vomiting, and, possibly, subsequent dehydration. Cardiovascular symptoms (variations in pulse rate, rise or fall of blood pressure, change in peripheral blood flow) and respiratory symptoms (increased ventilation, shallow breathing, sighing, yawning) may occur, as well as a variety of sensations, feelings, and performance changes. All this may result in anything from mild discomfort to incapacitation.

Prevention by Reduced Exposure and Nonpharmacologic Remedies

Various strategies have been recommended based on anecdotal observations. These include the following:

- Minimize exposure: sit in the middle of the plane, lying down or reclining, restricting head and neck movements.
- Restrict visual activity: match visual orientation with the horizon or keep the eyes closed if in an enclosed cabin; avoid reading or fixation on a moving object.
- Improve ventilation, ease pressure on the neck and abdomen by undoing buttons or belts.
- Engage in a distracting activity.

The effectiveness of plugging a piece of cotton into the right ear canal (or, if left-handed, vice versa), wrist bracelets resulting in acupressure, and a variety of diets and beverages, is questionable.

Chemoprophylaxis and Treatment

Many different agents presented as tablets (some sublingual), chewing gums, nasal sprays, transdermal patches, suppositories and injections have been used to prevent motion sickness. These include:

- antidopaminergics: promethazine hydrochloride, metoclopramide hydrochloride;
  anticholinergic: scopolamine hydrobromide;
- antihistamines: meclizine hydrochloride, diphenhydramine hydrochloride, dimenhydrinate, cyclizine, buclizine hydrochloride; also cinnarizine, possibly combined with domperidone; ginger with conflicting data on its effectiveness.

All have limited effectiveness and some side effects, mainly tiredness, dizziness, and dryness in the mouth. Scopolamine has been associated with visual blurring resulting in falls, particularly when the agent accidentally got into the eyes. Availability as prescription or over-the-counter medication varies between countries; many are not specifically approved for motion sickness by the national regulatory authorities. Since data on the comparative effectiveness of agents vary, and since there may be individual differences, it may be beneficial to recommend the medication that previously worked well for the individual seeking advice.

Most brands of prophylactic medication should be taken one hour before exposure, except for scopolamine and cinnarizine, which should be used at least 6 hours beforehand. Most drugs are contraindicated when driving or operating machines. In travelers who have already developed symptoms, chewing gums containing dimenhydrinate may bring quick relief in mild cases. For severe cases, an injection of promethazine (25 to 50 mg IV or rather IM. or 10 mg oral TID) should be considered. Recently, phenytoin has been suggested. Prophylaxis is preferred for those prone to motion sickness.

Additional Readings

Albert EG. Phenytoin for prevention of motion sickness. Med J Aust 2003;178:575–6.

Committee to Advise on Tropical Medicine and Travel (CATMAT). Statement on motion sickness. Canada Communicable Disease Report 2003;29(ACS11),1–12.

Flemmer M, Oldfield EC 3rd. The agony and the ecstasy. Am J Gastroenterol 2003;98:2098–9.

Golding JF, Gresty MA. Motion sickness. Curr Opinion Neurology 2005;18:29–34.

Sherman CR. Motion sickness: review of causes and preventive strategies. J Travel Med 2002;9:251–6.

POISONING

Accidents are common when drug runners smuggle illicit drugs in condoms or plastic containers, which they swallow or insert into the rectum or vagina. Condoms may get stuck in the esophagus and lead to obstruction. If such a container leaks or breaks, the contents are easily absorbed by the mucosa which, in the case of heroin, results in altered consciousness, myosis, vomiting, constipation, and sphincteric spasms in the bladder and pylorus. Respiratory depression may cause death. Cocaine, which is highly toxic, is rapidly hydrolyzed in the gastrointestinal tract. Although the rupture of balloons containing hashish oil or marijuana have resulted in severe intoxication, fatalities have not been recorded.

Fish Poisoning

Various fish carry various toxins. Scombroid poisoning is common and occurs worldwide. Fish rich in dark meat, most often mackerel, tuna, mahi-mahi, skipjack, sardines, and anchovies, may cause scombroid poisoning when preserved at temperatures above 15 °C. Histidine in the flesh of scombroid fish can then be transformed to histamine by bacteria. Histamine, not destroyed by cooking, and possibly other unidentified factors cause a syndrome resembling an acute allergic reaction within 10 to 90 minutes of ingestion. Flushing, headache, pruritus, urticaria, nausea, diarrhea, bronchospasm (occasionally), tachycardia, and hypotension occur. These symptoms usually resolve, even untreated, within 12 hours, and death is uncommon. Sensitization does not occur, and victims may consume the same type of fish later with no ill effect.

Ciguatera is common but limited to coral reef fish such as barracuda, grouper, sea bass, snapper, and jack. The attack rate in the Caribbean has been estimated to be 0.3%, which is more than that for hepatitis A. Ciguatoxin and various other toxins involved in ciguatera poisoning are produced by sporadic reef algae that are consumed by herbivorous fish, which are eaten by the carnivorous fish listed above. The toxin accumulates mainly in the viscera and roe. It is harmless to the fish but acts as a sodium channel poison in humans. Heat does not destroy the toxin. Symptoms occur 15 minutes to 24 hours (usually 1 to 6 hours) after ingestion. Gastroenteritis sets in initially, followed by various neurologic symptoms, such as paresthesia, pruritus, weakness and paralysis, fasciculations, tremor, seizures, and hallucinations. The reverse sensation of hot and cold is a pathognomonic symptom. Cardiovascular symptoms such as hypotension and bradycardia are less common. There are broad individual differences in susceptibility to the toxins. Ingesting alcohol or nuts may exacerbate the clinical picture. Symptoms persist for days to months, and the case fatality rate is usually > 1%.

Tetrodotoxin is found in puffer fish and porcupine fish, which are consumed in Japan as the delicacy "fugu" and prepared by trained chefs. Ingestion usually causes mild paresthesias and warmth. Initial signs of intoxication, occurring within 15 minutes to several hours, include nausea and dizziness, which progress to weakness and loss of coordination. By blocking neural sodium conductance, the toxins depress the medullary respiratory center, atrioventricular nodal conduction, and myocardial and skeletal muscle contractility. Symptoms persist for hours to days. Bronchospasm, hypotension, and coma are complications, which produce an overall case fatality rate of 10 to 50%. Most fatalities involve amateur cooks. Fugu consumed in restaurants is likely safe.

Tropical microalgae (eg, *Ostreopsis ovata*) prevalent in the Pacific and Caribbean, and, more recently, also on Italian coasts, produce neurotoxins resulting in high fever, dizziness, cough and diarrhea. Transmission occurs while swimming or after ingestion of contaminated fish or shellfish.

Food Poisoning

Bacterial toxins formed in foods before they are ingested may lead to a variety of symptoms. (See "Traveler's Diarrhea" in Part 2, "Infectious Health Risks and Their Prevention" for toxins produced in the patient after ingestion.)

Staphylococcus aureus causes an acute illness characterized by abdominal pain and nausea often with vomiting, possible diarrhea, and hypotension, with an onset 2 to 6 hours after consuming contaminated protein-rich foods. Low-grade fever and headache are observed in a minority of patients. The symptoms persist for 24 to 48 hours. The toxin usually originates in a cook with an infected finger or nasopharynx or in milk from a cow with mastitis. Contaminated food items may have been inadequately refrigerated (the toxin is heat stable). This form of food poisoning may occur anywhere; in the early 1970s, there was an outbreak aboard a long-distance flight.

Clostridium perfringens causes an acute illness with abdominal cramps and watery diarrhea 7 to 16 hours after consumption of contaminated meat or poultry. Nausea and fever are less-frequent symptoms. The illness usually persists for no longer than 24 hours. The toxin usually develops in food that is slowly cooled or kept warm on a steam table.

Bacillus cereus may produce two different syndromes. The first, caused by ingestion of a preformed toxin, is identical to *S. aureus* food poisoning, with vomiting and abdominal pain occurring 1 to 6 hours after eating contaminated food. The second syndrome resembles *C. perfringens* food-borne disease, with enterotoxin release leading to watery diarrhea 8 to 16 hours after consuming contaminated food. Fried rice is often the vehicle for *B. cereus* food-borne disease. Other foods may also be the source.

Clostridium botulinum toxins are the cause for rare, but life-threatening, botulism. After an incubation period of 12 to 36 hours (occasionally, 2 hours to 8 days), weakness and dizziness occur, followed by blurred vision, diplopia, photophobia, and descending paralysis, leading to dysarthria, dysphagia, and respiratory failure in severe cases. Early anticholinergic symptoms, including a dry mouth and sore throat, with various gastrointestinal symptoms are also possible. This is a rare disease in travelers, but several cases have been reported, usually following consumption of home-canned food and, in some instances, industrially produced food items.

Lead-glazed ceramic crockery is purchased as souvenirs in various countries in southern Europe and the developing world. The lead poisoning that may result presents a poorly defined clinical picture, with stomach pain, vomiting, loss of appetite, and neurologic symptoms.

Plant Poisoning

Travelers who venture away from the usual tourist destinations may be offered local products made from toxic plants or they might ingest ones that resemble nontoxic plants at home. Mushroom poisoning is a common problem. Herbal teas may be contaminated with anticholinergic compounds, hallucinogens, hepatotoxins, and heavy metals.

▌ Shellfish Poisoning

In addition to the many infections that can be transmitted by shellfish (eg, hepatitis A, Norwalk virus, *Vibrio parahaemolyticus*), paralytic shellfish poisoning (PSP), neurologic shellfish poisoning (NSP), diarrheal shellfish poisoning (DSP), and amnestic shellfish poisoning (ASP) may also result. Shellfish poisoning is rare compared with fish poisoning, although outbreaks have been reported in various parts of the world. It is caused by saxitoxins and other toxins produced by sporadically occurring algae, which shellfish feed upon. The toxins then become concentrated in the shellfish. Symptoms occur within minutes to 3 hours after ingestion. The most serious form is PSP, characterized by paresthesias, vomiting, diarrhea, and disequilibrium. Fatality resulting from respiratory arrest occurs in approximately 25% of cases. NSP and DSP, however, have a milder course without fatalities; ASP leads to gastroenteritis, headaches, loss of short-term memory, and, occasionally, to seizures and coma. The case fatality rate for ASP is 3%.

Adequate preservation will help prevent food, fish, and shellfish poisoning. Raw items must look and smell fresh.

Fish with an ammonia smell or a peppery or metallic taste may cause scombroid poisoning and should not be consumed. Carnivorous reef fish heavier than 3 kg should not be eaten because they may have accumulated large quantities of ciguatera toxins. Travelers should discard viscera of tropical marine fish and moray eels for the same reason. Several "stick" or "paddle" tests based on an immunoassay that can detect ciguatoxins in fish are not yet widely available.

Regulatory authorities routinely test for shellfish toxins. Avoid shellfish harvested outside regular commercial channels or during a red tide.

▌ Chemoprophylaxis

None

▌ Management Abroad

Medical treatment should be sought in cases of food, fish, or shellfish poisoning. Antihistamines are useful in scombroid poisoning, whereas treatment of other fish poisoning is mainly supportive.

Additional Readings

Barbier HM, Diaz JH. Prevention and treatment of toxic seafood borne diseases in travelers. J Travel Med 2003;10:29–37.

Ting JY, Brown AF. Ciguatera poisoning: a global issue with common management problems. Eur J Emerg Med 2001;8:295–300.

PSYCHIATRIC PROBLEMS

Risk Assessment for Travelers

Psychological disorder rates among World Bank consultants with varying degrees of experience in international travel demonstrate that inexperienced travelers are more at risk. Compared with their non-traveling counterparts, those with one trip were 2.1 times more likely to have psychological disorders while traveling, and those with two or more trips were 3.1 times more likely (see Figure 6).

The extent of psychiatric problems is underestimated in many cases, cases wherein diagnosis is made by non-psychiatrists. At the Hospital of Tropical Diseases in London, England, 2% of all patients were diagnosed as having a psychiatric disorder when a physician made the assessment. This rate rose to 32% when the same assessment was made by a psychiatrist, who found an additional 18% with personality disorders that could lead to breakdown. The most frequent psychiatric diagnoses included depression, manic depression, psychosomatic syndrome, anxiety, and alcoholism.

Many persons use travel or work abroad as an escape. Some seek adventure or a more interesting life, whereas some look for a higher salary or social status. Others wish to get away from family, restrictions, and boredom. Some think they will find "the land of milk and honey." Patients with schizophrenia, manic depression, or other psychiatric diseases may believe their illness will be less obvious in an exotic society. Persecution hallucinations may induce patients with chronic psychoses to flee their homes. Megalomaniac paranoids may feel an urge to tell politicians or organizations abroad about their ideas. Persons with schizophrenia may be found wandering aimlessly in airports. Finally, some travel to commit suicide in anonymity.

Travel is semantically linked to the French word for work: "travail." To carry luggage, to line up, to clear formalities, and to cope with an unknown language and culture all means work and stress.

This leads to exhaustion, particularly when exacerbated by delays, jet lag, or an inhospitable climate. Increased muscle tonus, headaches, insomnia, aggression, anxiety, and, sometimes, substance abuse may result. Trips of short duration may turn out to be bad experiences for travelers who lack coping skills.

Expatriates experience additional stresses. Moving to another country, which happens every few years in some professions, such as the diplomatic corps, means saying goodbye to friends and adjusting to a new culture and neighborhood. Preexisting depression tends to become more pronounced during travel; the only conditions that tend to improve are stresses related to feuds with neighbors.

The individual responsible for the move, usually male, tends to underplay the dissatisfaction expressed by other family members, which may cause conflict. In expatriates, mental breakdown can result, particularly when neurosis or other personality problems come into play.

Clinical Picture

The nature of the breakdown suffered depends on personality, surroundings, and cultural attitudes to illness. Many individuals panic, refusing to be left alone for fear of attempting suicide. Most cannot work. The "incubation period" in expatriates varies, with male employees tending to break down within the first 9 months and spouses in 9 months to 4 years.

Drug or alcohol abuse may be a problem among expatriates attempting to cope with the above stresses, especially where drugs are available at low cost.

Minimized Exposure in Travelers

Individuals who will serve abroad for long periods should undergo psychological screening. They should also be educated as to what to expect and to be aware of their own response to stress.

Management Abroad

Psychiatric problems are sometimes the reason for evacuating expatriates, although this is not common. Language and cultural differences abroad make psychiatric therapy difficult.

Additional Readings

Beny A, et al. Psychiatric problems in returning travelers. J Travel Med 2001;8:243–6.

Dimberg LA, et al. Mental health insurance claims among spouses of frequent business travelers. Occup Environ Med 2002;59:175–81.

Wood J. Psychological changes in hundred-day remote Antarctic field groups. Environ Behav 1999;31:299–337.

ULTRAVIOLET RAYS

Ultraviolet (UV) rays from the sun (UVA 320 to 400 nm and UVB 280 to 320 nm) can cause severe, incapacitating sunburn and other damage, particularly in lighter-skinned persons who are unused to the sun. The first days are particularly dangerous. In the summer, UVB is intense, especially at midday. Window glass will block UVB rays but not UVA.

There is public confusion over the use of multiple UV indices. International organizations recommended a Global Solar UV Index in 1995, which has been endorsed by the World Health Organization. The Global Solar UV Index is an estimate of maximum skin-damaging UV rays measured over a period of 10 to 30 minutes at solar noon. The higher the UV index, the less time it takes for damage to occur. In Europe, the maximum summer UV index is usually no more than 8 but can be higher at beach resorts. Close to the equator, index values may reach 20. Index values are categorized as low (1 to 2), moderate (3 to 4), high (5 to 6), very high (7 to 8), and extreme (≥ 9).

Risk Assessment for Travelers

Many tour guides will confirm that, at beach destinations, sunburn is the most frequent, or among the most frequent, of incapacitating health problems experienced by their clients. Risk of skin cancer, including malignant melanoma, is greatest with UVB. The eye may be damaged, causing "snow blindness" or, in the long term, cataracts.

Erythema is much less likely to be caused by UVA, but photoaging of the skin may be greater with UVA, because its skin penetration is higher.

UVB may trigger systemic lupus erythematosus. Various drugs, such as oral contraceptives, tetracyclines, sulfas, oral hypoglycemics (sulfonylureas), diuretics, tricyclic antidepressants, isotretinoin, and nonsteroidal anti-inflammatory agents may increase sensitivity to sunlight, particularly to UVA. Risk ultimately depends on exposure.

Clinical Picture

Erythema is noticeable 2 to 6 hours after exposure, peaks at 20 to 24 hours, and fades within 5 days. Note that a "healthy tan" is an oxymoron, as skin tan is a cutaneous response to ultraviolet injury.

Minimized Exposure in Travelers

Skin type I always burns and never tans, type IV rarely burns and always tans, and types V and VI, which are moderately or heavily pigmented, rarely burn. Skin type should not be equated with racial pigmentation; a very light-skinned person may just tan, whereas some dark-skinned person may burn readily.

Tightly-knit, dark-colored, dry fabrics are best for blocking UV rays. Snorkelers should use sunscreens and wear a T-shirt because UV rays can penetrate several centimeters of clear water. Use organic (formerly designated 'chemical') sunscreens that absorb UV rays or inorganic (physical) screens that reflect or scatter the rays. The chemical screens are invisible and usually preferred, whereas physical sunscreens resist being washed off. The latter are preferred by lifeguards and ski instructors and thus should be recommended to patients with photosensitivities. The most widely accepted rating of sunscreens is based on the sun protection factor (SPF), which is the ratio of minimum erythema-creating dose (MED) of protected skin to MED of unprotected skin.

In theory, the product with a SPF of 15 allows the traveler exposure to the sun with no burn for 15 times longer than with no screen. In practical life the time of protection is shorter, mostly due to inadequate application of the sunscreen. Most sunscreens labeled waterproof contain fat. They will wash off during swimming or other water sports.

There is a common misconception that sunscreens promote tanning, when, in fact, they simply prevent burning. Sufficient sunscreen (2 mg per cm^2) must be applied. For most tropical destinations or ski resorts, an SPF of 15 to 20 is sufficient, although type I skins require a higher SPF. Note that insect repellents may reduce sunscreen effectiveness.

Tans confer some protection against sunburn but no more than an SPF equivalent of 2 to 4.

Chemoprophylaxis

Oral photoprotection has been largely ineffective, with the exception of β-carotene for erythropoietic protoporphyria in some patients, chloroquine for lupus erythematosus, and psoralens for polymorphous light eruption. Corticosteroids are not a prophylaxis for sun exposure.

Management Abroad

Various ointments are offered over the counter for sunburn. Corticosteroid creams are usually not recommended.

Additional Readings

Argyriadou S, et al. Knowledge and behaviour of tourists towards the sun. Rural Remote Health 2005;5:367.

Kullavanja P and Lim HW. Photoprotection. J Am Acad Dermatol 2005;52:937–62.

Manning DL, Quigley P. Sunbathing intentions in Irish people travelling to Mediterranean summer holiday destinations. Eur J Cancer Prev 2002;11:159–63.

Thiden E, et al. Ultraviolet radiation exposure. Br J Dermatol 2006;154:133–8.

PART 4

DIAGNOSIS AND MANAGEMENT OF ILLNESS AFTER RETURN OR IMMIGRATION

DIAGNOSIS AND MANAGEMENT OF ILLNESS AFTER RETURN

Travelers returning from abroad often request a consultation for persisting health problems. The clinician should assess the following:

- Travel history, including destinations, potential exposure
- Preventive measures taken, such as immunizations, medication (and compliance)
- Symptoms and their chronology—consideration of the incubation period (see Part 2)
- Physical examination
- Blood sample in all febrile patients to promptly diagnose malaria (some nonimmune patients become febrile before parasites are visible; conversely, some patients, such as semi-immune individuals or persons with breakthroughs on chemoprophylaxis, may remain afebrile despite malaria infection)
- Other laboratory and technical evaluation as indicated under the circumstances

PERSISTENT DIARRHEA

Traveler's diarrhea will persist longer than 2 to 4 weeks in 1 to 2% of patients. Etiologic agents show some differences in persistent diarrhea (Table 32), compared with acute traveler's diarrhea. Consider the parasitic pathogens in travelers with persistent (> 14 days) or chronic diarrhea (> 30 days). A bacterial enteric infection may also cause prolonged diarrhea. Other causes include induced lactase deficiency or a transient small bowel bacterial overgrowth syndrome induced by small bowel motility stasis resulting from an earlier enteric infection. Some of these patients have Brainerd diarrhea, an idiopathic form of chronic diarrhea associated with consumption of untreated water or unpasteurized milk. Post infec-

Table 33 Etiology of Persistent Diarrhea (> 14 Days)*

Cause of Persistent Diarrhea	Comment
Parasitic agents including *Giardia*, *Cyclospora*, *Cryptosporidium*, *Microsporidium*, *Entamoeba histolytica*	Two freshly passed stools should be examined by a competent laboratory for each of the parasitic agents
Bacterial enteropathogens including Enterotoxigenic *Escherichia coli*, *Shigella*, *Salmonella*, *Aeromonas*, adherent or enteroaggregative *E. coli*, noncholera *Vibrios*	Special studies may be required to identify the enteropathogen
Lactase deficiency and other malabsorption syndromes	Diet alteration may lead to improved symptomatology
Bacterial overgrowth syndrome	Small bowel intubation or breath hydrogen testing is required to make the diagnosis
Idiopathic chronic diarrhea best classified as Brainerd diarrhea	This is an etiology of exclusion after a complete gastroenterologic evaluation fails to show other cause. Patients with a negative work-up should be reassured that the illness is likely to be self-limiting
Post-infectious irritable bowel syndrome (PI-IBS)	In infectioos diarrhea, particulary illness due to bacterial enteropathogens, functional bowel disease may result.
Inflammatory bowel disease (IBD)	Rarely, IBD may be unmasked by an acute bout of traveler's diarrhea

*In approximate order of importance according to the author's experience.

tious irritable bowel syndrome (PI-IBS) may ocur in subjects with travelers' diarrhea where diarrhea and bloating persist for months to years.

Approach the patient with persistent diarrhea sequentially (Figure 50). When seen in a general practice or travel clinic, these patients have usually not responded to at least one course of antimicrobial therapy. Adult patients, if they have not received antibacterial therapy, may be treated with a fluoroquinolone, as in the case of typical traveler's diarrhea. Those who have received one of these drugs before should not receive it again. Assess the etiology of the patient's diarrhea if they do not respond to antibacterial therapy. Ideally, two stool samples should be studied for the parasitic and bacterial pathogens listed in Table 32. Treat etiologic agents that are identified. Empiric Giardia therapy may

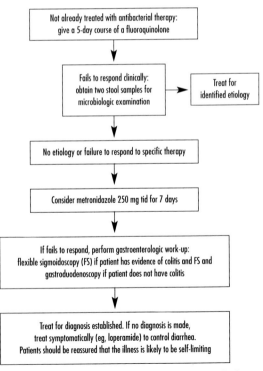

Figure 50 Evaluation and management of the traveler with persistent diarrhea

be justified if none is identified. Metronidazole may be given empirically for possible giardiasis or bacterial overgrowth. Failure to respond to metronidazole indicates the need for gastroenterologic evaluation. Evidence of colitis, such as fecal urgency and tenesmus, passage of many small-volume stools (which may contain blood and mucus), or the presence of fecal leukocytes in stool samples indicates the patient should have a flexible sigmoidoscopy with biopsy of any abnormal tissue. With no evidence of colitis, perform a flexible sigmoidoscopy and an upper gastroduodenoscopy with biopsy of abnormal tissue, study of duodenal material, and biopsy for Giardia and other intestinal parasites. With a negative work-up or only minimal focal colonic mucosal inflammation found (particularly chronic inflammation with lymphocytes), Brainerd diarrhea is suspected. Reassure patients that the illness will likely be prolonged but self-limited. In these cases, it is advisable to initiate symptomatic therapy with loperamide-like drugs. Chronic diarrhea associated with a post-infectious irritable bowel syndrome (PI-IBS) occurs in a subset of persons developing diarrhea during international travel, particularly following an enteric infection by bacterial enteropathogens. Less commonly, patients may progress to inflammatory bowel disease after a bout of traveler's diarrhea, making the diagnosis difficult to establish.

FEVER WITHOUT FOCAL FINDINGS

When fever is reported with focal findings (eg, respiratory symptoms, jaundice, or eosinophilia), its origin should be identified by carefully considering disorders of the specific organ system. When fever occurs without focal organ system involvement, the diagnosis is more difficult to develop. In the latter case, a systematic approach to evaluation should include the nature of the trip and places visited, with consideration of diseases endemic to regions visited, expected incubation period of a potential disorder and disorders that may make persons more susceptible. Table 34 lists disorders to consider in the patient with fever showing obvious organ system involvement. The laboratory is often the key to establishing the diagnosis. Blood culture, blood, or cerebrospinal fluid films for parasites, serologic studies, and bone marrow aspiration/biopsy with histologic and cultural study should be pursued. It is critical to develop an index of suspicion when considering potential diagnoses and ordering appropriate tests.

Table 34 Disorders to Consider in the Febrile Patient without Focal Disease Involvement

Disorders to Consider*	Diagnostic Approach
Bacterial endocarditis, bacterial sepsis, bartonellosis, brucellosis, leptospirosis, listeriosis, melioidosis, meningococcemia, plague, rat bite fever, typhoid fever	Blood cultures
Babesiosis, Borreliae, African and American trypanosomiasis, malaria, microfilariae, visceral leishmaniasis, loiasis	Blood or cerebrospinal films for parasites
Cytomegalovirus infection, Epstein-Barr virus infection, viral hepatitis, leptospirosis, rickettsial infections, viral hemorrhagic fevers, dengue, syphilis, relapsing fever, toxoplasmosis	Serologic procedure
Brucellosis, histoplasmosis, leishmaniasis, tuberculosis, typhoid fever	Bone marrow microscopy and culture

*Treatment of specific conditions may be found elsewhere in the manual or in other texts.

TREATMENT OF UNCOMPLICATED MALARIA

Because malaria is such an important disorder of travelers, we outline diagnosis and recommended therapy of uncomplicated malaria separately. The keys to diagnosing malaria are (1) if the traveler stayed in an endemic area or other possible exposure to malaria at least 6 days before onset of illness and (2) a positive blood film for plasmodia. Perform thick and thin smears to ascertain the degree of parasitemia and the type of infection: *Plasmodium falciparum*, *Plasmodium vivax*, *Plasmodium ovale*, *Plasmodium malariae*. Use of rapid diagnostic tests as a diagnostic auxiliary is increasing, but this does not replace traditional blood films. Fever is usually, but not always, present when patients present with malaria. A periodic fever pattern is helpful but not required in making the diagnosis and is rarely seen in travelers. If malaria is suspected because of the traveler's itinerary and if the blood film is negative, it should be repeated in 12 to 24 hours.

Initially, uncomplicated and severe malaria should be differentiated. Severe malaria is defined by

- impairment of consciousness
- prostration: inability to sit unassisted in a child who was able to do so
- severe anemia, hematocrit < 15% or hemoglobin < 5 g/dL
- hyperparasitemia, > 4% in nonimmune children, > 20% under any circumstances—to be on the safe side, a suggested > 2%
- renal failure, defined as urinary output < 400 mL per 24 hours in adults, or < 12 mL per kg per 24 hours in children
- pulmonary edema or adult respiratory stress syndrome
- hypoglycemia with whole blood glucose < 2.2 mmol/L (40 mg/dL)
- circulatory collapse or shock with systolic value < 70 mm Hg in adults, < 50 mm Hg in children
- spontaneous bleeding from mucosal tissues and/or laboratory evidence of disseminated intravascular coagulation
- convulsions
- acidemia with pH < 7.35, or acidosis with plasma bicarbonate levels < 15 mmol/L
- macroscopic hemoglobinuria

This clearly requires hospital treatment under the guidance of experienced specialists. Uncomplicated falciparum malaria (parasitemia < 2%) usually requires hospital treatment, except in some countries where home treatment is an option under specific circumstances.

Table 35 provides recommended treatment for documented uncomplicated malaria. In Table 36, alternative treatments for uncomplicated malaria are provided. For malaria acquired in the few remaining areas without chloroquine resistance, chloroquine is the drug of choice for therapy. Most cases of malaria in international travelers are acquired during travel to sub-Saharan Africa, where chloroquine-resistant *P. falciparum* is the most frequent etiologic agent. Standard therapy for chloroquine-resistant malaria is quinine sulfate given for 3 days, along with doxycycline. In Southeast Asia and in South America, relative resistance to quinine has been seen, so when malaria is acquired in these areas, quinine is continued for 7 days. When *P. vivax* or *P. ovale* is diagnosed based on blood film examination, give primaquine phosphate (15 mg base) by mouth daily for 14 days to prevent relapses. The pediatric dose is base 0.3 mg/kg/daily for 14 days. It is necessary to screen patients for presence of G-6P-D deficiency if primaquine is to be used. G-6P-D-deficient patients should not receive primaquine. *P. vivax* occurs characteristically during travel to Asia or Latin America.

Table 35 Evaluation and Treatment for Uncomplicated Malaria

Expected Chloroquine Susceptibility Based on Place of Travel	Drug and Dose in Adults	Drug and Dose in Children
Susceptible (Central America and Middle East)	Chloroquine base 25 mg/kg over 3 days (10 mg, 10 mg after 24 hrs, 5 mg after 48 hrs)	Chloroquine 10 mg base/kg initial dose followed by 5 mg/kg/base 12, 24, and 36 hrs later
Resistant (Africa, Southern Asia, South America)	Quinine 8 mg base/kg orally 3 times daily for 7 days, plus doxycycline 100 mg bid for 7 days	Quinine 8 mg base/kg orally 3 times daily for 7 days, plus in areas of high levels of resistance and if age > 8 yrs, doxycycline 2 mg/kg/d for 7 days

Table 36 Alternative Therapy for Uncomplicated *Falciparum* Malaria (parasitemia < 2%)

	Drug and Dose in Adults	Drug and Dose in Children
Alternative drugs for areas with resistance	Mefloquine 25 mg base split dosage (15 mg base /kg initial dose, followed by 10 mg base/kg 6–24 hrs later)	Mefloquine 25 mg base split dosage (15 mg base /kg initial dose, followed by 10 mg base /kg 6–24 hrs later)
	Artemeter-lumefantrine (Riamet, Co-artem) 4 tablets, each at 0, 8, 24, 36, 48, 60 hrs in semi-immune persons only at 0, 8, 24, 48 hrs with food	Artemeter-lumefantrine 1.5/9 mg twice daily for 3 days with food
	Atovaquone-proguanil (Malarone) 4 tablets each at 0, 24, 48 hrs with food	Atovaquone-proguanil (Malarone pediatric tablet with 62.5/25 mg) 1 for 11–20 kg, 2 for 21–30 kg, 3 for 31–40 kg, 1 adult tablet if > 40 kg each at 0, 24, 48 hrs with food
	Pyrimethamine-sulfadoxine (Fansidar)3 tablets, single dose	Pyrimethamine-sulfadoxine single dose depending on weight

Repeat medication if vomiting occurs within 1 hour

Never use halofantrin (Halfan) in view of risk of fatal QTc-prolongation.

DERMATOLOGIC DISORDERS

Skin involvement may be generalized or localized, macular, papular, or ulcerative. The appearance of the cutaneous process will provide clues to the cause of the condition. Table 36 provides a partial list of potential causes of cutaneous eruption.

Generalized eruption usually signals systemic disease, often an infection (usually viral). Serologic studies may assist in establishing an etiologic diagnosis. With a petechial or ecchymotic skin eruption, dengue or other hemorrhagic fever viruses, meningococcemia, disseminated intravascular coagulation associated with sepsis, and advanced rickettsial infection should all be suspected. With a localized skin eruption, especially if the condition is ulcerative, biopsy and histologic examination and, in selected cases, culture may establish the etiology.

Table 37 Cutaneous Process in a Returning Traveler: Differential Diagnosis

Pattern of Skin Eruption	Differential Diagnosis (Partial List)
Generalized skin rash	Systemic viral infection: measles, rubella, chickenpox, arbovirus, filovirus or Sindbis fever, rickettsial infection, leptospirosis, relapsing fever
Petechial or ecchymotic rash	Viral hemorrhagic fever including dengue, arenaviral infection, meningococcemia and other septicemias, advanced Rocky Mountain spotted fever
Localized maculopapular rash	Onchocerciasis, strongyloidiasis, scabies, lice, cercarial dermatitis in schistosomiasis
Nodular skin lesions	Furuncles, tungiasis, myiasis
Ulcerative or crusted process	Impetigo, primary chancre of African trypanosomiasis, chagoma in Chagas' disease, cutaneous anthrax, fungal, nocardial, or mycobacterial infection, cutaneous leishmaniasis, cutaneous amoebiasis
Serpiginous and migratory processes	Cutaneous larva migrans, loiasis, strongyloidiasis

EOSINOPHILIA

Patients showing > 450 eosinophils per microliter of blood have a peripheral eosinophilia. This finding, together with a history of international travel, suggests a parasitic infection (Table 38). With the exception of *Isospora belli* and *Dientamoeba fragilis*, protozoal parasites do not produce a peripheral eosinophilia. When other protozoal infections are diagnosed (eg, giardiasis and malaria) in the presence of an eosinophilia, suspect a second parasitic infection. The nonprotozoal parasites with an extraintestinal migration phase, particularly in association with tissue infection, produce the most intense eosinophilia.

The incubation period of eosinophilia causes varies widely. Certain agents may produce illness and eosinophilia years after the traveler leaves the endemic area (eg, onchocerciasis and loiasis) so that a history of remote travel may be important. The traveler who lived under primitive conditions with local populations is at greater risk of parasitic infection. Those exposed to local water sources (local drinking water or an unchlorinated or poorly chlorinated pool) may have schistosomiasis. Diagnosis is suggested by history and place of travel and is confirmed by examination of stool and blood, or tissue biopsy. Treatment depends on the diagnosis.

Table 38 Major Causes of Peripheral Eosinophilia in International Travelers

Clinical Condition	Symptoms and Geographic Region of Occurrence	Diagnosis
Allergic disorder	Rhinitis, respiratory symptoms, hives, (worldwide)	History
Bronchopulmonary aspergillosis	Asthma and respiratory symptoms (worldwide)	History plus tissue biopsy
Isospora belli infection	Intestinal symptoms (worldwide)	Stool examination
Dientamoeba fragilis infection	Intestinal symptoms (worldwide)	Stool examination
Ascariasis	Intestinal symptoms, asymptomatic (worldwide)	Stool examination
Hookworm infection	Intestinal symptoms, asymptomatic (worldwide)	Stool examination
Strongyloidiasis	Intestinal symptoms, skin lesion (worldwide)	Stool examination, sputum examination, serology

Table 38 (continued) Major Causes of Peripheral Eosinophilia in International Travelers

Clinical Condition	Symptoms and Geographic Region of Occurrence	Diagnosis
Myalgias, intestinal symptoms, periorbital edema (worldwide)		Trichinosis Serology, muscle biopsy
Lymphatic filariasis	Lymphangitis, lymphedema, asymptomatic (tropical regions)	Blood smears, serology, skin biopsy
Onchocerciasis	Nodular skin lesions (Africa and Central and South America)	Skin biopsy,
Loiasis	Nodular skin lesions, subconjunctival worm (West and Central Africa)	Blood smear, worm, identified in eye examination
Mansonellosis	Dermatitis, asymptomatic(Africa and Central and South America)	Blood smear or skin biopsy
Dracunculiasis	Blister or ulcer of skin, fever, generalized urticaria, periorbital edema, and wheezing (Africa, the Middle East, and the Indian Subcontinent)	Clinical diagnosis: visual and microscopic identification of worm or larvae
Tropical pulmonary eosinophilia,	Respiratory symptoms (tropical areas, especially Africa)	Serology, clinical history

SEXUALLY TRANSMITTED DISEASES

Approximately 5% of short-term travelers and up to 50% of expatriates engage in sexual activities with local persons while outside their own home region. Sexually transmitted diseases (STDs) are common among young, sexually active international travelers. Diagnosis and recommended treatment for sexually active adults with common STDs are given in the Table 39.

Table 39 Sexually Transmitted Diseases of International Travelers and Expatriates — Diagnosis and Management

Sexually Transmitted Diseases	Diagnosis	Recommended Therapy
Primary syphilis	Finding *Treponema pallidum* on darkfield exam of chancre or ulcer or serodiagnosis	Benzathine penicllin G, 2.4 million units IM weekly for 2 or 3 doses or amoxicillin 3 g PO bid, plus probenecid 1 g PO qd for 14 days
Genital herpes simplex	Clinical diagnosis, can be confirmed by viral culture	Acyclovir 400 mg PO tid for 7–10 days or famciclovir 250 mg PO tid for 7–10 days
Granuloma inguinale (Donovanosis)	Identification of dark-staining Donovan bodies on tissue crush preparation or biopsy	Doxycycline 100 mg PO bid for at least 3 weeks or trimethoprim sulfamethoxazole 800 mg 160 mg bid for at least three weeks
Lymphogranuloma venereum	Serologic study with CF titers $\geq$ 1:64 and exclusion of other causes of inguinal adenopathy	Doxycycline 100 mg bid for 21 days or erythromycin base 500 mg PO qid for 21 days
Chancroid	Darkfield exam on ulcer exudate of serologic test > 7 days after onset of ulcer	Azithromycin 1 g PO or ceftriazone 250 mg IM or ciprofloxacin 500 mg PO bid for 3 days with follow-up exam in 3–7 days

Table 39 (continued)

Sexually Transmitted Diseases	Diagnosis	Recommended Therapy
Urethritis in a male	Consider *Clamydia trachomatis* and *Neisseria gonorrhoeae* in Gram stain positive smears of exudates showing ≥ 5 white blood cells per oil immersion field. Intracellular Gram-negative diplococci confirms gonococcal infection. Employ culture and diagnostic tests to establish a diagnosis	For *C. trachomatis:* azithromycin 1 g PO in a single dose or doxycycline 100 mg PO bid for 7 days; for *N. gonorrhoeae:* ceftriaxone 125 mg IM once or cefixime 400 mg PO once. For uncertain diagnoses or when follow-up is not possible, treat for both conditions
Acute proctitis in a homosexual male	History of receptive anal intercourse, rectal pain, and tenesmus	Ceftriaxone 125 mg IM plus doxycycline 100 mg bid for 7 days
Epididymitis	Unilateral testicular pain and tenderness, hydrocele and palpable swelling of the epididymis or symptoms of urethritis	Ceftriaxone 250 mg IM once and doxycyline 100 mg PO bid for 10 days
Bacterial vaginosis	Vaginal discharge showing clue cells microscopically, pH of > 4.5 and fishy odor (whiff test)	Metronidazole 500 mg bid PO for 7 days or intravaginal metronidazole gel or clindamycin cream
Human papillomavirus infection	Genital warts (diagnosis can be confirmed by biopsy, but clinical diagnosis is usually sufficient	Patient applied podofilox 0.5% solution or gel bid for 3 days (cycle may be repeated), or cryotherapy with liquid nitrogen, or cryoprobe with repeat application each 1–2 weeks

Table 39 (continued)

Sexually Transmitted Diseases	Diagnosis	Recommended Therapy
Pubic lice	Pruritis and noticing of lice or nits on pubic hair	Permethrin 1% crème rinse. Apply to affected areas and wash off after 19 minutes. Or Lindane 1% shampoo. Apply for 4 minutes to affected area, and then wash off.
Scabies	Pruritis due to sensitization to *Sarcoptes scabiei*	Permethrin cream 5%. Apply to all areas of the body from the neck down, and wash off after 8–14 hours or Lindane lotion 1% one oz or 39 g cream. Apply in a thin layer to all body areas from neck down and thoroughly wash off after 8 hours.

SCREENING OF EXPATRIATES AFTER PROLONGED STAY IN TROPICAL REGIONS

Persons who spend considerable time (> 1 year) in a tropical region are invariably exposed recurrently to infectious and noninfectious health threats. Accidents are common, exposure to blood products may occur secondary to sexual contact, use of intravenous drugs or receipt of blood products and infectious agents are found in food, drinking or recreational water, air, or insects. It is important to evaluate such expatriates upon return to their home country for acquired illnesses and infecting agents; often such evaluation is required by occupational regulations. For all returning expatriates, a careful history (Table 40), physical examination (Table 41), and routine laboratory tests (Table 42) should be carried out as a routine. Address abnormalities and treat. Table 43 provides specific treatment for identified tropical diseases.

Table 40 History to Obtain from All Expatriates after Leaving Tropical Regions

Finding Identified by History	Comment
Fever and chills	See Table 37
Unintentional weight loss (> 5% body weight)	Consider a chronic illness, including parasitic infection (eg, amebic liver disease) or malignancy
Chronic diarrhea	See Table 36 and consider tropical sprue or chronic intestinal parasitic infection
Psychoneurologic problems	Neurologic and psychologic exam is needed to pinpoint the disorder and suggest therapy
Sore throat	Diphtheria, group A *Streptococcus*, hemorrhagic fever, HIV infection
Cough or shortness of breath	Perform a chest radiograph, and screen for tuberculosis and other forms of acute and chronic pneumonia; serologic studies may confirm Q fever or psitticosis, and certain parasitic infections may have a pulmonary phase, either directly or through hypersensitivity reaction
Cough or shortness of breath	(Loeffler's syndrome), where presence of eosinophilia, serology or fecal ova and parasite examination may lead to the diagnosis

Table 40 (continued)

Finding Identified by History	Comment
Rafting or swimming in recreational lakes and rivers	Stool exam for ova and serology test for schistosomiasis is indicated, consider risk for leptospirosis where serology should be obtained
Contact with farm or wild animals	Enteric infection with *Salmonella* or *Campylobacter* strains (stool culture), rabies (serology)
Sexual contact with local persons, IV use of illicit drugs or receipt of blood products	Screen for HIV (with informed consent and counseling), hepatitis B and STDs (see Table 42)
Abdominal pain	Amebic liver abscess (computed tomography and serology), typhoid fever (blood culture), various enteric infections (stool culture), mesenteric adenitis, appendicitis or vascular disease (clinical diagnosis)
Consumption of unpasteurized diary products	Consider this a source of *Brucella* (blood culture and serology), *Salmonella* (culture), *Campylobacter* (culture) infection, or Brainerd agent (clinical diagnosis) in patients with chronic diarrhea
Recent insect or animal bites	Consider insectborne illness: malaria (blood film), arboviruses including dengue (serology), *Pasteurella* (culture) infection
Important accidents, surgery or illnesses while abroad	Review what transpired and how it might relate to current health, consider HIV serotesting (with informed consent and counseling)

Table 41   Physical Examination to be Performed on all Expatriates after Leaving Tropical Regions

Finding Identified by Physical Examination	Comment and Follow-up Studies
Fever (oral temperature > 37.8°C)	See Table 37
Jaundice	Evaluate serologically for leptospirosis, relapsing fever, hepatitis A, B, C, E, rickettsial infection, dengue hemorrhagic fever and or yellow fever, blood cultures for typhoid, stool examination, blood film for malaria and serology for liver flukes
Rash, petechiae, echymoses	Serology for rickettsial, viral hemorrhagic fevers and dengue and other arboviral infections, blood culture for meningococcemia or *Salmonella typhi*, blood smear and serology for relapsing fever
Ulcerative process involving skin, genitals or mucous membranes	Evaluate for STD (see Table 42), cutaneous leishmaniasis, American trypansomiasis, mycobacterial, fungal rickettsial or nocardial infection, plague, creeping eryption, insect bite, tungiasis, Tumbu fly or Bot fly infection
Hepatomegaly or splenomegaly	Blood culture for typhoid fever, blood film for malaria, serology for leptospirosis, serology for visceral leishmaniasis, serology for amebic liver abscess, stool exam and serology for liver flukes
Pharyngitis or pharyngeal exudate	Thrush suggests HIV infection (serology done with informed consent and counseling), culture and smear for diphtheria, *Neisseria gonorrhoeae* (gay male), hemorrhagic fevers

Table 42 Routine Tests and Procedures to Perform on all Expatriates after Leaving Tropical Regions

Hematology: Complete blood count (CBC), white blood count, white blood cell differential, hemoglobin and hematocrit, red blood cell indices, platelet count

Liver Function Studies: bilirubin, alkaline phosphatase, SGOT, SGPT, albumin, globulin

Tuberculin skin test and chest x-ray if positive

Urinalysis

Stool ova and parasite examination done on two different samples

Special studies as suggested by history and or physical

SGOT=serum glutanic-oxaloacetic transaminase
SGPT=serum glutamate pyruvate transaminase

Table 43 Specific Therapy for Selected Tropical Infectious Diseases in Adults Identified During Screening

Etiologic Diagnosis	*Recommended Therapy*
Ascariasis	Mebendazole 100 mg bid for 3 days
Trichuriasis	Same as ascariasis
Hookworm	Same as ascariasis
Strongyloidiasis	Thiabendazole 25 mg/kg bid for 2 days (max 3 g/d)
Leptospirosis	Doxycycline 100 mg PO bid or pencillin G 1.5 million U IV q 6 hr for 7–10 days
Typhoid fever	Ciprofloxacin 500 mg bid or levofloxacin 500 mg qd for 7–10 days
Brucellosis	Doxycycline 100 mg bid together with rifampin (600–900 mg/d) for 6 weeks
Amoebic liver abscess	Metronidazole 750 mg tid for 5–10 days, plus one of the following: diiodohydroxyquin 650 mg tid for 20 days, diloxanide furoate 500 mg tid for 10 days or paromomycin 500 mg tid for 10 days
Cutaneous larva migrans	Topical Thiabendazole 25 mg/kg/bid PO for 2–5 days
Schistosomiasis	Praziquantel 40 mg/kg/d in 2 divided doses for 1 day

Additional Readings

Al-Zurba F, Saab B, Musharrafieh U. Medical problems encountered among travelers in Bahrain International Airport clinic. J Travel Med. 2007;14(1):37-41.

Behrens RH, Hatz CH, Gushulak BD, MacPherson DW. Illness in travelers visiting friends and relatives: what can be concluded? Clin Infect Dis. 2007;44(5):761-2; author reply 762-3.

Bottieau E, Clerinx J, Van den Enden E, et al. Fever after a stay in the tropics: diagnostic predictors of the leading tropical conditions. Medicine (Baltimore). 2007;86(1):18-25.

O'Brien DP, Leder K, Matchett E, Brown GV, Torresi J. Illness in returned travelers and immigrants/refugees: the 6-year experience of two Australian infectious diseases units. J Travel Med. 2006;13(3):145-52.

Sohail MR, Fischer PR. Blastocystis hominis and travelers. Travel Med Infect Dis. 2005;3(1):33-8.

Toovey S, Moerman F, van Gompel A. Special infectious disease risks of expatriates and long-term travelers in tropical countries. Part I: malaria. J Travel Med. 2007;14(1):42-9.

Toovey S, Moerman F, van Gompel A. Special infectious disease risks of expatriates and long-term travelers in tropical countries. Part II: infections other than malaria. J Travel Med. 2007;14(1):50-60.

APPENDICES

APPENDIX A:
ABBREVIATIONS

AIDS	acquired immunodeficiency syndrome
CDC	Centers for Disease Control and Prevention, Atlanta, GA, USA
CFR	case fatality rate
CRPF	chloroquine-resistant *Plasmodium falciparum*
DEC	diethylcarbamazine
DCS	decompression sickness
G-6-PD	glucose-6-phosphatedehydrogenase
IAMAT	International Association for Medical Assistance to Travelers
IATA	International Air Transport Association
ID	intradermal (injection)
IHR	International Health Regulations (WHO)
IM	intramuscular (injection)
IV	intravenous (injection)
MMR	measles, mumps, rubella (vaccine)
MMWR	Morbidity Mortality Weekly Report (CDC)
MSM	men who have sex with men
ORS	oral rehydration solution (or salt)
PAX	passenger (airline, ship)
PPM	personal protection measures (against mosquitoes)
RCT	randomized controlled trial
SBT/SBET	stand-by (emergency) treatment
SC	subcutaneous (injection)
TB	tuberculosis
TD	travelers' diarrhea
TIM	Travel Information Manual (IATA publication)
UC	unaccompanied children
UK	United Kingdom
USA	United States of America
WER	Weekly Epidemiological Record (WHO)
WHO	World Health Organization, Geneva, Switzerland
WTO	World Tourism Organization, Madrid

APPENDIX B: RECOMMENDATIONS AND MALARIA ENDEMICITY MAPS

Country N = North S = South W = West E = East	Malaria	Yellow Fever	Hepatitis A	Hepatitis B	Typhoid	Rabies	Meningococcal Disease	Japanese Encephalitis	Tetanus/Diphtheria	Poliomyelitis	TBE	Miscellaneous
AFRICA												
Algeria	—: minimal risk: SE	T1	+	R	R	R			+			
Angola	MP (1–12)	+T2	+	R	+	R			+	+		
Benin	MP (1–12)	required	+	R	+	R	R:N		+	+		
Botswana	MP (11–6), MT (or MP) (7–10) Boteti, Okavango, Chobe, Ngamiland, Tutume districts		+	R	R	R			+	+		
Burkina Faso	MP (1–12)	required	+	R	+	R	R		+	+		
Burundi	MP (1–12)	+T1	+	R	R	R			+	+		
Cameroon	MP (1–12)	required	+	R	+	R	R:N		+	+		
Cape Verde Islands	—: minimal risk (9–11) São Tiago Island	T1	+	R	-				+	+		
Central African Republic	MP (1–12)	required‡	+	R	+	R	R		+	+		

Country (N = North, S = South, W = West, E = East)	Malaria	Yellow Fever	Hepatitis A	Hepatitis B	Typhoid	Rabies	Meningococcal Disease	Japanese Encephalitis	Tetanus/Diphtheria	Poliomyelitis	TBE	Miscellaneous
Chad	MP (1–12)	required	+	R	+	R	R		+	+		
Congo- Brazzaville	MP (1–12)	required	+	R	+	R			+	+		
Congo-Kinshasa (Zaïre)	MP (1–12)	required	+	R	+	R			+	+		
Comores	MP (1–12)		+	R	R	R			+	+		
Djibouti	MP (1–12)	T1	+	R	R	R			+	+		
Egypt	Ø. no cases since 1998	T1	+	R	+	R			+	+		
Equatorial Guinea	MP (1–12)	+T1	+	R	+	R			+	+		
Eritrea	MP (1–12) <2000m; ø Asmara	T1	+	R	R	R			+	+		
Ethiopia	MP (1–12) <2000m; ø Addis Ababa	+T1	+	R	+	R	R		+	+		
Gabon	MP (1–12)	required	+	R	+	R			+	+		
Gambia	MP (1–12)	+T1	+	R	+	R	R		+	+		
Ghana	MP (1–12)	required	+	R	+	R	R:N		+	+		
Guinea	MP (1–12)	required	+	R	+	R			+	+		

Guinea-Bissau	MP (1–12)			R	R			+	+
Ivory Coast	MP (1–12)	required	+	R	+	R	R:N	+	+
Kenya	MP (1–12) <2500m; ø Nairobi-City	+T1	+	R	+	R		+	+
Lesotho	ø	T2	+	R	R			+	+
Liberia	MP (1–12)	required	+	R	+	R		+	+
Libya	—	T1	+	R	R			+	+
Madagascar	MP (1–12) <1100m	T1	+	R	R	R		+	+
Malawi	MP (1–12)	T2	+	R	R	R		+	+
Mali	MP (1–12)	required	+	R	+	R	R	+	+
Mauritania	MP (1–12) S; MP (7–10) Adrar, Inchiri	+T2, >2w required	+	R	+	R	R	+	+
Mauritius	ø. no cases since 1998	T1	+	R	–			+	
Mayotte	MP (1–12)		+	R	R	R		+	+
Morocco	—: minimal risk (5–10) in Chefchaouen province		R	R	R			+	
Mozambique	MP (1–12)	T1	+	R	R	R		+	+

Country (N = North, S = South, W = West, E = East)	Malaria	Yellow Fever	Hepatitis A	Hepatitis B	Typhoid	Rabies	Meningococcal Disease	Japanese Encephalitis	Tetanus/Diphtheria	Poliomyelitis	TBE	Miscellaneous
Namibia	MP (1–12) Cubango (Kavango) Valley, Kunene Valley, Caprivi Strip; XP (11–6), MT (or XP) (7–10) other in the N; —: minimal risk S of above areas	T2	+	R	R	R			+	+		
Niger	MP (1–12)	required	+	R	+	R	R		+	+		
Nigeria	MP (1–12)	+T2	+	R	+	R	R:N		+	+		
Réunion (La)	ø	T1	+		R	R			+			
Rwanda	MP (1–12)	required	+	R	R	R			+	+		
São Tomé & Principe	MP (1–12)	required	+	R	+	R			+	+		
Senegal	MP (1–12)	+T1	+	R	R	R	R		+	+		
Seychelles	ø	T2	+	R	ı				+			
Sierra Leone	MP (1–12)	+T2	+	R	+	R			+	+		

Country	Distribution	+T2							
Somalia	MP (1–12)		+	R	+	R		+	+
South Africa	MP (10–5), MT (or MP) (6–9) provinces Mpumalanga, Limpopo; MP (11–6), MT (or MP) (7–10) Kwazulu-Natal (N of Tugela River)	T2	+	R	R	R	R	+	+
St. Helena	ø	T1	+	R	–			+	+
Sudan	MP (1–12); MT (or MP) Red Sea shores in the northern half	+T2	+	R	+	R	R	+	+
Swaziland	MP (11–6), MT (or MP) (7–10) mainly lowlands	T2	+		R	R		+	
Tanzania	MP (1–12) <1800m	+ / ø (Zanzibar, coast)	+	R	R	R		+	+
Togo	MP (1–12)	required	+	R	+	R	R:N	+	+
Tunisia	ø	T1	+	R	R	R			+
Uganda	MP (1–12)	required	+	R	R	R	R:N	+	+
Zambia	MP (1–12) <1000m	–	+	R	R	R		+	+

Country N = North S = South W = West E = East	Zimbabwe	AMERICAS	Argentina	Bahamas	Belize	Bermuda	Bolivia
Miscellaneous							
TBE							
Poliomyelitis	+						
Tetanus/Diphtheria	+		+	+	+	+	+
Japanese Encephalitis							
Meningococcal Disease							
Rabies	R		R	R	R		R
Typhoid	R		ı	ı	R	ı	R
Hepatitis B	R		R	R	R	R	R
Hepatitis A	+		+	+	+	+	+
Yellow Fever	T2			T1	T1		+T1
Malaria	MP (1–12) N, Victoria Falls, Zambezi River valley; MP (11–6), MT (or MP) (7–10) elsewhere <1200m; ø Harare, Bulawayo		–; minimal risk (10–5) N <1200m	ø	CT (or CP) (1–12); ø Belize-District	Ø	MT (or MP) (1–12) N <2500m; MT (or CP) (1–12) rest of country <2500m; ø cities and provinces of Oruro and Potosi

		+T1	+	R	R	R		+	+
Brazil	MP or MT (1–12) forested areas of Legal Amazonia, <900m, see map; ø E, NE coast, Iguassu							+	
Caribbean (excl. Haiti and Dominican Republic)	ø	T1	+	R	R	R		+	
Chile	ø	T2 for Easter Islands	+	R	-	R		+	
Colombia	MT (or MP) (1–12) rural areas of Urabá-Bajo Cauca, Pacífico, Amazonia; MT (or XP) (1–12) other risk areas; ø Bogotá, Caribbean islands (San Andres and Providencia)	+T2	+	R		R		+	
Costa Rica	CT (or CP) (1–12) <700m; ø San Jose	T2	+	R	R	R		+	
Cuba	ø		+	R	R	R		+	+

Country N = North S = South W = West E = East	Malaria	Yellow Fever	Hepatitis A	Hepatitis B	Typhoid	Rabies	Meningococcal Disease	Japanese Encephalitis	Tetanus/Diphtheria	Poliomyelitis	TBE	Miscellaneous
Dominican Republic	CT (or CP) (1–12) central border with Haiti, Altagracia in the E		+	R	R	R			+			
Ecuador	MT (or MP) (1–12) <1500m; ø Andes highlands, Galapagos	+T1	+	R	R	R			+			
El Salvador	CT (or CP) (1–12) Santa Ana province only <600m	T1	+	R	R	R			+			
French Guiana	MP (1–12): border areas facing Surinam and Brazil; MT (or MP) (1–12) rest of country; ø coastal areas required	required	+	R	R	R			+			
Guatemala	CT (or CP) (1–12) <1500m; ø Guatemala City, Lake Atitlán	T1	+	R	R	R			+			
Guyana	MT (or MP) (1–12) coastal areas; MP (rest of the country ø Georgetown, New Amsterdam	+T1	+	R	R	R						

Haiti	CT (or CP) (1–12)	T1	+	R	R	R	+
Honduras	CT (or CP) (1–12) <1000m; ø Tegucigalpa	T1	+	R	R	R	+
Jamaica	CT (or CP): Cases 2006/7 in Kingston	T2	+	R	R	–	+
Mexico	CT (or CP) (1–12) <1000m, minimal risk in S border areas only; Ø main archeological sites, Yucatan		+	R	R	R	+
Nicaragua	CT (or CP) (1–12); ø Managua	T1	+	R	R	R	+
Panama	CT (or CP) (1–12) <800m; MT (or MP) (1-12) Darien and Kuna Yala; ø Panama, Colon	+T1	+	R	R	R	+
Paraguay	CT (or CP) (10–5) E; ø Iguassu falls	T1	+	R	R	R	+
Peru	MT (or MP) (1–12) Luciano Castillo, Loreto, Piura; MT (or XP) (1–12) rest of the country <1500m; ø Lima, Cuzco, Machu Picchu, Ayacucho	+T1	+	R	+	R	
Surinam	MP (1–12) most of the country; ø Paramaribo and coast	+T1	+	R	R	R	+

Country (N = North, S = South, W = West, E = East)	Malaria	Yellow Fever	Hepatitis A	Hepatitis B	Typhoid	Rabies	Meningococcal Disease	Japanese Encephalitis	Tetanus/Diphtheria	Poliomyelitis	TBE	Miscellaneous
Trinidad, Tobago	ø	+T1	+	R	R	R			+			
Uruguay	ø	T1	+	R	-				+			
Venezuela	MT (or MP) (1–12) jungle areas of the Amazonas; MT (or XP) (1–12) rest of the country; ø NW coast	+T2	+	R	R	R			+			
ASIA												
Afghanistan	MT (or MP) (5–11) <2000m	T1	+	R	+	R			+	+		
Armenia	CT (or CP) (6-10) minimal risk Masis district		+	R	R				+			
Azerbaijan	CT (or CP) (6-10) low risk in S borders and N Khachmas region		+	R	R	R			+			
Bahrein	ø		+	R	-				+			
Bangladesh	MP (7-11), MT (or MP) (12-6) rural areas; ø Dhaka	T1	+	R	+	R			+	+		

Country		T2	+	R	+	R	R:S	+	+	(R)
Bhutan	MT (or MP) (1–12) S <1700m	T2	+		+		R	+	+	
Brunei Darussalam	ø		+	R	R		R	+	+	
Cambodia	MT (or MP) (1–12); ø Phnom Penh.	T2	+	R	R	R	R	+	+	
China	MT (or MP) (1–12) S half of the country <1500m; ø Beijing and other major cities. E and NE coast	T2	+	R	R	R	R	+	+	(R)
Georgia	—: minimal risk in the SE		+	R	R	R	R			
India	MP (7-11), MT (or MP) (12-6) rural areas in the NE (W.Bengal, Assam etc); MT (or MP) (1–12) rest of the country <2000m; Malaria is also present in major cities (Delhi, Mumbai, |Kolkata, etc) and Goa; ø Himachal Pradesh, Jammu & Kashmir, Sikkim	T2	+	R	+	R	R	+	+	

Country N = North S = South W = West E = East	Malaria	Yellow Fever	Hepatitis A	Hepatitis B	Typhoid	Rabies	Meningococcal Disease	Japanese Encephalitis	Tetanus/Diphtheria	Poliomyelitis	TBE	Miscellaneous
Indonesia	MP: islands and areas E of Bali; MT (or MP) (1–12) rest of the country; ø Jakarta or other major cities and main tourist resorts in Java and Bali	T1	+	R	+	R		R	+	+		
Iran	CT (or CP) (6–9) Ardebil, E Azerbijan <1500m; MT (or MP) (3–11) rural areas in the S and SE	–	+	R	R	R			+			
Iraq	CT (or CP) (5–11) <1500m	T1	+	R	+	R			+	+		B
Israel	ø								+			
Japan	ø				–				+			
Jordan	ø	T1	+	R	R	R			+			B
Kazakstan	ø	T1	+	R	R	R			+		(R)	B
Korea (North)	—: minimal risk in border areas facing S Korea		+	R	+	R		R	+			

Country	Notes									
Korea (South)	—: minimal risk in border areas facing N Korea		+		−		R		+	
Kuwait	ø		+	R	−				+	
Kyrgyzstan	CT (or CP) rural areas of SE		+	R		R		R	+	
Laos	MT (or MP) (1–12); ø Vientiane	T1	+	R	R	R			+	
Lebanon	ø	T1	+	R	R	R			+	
Malaysia	MT (or MP) (1–12) limited risk in the hinterland only; ø major cities, coasts	T1	+	R	R	R		R	+	
Maldives	ø	T1	+	R	−				+	
Mongolia	ø		+	R	−	R			+	R:N
Myanmar (Burma)	MT (or MP) (1–12) most of the country <1000m; YT (or YP) (1–12) NE border facing Thailand; ø Yangoon, Mandalay (City)	T1	+	R	R	R	R	R	+	+
Nepal	XT (or XP)(1–12) rural areas of the S (Terai) <1300m; Ø Kathmandu	T1	+	R	+	R	R	R	+	+

Country N = North S = South W = West E = East	Malaria	Yellow Fever	Hepatitis A	Hepatitis B	Typhoid	Rabies	Meningococcal Disease	Japanese Encephalitis	Tetanus/Diphtheria	Poliomyelitis	TBE	Miscellaneous
Oman	Ø. no cases since 2001	T2	+	R	-	R			+			
Pakistan	MT (or MP) (1–12) <2000m	T1	+	R	+	R		R:SE	+	+		
Philippines	MT (or MP) (1–12) <600m; ø Manila City, Aklan, Benguet, Bilaran, Bohol, Camiguin, Capiz, Catanduanes, Cebu, Guimaras, Iloilo, Leyte, Masbate, N Samar, Sequijor	T1	+	R	R	R		R	+			
Qatar	ø		+	R								
Russian Federation	ø		+	R	R	R			+			
Saudi Arabia	MT (or MP) (1–12) SW; ø Jeddah, Mecca, Medina, Riyadh, Taif	T1	+	R	-	R	A		+	+*		B
Singapore	ø	T1		R					+			

Country	Malaria prophylaxis									
Sri Lanka	MT (or XP) (1–12); ø District of Colombo, Galle, Gampaha, Kalutara, Matara, Nuwara Eliya	T1	+	R	+	R	+	R	+	
Syria	CT (5–10) minimal risk in the NE border areas only	T1	+	R	R	+		R	+	B
Taiwan	ø		+	R	R	-	R	+		B
Tajikistan	CT (or CP) (6-10) rural areas of SW (Kathlon area), N (Leninabad-Khujand area)	+	R	R	R			R	+	
Thailand	MT (or MP) (1–12) most of the country; YT (or YP) (1–12) border areas facing Myanmar in the NW; ø Bangkok, Phuket, Pattaya, Chiang Mai, Chiang Rai, Samui	T2	+	R	R	R		R:N	+	
Timor Leste	MP (1–12)		+	R	+	R		R	+	
Turkey	CT (or CP) (3–11) SE Anatolia, Amicova and Cucurova plains; ø main tourist areas in the SW		+	R	R	R	R	R	+	
Turkmenistan	— : minimal risk in the SE		+	R	R	R			+	

Country (N = North, S = South, W = West, E = East)	Malaria	Yellow Fever	Hepatitis A	Hepatitis B	Typhoid	Rabies	Meningococcal Disease	Japanese Encephalitis	Tetanus/Diphtheria	Poliomyelitis	TBE	Miscellaneous
Uzbekistan	—: minimal risk in the S		+	R	R	R			+			
United Arab Emirates	ø		+	R	R	R			+			
Vietnam	MT (or MP) (1–12); ø Red River delta, central coast; cities	T1	+	R	R	R		R	+			
Yemen	MT (or MP) (1–12); ø Sana'a City	T1	+	R	R	R			+	+		
OCEANIA												
Australia	ø	T1	+	R					+			
Fiji	ø	T1	+	R	R				+			
French Polynesia	ø	T1	+	R	R				+			
Kiribati	ø	T2	+	R	-				+			
Nauru	ø	T2	+	R	R				+			
New Caledonia	ø	T1	+	R	-				+			
New Zealand	ø	T1		R					+			

Niue	ø	T1	+	R	-	+	
Palau	ø	T2	+	R	R	+	B
Papua New Guinea	MP (1–12) <1800m, also Port Moresby	T2	+	R	+	+	
Pitcairn	ø	T1	+	R	-	+	
Samoa / US Samoa	ø	T2	+	R	-	+	
Solomon Islands	XP (1–12)	T2	+	R	R	+	
Tonga	ø	T2	+	R	R	+	
Vanuatu	XP (1–12)		+	R	R	+	
Wallis and Futuna	ø	T1	+	R	-	+	
EUROPE							
Albania	ø	T2	+	R	-		R
Austria	ø			R		+	R
Belarus	ø		+	R	R	+	R
Bosnia	ø			R		+	R
Czechia	ø			R		+	R
Croatia	ø					+	R
Danmark	ø			R		+	R

Country N = North S = South W = West E = East	Estonia	Finland	France	Germany	Greece	Hungary	Italy	Latvia	Liechtenstein	Lithuania	Malta	Moldova	Norway
Miscellaneous													
TBE	R	R	R	R	(R)	R	R	R	R	R		R	R
Poliomyelitis				ı							ı	ı	
Tetanus/Diphtheria	+	+	+	+	+	+	+	+	+	+	+	+	+
Japanese Encephalitis													
Meningococcal Disease													
Rabies													
Typhoid												R	
Hepatitis B	R	R	R	R	R	R	R	R	R	R	R	R	R
Hepatitis A	+							+		+		+	
Yellow Fever											T2		
Malaria	Ø	Ø	Ø	Ø	Ø	Ø	Ø	Ø	Ø	Ø	Ø	Ø	Ø

Country										
Poland	ø			R				+		R
Portugal (Azores only, Madeira)	ø	T1		R				+	-	
Romania	ø		+	R	R	R		+		R
Russian Fed.	ø		+	R	R	R		+		R
Serbia	ø			R				+		R
Sweden	ø			R				+		R
Slovakia	ø			R				+		R
Slovenia	ø			R				+		R
Spain	ø			R				+		
Switzerland	ø			R				+		R
Turkey	ø		+	R	R	R		+		
Ukraine	ø		+	R	R	R		+		R

Adapted from WHO and from Travel Information Manual for required vaccinations. Status is current as of June 2007. Consult current recommendations in home country.

MALARIA

Periods of risk: January–December = (1–12)

Limits of altitude for malaria transmission, in meters = (m)

Chemoprophylaxis, first choice (Zones Type I, II, III, IV as per WHO, see figure 13):

Zone Type I: Mosquito bite prevention (valid also for other zones!) only

Zone Type II: CP = Chloroquine

Zone Type III: XP = Chloroquine plus Proguanil. Note: Proguanil is not marketed in the US; therefore, the CDC recommends MP instead.

Zone Type IV: MP = Mefloquine or Doxycycline or Atovaquone-Proguanil

Special zones, mefloquine resistant areas in Thailand, Myanmar and Cambodia:

YP = Doxycycline or Atovaquone-Proguanil

Stand-by emergency treatment (Note: In the US, CDC does not recommend stand-by emergency treatment as an option, but only CP or MP or YP, respectively. The same applies for various other national expert groups.):

CT   Chloroquine

MT   Mefloquine or Atovaquone-Proguanil

YT   Atovaquone-Proguanil (or in some countries where available, artemisinin/lumefantrin (Coartem®, Riamet®)

—   No chemoprophylaxis, no stand-by treatment recommended:

ø   No malaria risk

VACCINE PREVENTABLE DISEASES

Yellow Fever: Infected areas are countries that have "required" or "+" in the yellow fever column

required   vaccination required (except for airport transits within country)

requ*‡   vaccination required (including for airport transit within country)

+   vaccination recommended

T1   vaccination required if arriving within 6 days after leaving or transiting infected areas (airport transits exempt)

T2   vaccination required if arriving within 6 days after leaving or transiting infected areas (including airport transits).

Hepatitis A

+ = vaccination recommended for non-immunes

Hepatitis B

R = additionally to routine vaccination in many countries recommended for all travelers and for special risk groups, such as health care personnel, social workers, MSM, frequent travelers, travelers likely to engage in casual sex, tattooing, piercing, or needle-sharing, and travelers who may need to undergo medical or dental procedures

Typhoid Fever

+   vaccination recommended

R   vaccination recommended for risk groups, mainly those eating and drinking under poor hygienic conditions (e.g. VFR) and those staying longer than 1 month

Rabies

R   vaccination recommended for risk groups, mainly those with occupational exposure to animals, and those staying longer than 1 month, particularly bicyclists

Meningococcal Meningitis

R   vaccination recommended for risk groups: in sub-Saharan Africa during the season of transmission (12-6), for persons with close contact to the local population staying over 1 month, during epidemics also for short stays (? 1 week).

A   vaccination required for pilgrims (Hajj, Umra) and seasonal workers

Japanese Encephalitis

R   vaccination recommended for risk groups: >1 month stay in rural areas. For seasonal information, see Figure 30.

Tetanus and Diphtheria

+   vaccination recommended for non-immunes

Poliomyelitis

+   vaccination recommended for non-immune travelers, i.e. booster every +10 years.

*   vaccination required for pilgrims <15 years.

TBE (Tickborne Encephalitis)

R   vaccination recommended for risk groups (outdooring).

(R)   minimal risk, only single cases reported. No transmission in cities (except Riga). Distribution mostly focally. Information at http://www.eurosurveillance.org/ew/2004/040715.asp and http://www.bag.admin.ch/themen/medizin/00682/00685/03062/index.html?lang=de (German or French)

Miscellaneous

Countries omitted: no special recommendations or requirements

B   HIV test may be required for some individuals (information may be obtained at respective embassy)

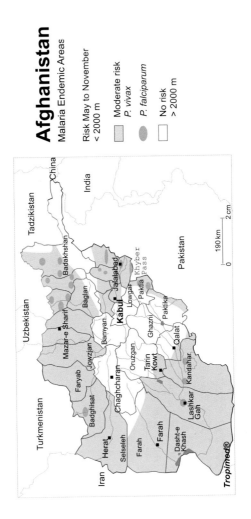

Afghanistan

Malaria Endemic Areas

Risk May to November
< 2000 m

Moderate risk
P. vivax

P. falciparum

No risk
> 2000 m

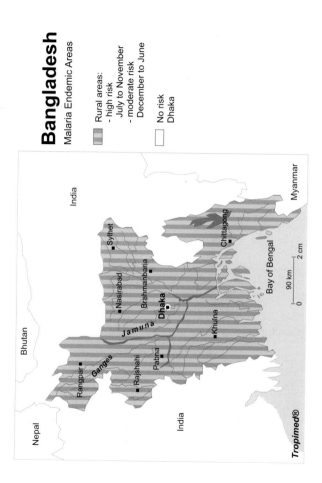

Bangladesh
Malaria Endemic Areas

Rural areas:
- high risk
  July to November
- moderate risk
  December to June

No risk
Dhaka

Tropimed®

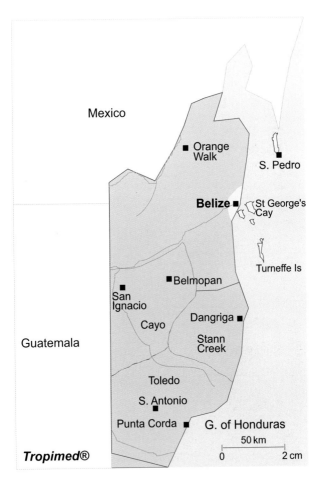

Mexico

Orange Walk

S. Pedro

Belize

St George's Cay

Turneffe Is

Belmopan

San Ignacio

Cayo

Dangriga

Stann Creek

Guatemala

Toledo

S. Antonio

Punta Corda

G. of Honduras

50 km

0   2 cm

Tropimed®

Belize

Malaria Endemic Areas

Moderate risk
main risk in Cayo and Toledo

Minimal risk
Belize City and most Cays (Islands)

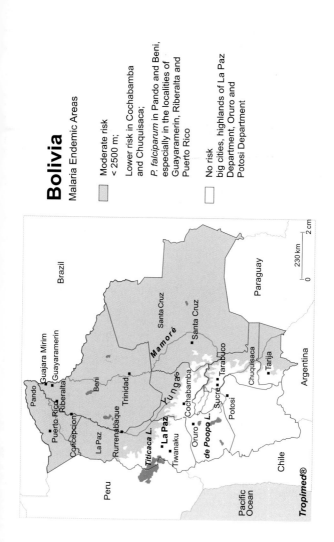

Bolivia

Malaria Endemic Areas

Moderate risk
< 2500 m;

Lower risk in Cochabamba
and Chuquisaca;

P. falciparum in Pando and Beni,
especially in the localities of
Guayaramerin, Riberalta and
Puerto Rico

No risk
big cities, highlands of La Paz
Department, Oruro and
Potosi Department

Tropimed®

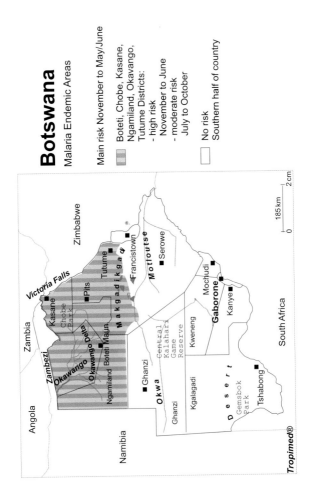

Botswana

Malaria Endemic Areas

Main risk November to May/June

Boteti, Chobe, Kasane, Ngamiland, Okavango, Tutume Districts:
- high risk
  November to June
- moderate risk
  July to October

No risk
Southern half of country

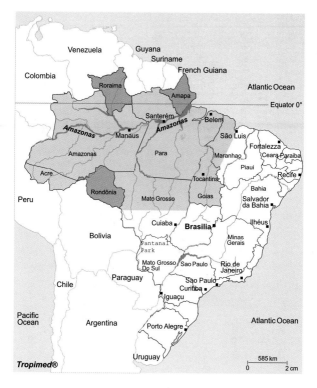

Brazil

Malaria Endemic Areas

High risk
Rondônia, Roraima
and Amapa States

Moderate risk
all other States of
the Amazon basin

No risk
east coast and cities
outside the Amazon basin,
including Iguassu Falls

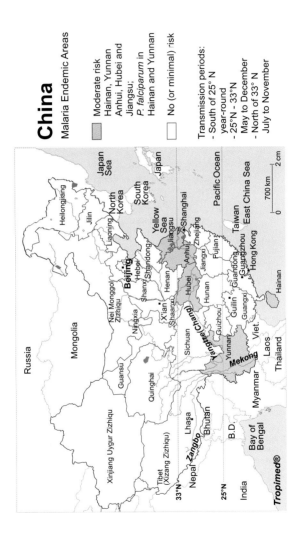

China

Malaria Endemic Areas

Moderate risk
Hainan, Yunnan
Anhui, Hubei and
Jiangsu;
P. falciparum in
Hainan and Yunnan

No (or minimal) risk

Transmission periods:
- South of 25° N
  year-round
- 25°N - 33°N
  May to December
- North of 33° N
  July to November

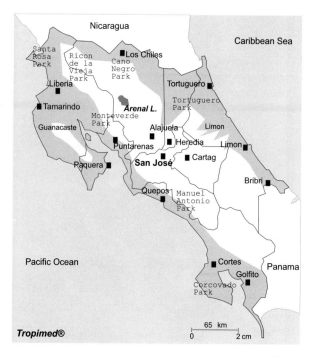

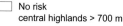

Costa Rica

Malaria Endemic Areas

Moderate risk
rural areas

No risk
central highlands > 700 m

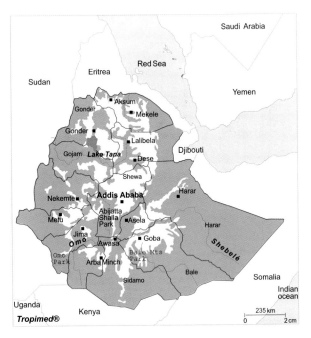

Ethiopia

Malaria Endemic Areas

High risk
< 2200 m

No (or minimal) risk
> 2200 m

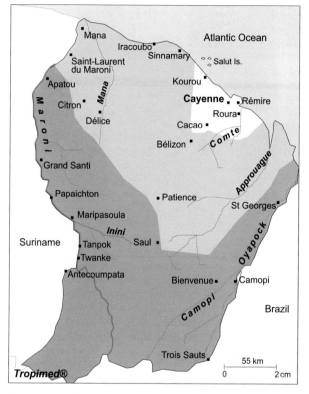

French Guiana

Malaria Endemic Areas

High risk
mainly in the areas of
Maroni and Oyapock Rivers

Moderate risk

No risk

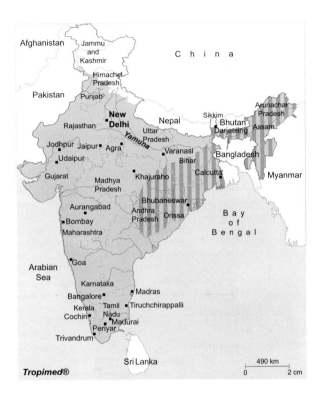

India

Malaria Endemic Areas

Risk < 2000 m

Westbengal, Orissa, Jharkand, Chhattisgarh and in the East of these areas (Assam, Tripura, Darjeeling, Meghalaya, Mizoram etc):
- high risk
  July to November
- moderate risk
  December to June

Moderate risk
all year

No risk
montainous areas of Jammu, Kashmir, Himachal Pradesh, Sikkim

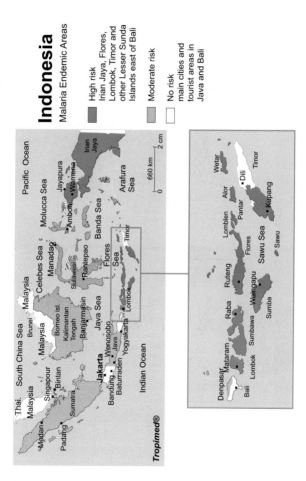

Indonesia
Malaria Endemic Areas

High risk
Irian Jaya, Flores,
Lombok, Timor and
other Lesser Sunda
Islands east of Bali

Moderate risk

No risk
main cities and
tourist areas in
Java and Bali

Tropimed®

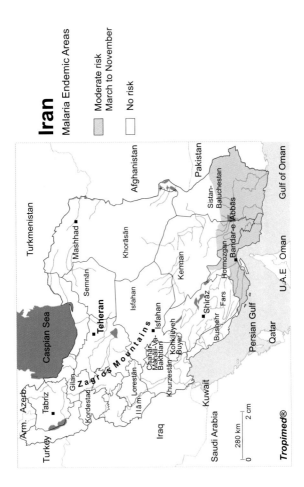

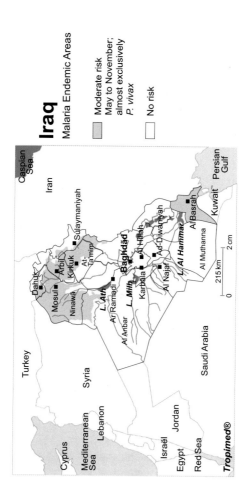

Iraq

Malaria Endemic Areas

Moderate risk
May to November;
almost exclusively
P. vivax

No risk

Tropimed®

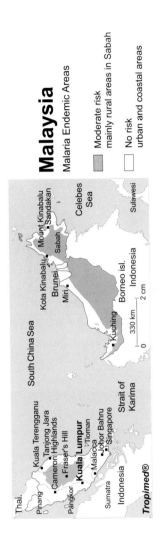

Malaysia

Malaria Endemic Areas

Moderate risk
mainly rural areas in Sabah

No risk
urban and coastal areas

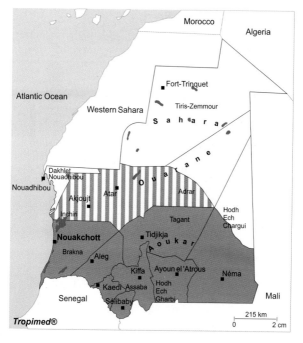

Mauritania

Malaria Endemic areas

High risk
all year

Adrar and Inchiri:
- high risk
July to October
- no (or minimal) risk
November to June

No (or minimal) risk

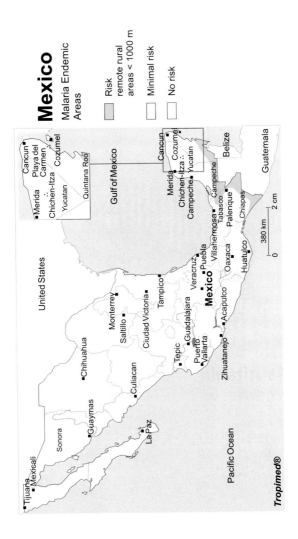

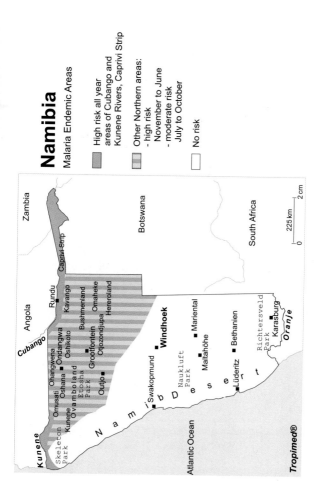

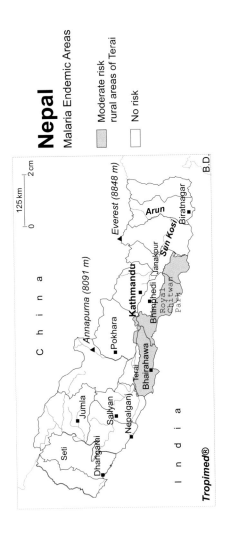

Nepal

Malaria Endemic Areas

Moderate risk
rural areas of Terai

No risk

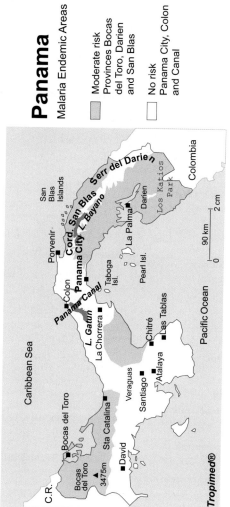

Panama

Malaria Endemic Areas

Moderate risk
Provinces Bocas
del Toro, Darien
and San Blas

No risk
Panama City, Colon
and Canal

Tropimed®

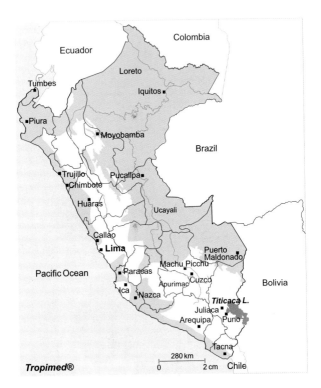

Peru

Malaria Endemic Areas

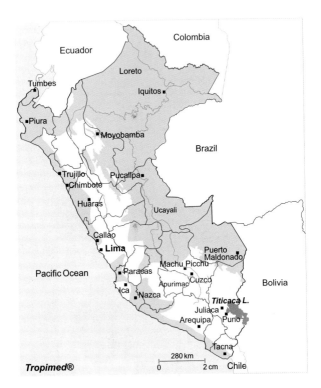 Moderate risk

No risk
Lima and Andean highlands

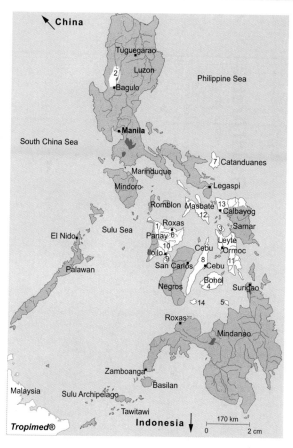

Philippines

Malaria Endemic Areas

▨ Moderate risk
rural areas < 600 m

☐ No risk
Manila and Provinces

1. Aklan
2. Benquet
3. Bilaran
4. Bohol
5. Camiguin
6. Capiz
7. Catanduanes
8. Cebu
9. Guimaras
10. Iloilo
11. Leyte
12. Masbate
13. N Samar
14. Sequijor

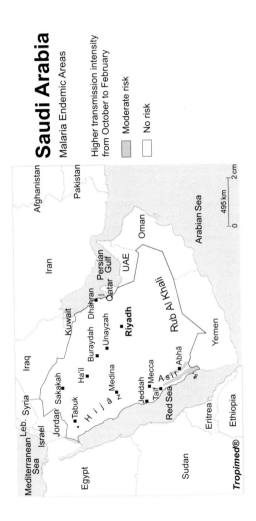

Saudi Arabia

Malaria Endemic Areas

Higher transmission intensity
from October to February

Moderate risk

No risk

Tropimed®

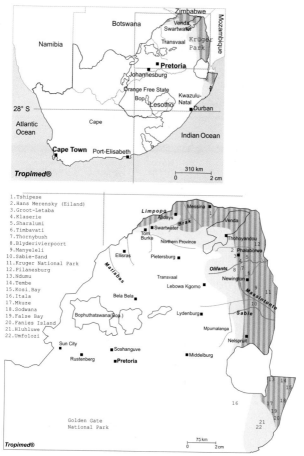

1. Tshipese
2. Hans Merensky (Eiland)
3. Groot-Letaba
4. Klaserie
5. Sharalumi
6. Timbavati
7. Thornybush
8. Blyderivierpoort
9. Manyeleli
10. Sabie-Sand
11. Kruger National Park
12. Pilanesburg
13. Ndumu
14. Tembe
15. Kosi Bay
16. Itala
17. Mkuze
18. Sodwana
19. False Bay
20. Fanies Island
21. Hluhluwe
22. Umfolozi

South Africa

Malaria Endemic Areas

▨ Province Mpumalanga (E, Krüger
including neighbouring parks),
Northern Province (N),
Kwazulu-Natal (NE coast):
- high risk
  September to June
- moderate risk
  July to August

☐ Minimal risk
other Northern parts as far as
Tugela River and Swartwater

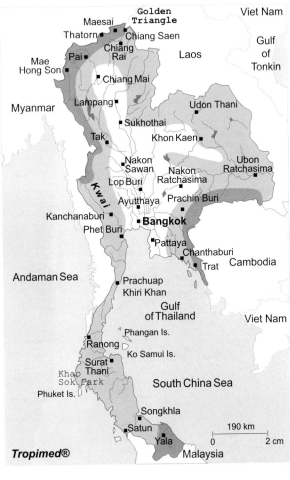

Thailand

Malaria Endemic Areas

High risk
border areas to Myanmar, Cambodia
and Malaysia

No (or minimal risk)
cities and major tourist areas including
Bangkok, Chiang Mai, Chanthaburi,
Ko Samui, Pattaya, Phuket, Songkhla

Venezuela

Malaria Endemic Areas

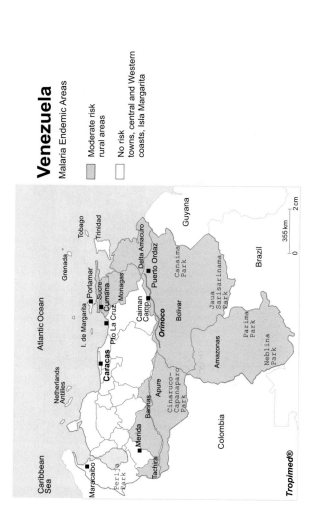

Moderate risk
rural areas

No risk
towns, central and Western
coasts, Isla Margarita

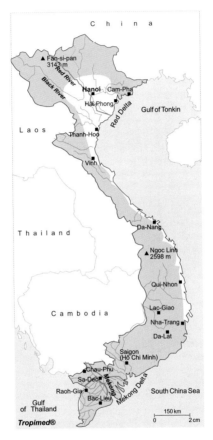

Viet Nam

Malaria Endemic Areas

Moderate risk
rural areas

No risk
main cities, Red River Delta,
coast North of Nha-Trang

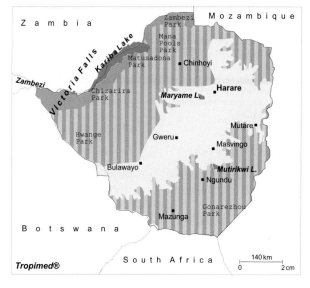

Zimbabwe

Malaria Endemic Areas

 High risk all year
along Zambesi River
and at Victoria Falls

 - High risk
November to June
- Moderate risk
July to October

Minimal risk
> 1200 m

INDEX